Current Medical Terminology

Fourth Edition

Vera Pyle, CMT

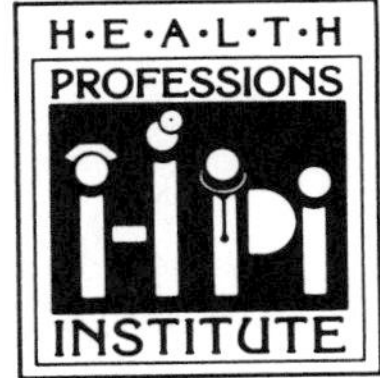

Health Professions Institute · Modesto, California · 1992

Current Medical Terminology
Fourth Edition

First Edition published 1985 by Prima Vera Publications.
Second Edition published 1987 by Prima Vera Publications.
Third Edition published 1990 by Health Professions Institute.

Published by:

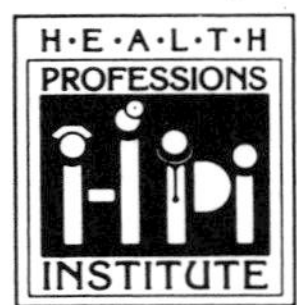

Health Professions Institute
P. O. Box 801
Modesto, California 95353
Phone (209) 551-2112
Fax (209) 551-0404
Sally Crenshaw Pitman, Editor & Publisher

Printed by:
Parks Printing & Lithograph
Modesto, California

Bound by:
Cardoza-James Binding Company
San Francisco, California

ISBN: 0-934385-54-8

Last digit is the print number: 9 8 7 6 5 4 3 2 1

To those who have contributed to this book,
To those who read it and find it useful,
To all who love words.

and

To Dan Pae, who passed through life—
and made a difference.

''What is the use of a book,'' thought Alice, ''without pictures or conversations?''

Lewis Carroll
Alice's Adventures in Wonderland

Contents

Page

Acknowledgments

The fourth edition of *Current Medical Terminology* is the product of the love, enthusiasm, unbelievably hard work, determination, and generosity of many talented people.

To these wonderful people, and to those medical transcriptionists who have sent in words, offered suggestions, asked questions, praised and appreciated the previous editions of the book, my gratitude and affection.

Special thanks are due to those who contributed most to the new edition—Susan M. Turley, MA, CMT, RN, Baltimore; Bron Taylor, San Francisco; Catherine Gilliam, CMT, Houston; John H. Dirckx, M.D., Dayton; and the Health Professions Institute staff members in Modesto—Elaine Aamodt and Linda Campbell, CMT. And the greatest thanks of all to the editor and publisher, Sally C. Pitman, MA, CMT, without whom the book would not exist.

Vera Pyle, CMT
July 1992

Preface

Words are a large part of the stock-in-trade of the medical transcriptionist, and we encounter new ones every day. There is the usual flurry of identifying the new word: "What do you hear? Yes, that's what I heard. What is it? What does it mean? How do you spell it? What's your source?"

Much has happened in medicine in the last ten years—monoclonal antibodies, magnetic resonance imaging (MRI), DNA recombinant method of producing biosynthetic hormones and other products, breakthroughs in our knowledge of cell function and reproduction, new methods of treatment without resorting to surgery, investigational drugs for treatment of AIDS and cancer. With all of these innovations, there are thousands of new words which, if you haven't yet heard, you soon will. In medicine, we can hardly say "current" for very long; thus, it is necessary to update *Current Medical Terminology* every two years.

New features include definitions of many specialized terms used in surgery and radiology. Under the entry *medication* is a quick-reference list of all the pharmaceuticals defined in main entries throughout the book, including drugs used to treat AIDS, chemicals, chemotherapy drugs and protocols, classes of drugs, contrast media, investigational drugs, natural substances, prescription and over-the-counter drugs, monoclonal antibodies, orphan drugs, radioisotopes, and solutions. In most cases we have listed both generic and brand name, the latter with capitalization where needed.

Extensive cross-referencing has been done. In most cases, the definition will appear with the form of the word most often used in dictation. That is, if the acronym, abbreviation, or brief form of the word is that most often dictated, then the definition will appear under that term, with a cross-reference to the other form. Sometimes a medical transcriptionist can hear or understand only one word of a phrase dictated by a physician; thus, cross-referencing under other important words of a phrase is provided.

I hope you will find this book even more useful than the earlier editions, which I know you all took to your hearts.

Vera Pyle, CMT
July 1992

Introduction

This book is intended primarily for medical transcriptionists, but now I find that it is also being used by court reporters, medical record technicians, medical record administrators, coders, legal secretaries, nurses, and students in the allied health professions. Also, with the continued importance of the patients' medical record in reimbursement systems, insurance claims examiners and Medicare evaluators refer to it as well. The recent increase in medico-legal cases has driven court reporters to expand their medical knowledge and reference libraries, and many have found this book to be a valuable tool. So it now becomes necessary to keep a diverse group of readers in mind.

Most medical transcriptionists are either hospital-based or work for off-site transcription services. They transcribe and edit the very detailed and highly technical medical and surgical reports that are used in the delivery of medical care. These written reports assure that everyone involved in that care knows the patient's medical history, what was found on physical examination and on laboratory examinations, the pathology discovered, the treatment given, the medications administered, and the response to therapy noted.

These reports are of importance medically and legally, and in research. They are valued by everyone who uses them (they are often the only legible documents in a patient's record), but the people who transcribe them are largely unknown, individually and as a profession.

New medical terms crop up daily—new medications, new operative procedures, new instruments, new equipment, new techniques, new research terms, new laboratory tests, new abbreviations—many of them—and with little documentation except for a physician's occasional attempt at spelling. It therefore becomes necessary to provide a reliable and *immediate* source of information to tens of thousands of medical transcriptionists.

References are made throughout the book to "the dictator." These definitions were originally written for an "in-group" of medical transcriptionists who know that the dictator refers to the physician or medical student who dictates the medical and surgical reports.

Perhaps an explanation is in order at this time to help familiarize new readers with how I research terms, and how I arrive at conclusions (or decisions) when research fails.

Many years ago when my younger daughter was five or six, I overheard an argument she was having with one of her playmates. I don't now recall what it was all about, but I do remember my daughter's clinching argument—"My mother says . . ." Her friend was not prepared to challenge Taffy's mother; end of argument.

No one since then has appointed me The Higher Authority, and the self-appointed are setting themselves up for being leaders with no followers. So I feel that ours must be a collaborative venture. We give our opinions, our reasons for them, and our sources. Our readers may evaluate our conclusions, discuss their differences of opinion, and decide to accept them or not. I hasten to add that we all have a strong instinct for self-preservation and try to make certain that our sources are generally respected and accepted and that our conclusions are those we can defend.

Where do we find entries for *Current Medical Terminology*? From words encountered in medical transcription, from questions from medical transcriptionists, from dozens of medical journals we read regularly. We consult medical textbooks, talk to physicians, and have friends in central supply. Over the years we have learned to be less trusting of the written, as well as the spoken, word.

Of all sources, dictionaries are perhaps my most trusted, although I have found errors in even the most respected. Next are books, although I am finding that they, too, often have errors; apparently proofreading is considered an expendable luxury. I should mention that books do have the disadvantage of being dated, even when newly published. Somewhere at the top of the list would be the trusted person in central supply who will *read* the label on the equipment, instrument, or medication container, although there are times when there may be more than one spelling, as in Tycron and Ti-Cron. Next are journals, in which I find the most current information available, but I do find errors in even the most prestigious.

A close tie for last place on my list of trusted sources would be catalogs of instrument manufacturers and the spelling given us by physicians. An old newspaperman once told me that typesetters were given instructions to "follow the copy, even if it goes out the window." There are a few physicians whose spelling *is* impeccable and whose dictation I *would* "follow out the window," but, unfortunately, they are all too few.

In researching words, sometimes hunches and the educated guess based on experience and the knowledge of analogous words or terms are all one has to go on and are useful. Here is an example: I came across the word *Versatex* as a cardiac pacemaker. I should tell you that it is fatal in this situation to trust; it is *essential* that one question—everything and always. At any rate I felt uncomfortable with that spelling (it was guilty until proven innocent), and I decided to pursue it further. Unable to document it, but finding analogous terms (Activitrax and Spectrax), I felt quite comfortable with the spelling *Versatrax* and that is what has been used in this book.

A reader inquired about *Angiocath PRN* and wanted to know the meaning of PRN. My first information about Angiocath PRN, trade name of a catheter manufactured by Siemens Medical Systems, came from the *Journal of Neurosurgery.* I can only hazard a more-or-less educated guess as to what is meant. As you know, p.r.n. (L. *pro re nata)* means "as circumstances may require." This catheter has many different uses and the PRN may *perhaps* make reference to that.

Medical equipment manufacturers and pharmaceutical companies are most imaginative in creating names for their products. They are *so* clever, and running these things to earth is *so* frustrating. Sometimes they provide clues, e.g., Cefobid is a third-generation cephalosporin medication (which accounts for the first syllable) and is to be taken twice a day (b.i.d.), which accounts for the last syllable.

Sometimes there is no clue; one has to know what the device or medication is used for to know what the abbreviation means, e.g., the EID percutaneous central venous large-bore catheter manufactured by Arrow International, Inc. The EID turns out to mean *e*mergency *i*nfusion *d*evice! Or how about the SRT vaginal speculum manufactured by Amko Manufacturing Company? The SRT is from *s*moke *r*emoval *t*ube; the device has a supplementary tube used when smoke evacuation is necessary in laser-induced tissue vaporization.

A few years ago I searched for the definitive spelling of a needle we've been spelling *Verres* for many years. I got a letter from a medical transcriptionist who said she had been told by a physician that that spelling was in error, that it should be *Veress.* She said that she had looked in a dozen different textbooks and the spelling she found was indeed *Veress,* and she also sent me a photocopy of an article about this needle, written by the physician who had developed it, a Dr. Veress. We must assume that Dr. Veress knows how to spell his name, so we have now changed our spelling of this instrument to *Veress.*

In the medical field we don't have to look far or wait long for new words, abbreviations, and acronyms to appear. Just stand still for a couple of hours and a dozen new ones will have been born!

Vera Pyle, CMT
July 1992

A Medical Transcriptionist's Fantasy

A letter from a reader came in yesterday's mail. I thought about it during a sleepless night and at 3 a.m. arose from my bed, sat down in front of the typewriter, and ventilated.

Prices on many things have gone through the roof; dinner out, a play, even a film, are now rare treats. But there is something we can still afford—fantasy.

First, let me quote from the letter:

> *I will again bring to your attention an item I mentioned in a previous survey, to which I have never received a response either directly or indirectly. That is—the providing of information, be it names of newly approved drugs, newly developed prostheses, etc. I recently noted a reprint in one of the local newsletters from another professional journal. It contained "new" items. Although our present Notebook is terrific, it is just too limited to provide us with the information we require; that is, we need to "know" when the dictator "knows," not after the fact. Every time a "new" word is dictated, it involves excessive time and effort not only on the part of the transcriptionists, but on the part of the people they ask for help in listening, only to determine in the end that the spelling is not available to them because it is a "new" item, at which point either the word is researched or left blank for fill-in. If we knew the "new" words by preview, the time and effort saved could be tremendous!*

Now, let us fantasize. Wouldn't it be marvelous if we had a modern-day Paul Revere who would ride through the countryside shouting, not "The British are coming!" but instead "lithotriptor!—a new extracorporeal stone-disintegrating machine! First used in Europe, now being brought to the United States! Generates shock that breaks up kidney stones! Lowercase 'L'!"—as he rides off into the cold, starry night. Or how about "Kim-Ray Greenfield filter—used in prevention of pulmonary emboli! Kim-Ray is capitalized and hyphenated!" as he gallops, on his panting, snorting, sweating horse, to the next darkened village.

Let's fantasize further. Wouldn't it be wonderful if Dr. Andreas Gruentzig had called us and said: "Just wanted to let you know that I'm inventing a new balloon catheter; it will be a very nice thing to use in transluminal dilatation and in performing angioplasties. And, by the way, my name is spelled *G-r-ü-* (with an umlaut) *n-t-z-i-g,* in which case don't forget the umlaut over the *u*; or else, you can spell it *Gruentzig,* but in that case, don't use the umlaut. However, I *will* answer to either."

Or—if Dr. Richard Osgood had written, "You may be interested in being among the first to know that my colleague, Dr. Carl Schlatter (that's spelled *Schlatter;* don't forget the c, and remember there are two t's), and I have just identified a new disease entity—osteochondrosis of the tuberosity of the tibia; also called apophysitis tibialis adolescentium, which we are going to call 'Osgood-Schlatter disease.' If he should call you and tell you about this and tells you it is 'Schlatter-Osgood' disease, remember you heard it from me first, and correctly!"

There has been the time or two—or three—that I have rushed to press, triumphantly, with a word hot out of the operating room, newly born, nowhere else to be found, a real scoop—only to find it in print at a later date, and to learn that it had been given us—wrong.

Paul Revere, where are you now that we need you?

Adapted from Vera Pyle, "A Medical Transcriptionist's Fantasy," *Journal of the American Association for Medical Transcription,* Winter 1983-84, p. 3.

In Defense of "Sterilely"

A question from a medical transcriptionist about the word *sterilely* prompted the following responses. They are quoted here to illustrate the dilemma medical transcriptionists face in striving for accuracy, and a warning about what might happen if they forget that *physicians dictate and medical transcriptionists transcribe.*

The question was how to spell the adverb form of the word *sterile.* The inquirer wrote:

> *I say that if you use this word as an adverb, you retain the original form of the word and add "-ly," making the spelling sterilely, as it is in futile, puerile, hostile, etc. My colleagues see no point in dragging grammar into this and spell the word sterilly, as in "Sterilly we roll along."*

This is one of the questions to which I can say, with confidence, there is one and only one correct answer. The word is *sterilely.* I refer you to *Webster's Third International Dictionary, Unabridged* (1981), and to the *Random House Dictionary of the English Language, Unabridged,* 2nd ed. (1987); this is the *only* spelling given for this word.

I have just finished reading a book (in the nonmedical part of my life) about the people who colonized New England in the early 1600s, the Pilgrims and Puritans. Much of the journal written by Governor William Bradford of Plymouth was quoted, as well as letters written by many of the other men involved in the affairs of the Colony. Many of them were men of education, men who had studied at Cambridge. It was most interesting to see their spelling. In Elizabethan times there were no hard and fast spelling rules, and each person spelled as the spirit moved him, not even consistently with any individual. Shakespeare himself spelled his name a number of different ways. In those days this was not considered flouting of rules, since there were few if any rules. But that was then, and this is now.

Now there are dictionaries and rules. Sometimes there is more than one spelling of a word, and dictionaries will give preferred ones and acceptable ones. However, now, if one were to spell in a very personal manner, disregarding the rules, one would be open to criticism. And here I might give you Pyle's observation: Praise and credit rise to the highest person on the totem pole; criticism and blame fall on the lowest. So you see, we can ill afford to be cavalier about such things as correct spelling and grammar. Remember, we are judged and evaluated by people who know the rules and play by them, and they expect us to observe them as well.

A few months later I received the following comment, and apparently it struck a nerve; hence, the following response:

> *It was interesting to read the debate on the spelling of the word sterilely. Occasionally, due to progress in the English language, certain words or versions of certain words become outdated. Sterilely is one of them. I feel that proper grammar would dictate that we transcriptionists use the present-day terminology "in a sterile manner."*

Sterilely is not among my very favorite words. "I love you" and "I love your book" are higher on my list. Not too far behind comes ". . . the patient was taken to the recovery room in good condition." But I rise to the defense of *sterilely* for several reasons. First of all, there is nothing wrong with the word. Where has it been decreed that it is "outdated"? Words die when they are no longer viable and therefore no longer used. *Sterilely* is very much alive. If you don't believe it, transcribe operative reports in any hospital. If you don't want to believe it, just tell every surgeon in the country that it may no longer be used, that it is a forbidden word.

Imagine the unleashed fury of fifty thousand surgeons when they are told they may no longer say the WORD. I can see the backlash now—thousands of angry surgeons under the cover of night surging into the streets, chalking on fences and spray-painting on walls the naughty word—STERILELY, or possibly even (perish the thought) *sterilly.*

Carried to its logical conclusion, this stance puts us in the position of saying that physicians are permitted to use only those words that all transcriptionists can spell. Carried further there will then be no need for dictionaries, for drug books, for word books. Sounds like a dream, doesn't it? Now comes the alarm clock, shrilling the end of the dream. *Medical transcriptionists don't dictate, physicians do.*

I urge you—cease and desist. Don't type "The patient was draped in a sterile manner" when the surgeon dictates "The patient was sterilely draped," or the fence-chalking, spray-painting surgeons are likely to burn us in effigy.

Adapted from Vera Pyle, "A Question of Style," *Journal of the American Association for Medical Transcription,* Winter 1984-85, Fall 1985.

Medical Slang—Its Use and Abuse

The language of medicine is an "in-language." It is the means of communication for a comparatively small, select group in a world divided into "us" and "them." Its use makes one feel part of that group of "us's." Medical abbreviations and medical slang are subspecies of this language (slanguage?) and are particularly dear to the hearts of the newest members of the in-group.

Its use makes medical students feel that they sound "professional." It has much the same effect as wearing a stethoscope. To only a slightly lesser degree, this applies also to the intern and resident. I once asked a resident in surgery the reason for this. He thought about it for a while, grinned, and replied, "Well, when you've just learned all these new long words, it's a pity not to use them, and you must admit that some of them *are* pretty impressive." Interestingly enough, the truly impressive people in medicine speak simply, almost in lay language.

Language changes. It is far from static. The English we speak now is far from the English of Chaucer or Shakespeare. The language of medicine also changes. Many of these changes fill a real need, in which case they are likely to last. Some of this change is frivolous, "trendy," highly personal, and likely to be understood by few. Much of this language is not yet found in dictionaries for these reasons. Dictionaries, after all, are *de*scriptive, not *pre*scriptive, and many of these words are too new, too ephemeral, too localized to make their way into dictionaries. And for these same reasons, we cannot be certain that we can use them safely in reports which are considered legal documents.

I think we must take a long look at what is now being dictated, and we may find it necessary to accept terms that have been frowned on in the past, that have not yet been accepted in dictionaries but are used constantly by physicians because they fill a need.

Some twenty years ago, we began hearing the word "bovied" but were told, "You can't make a verb of a noun." So we would type, "Bleeders were electrocoagulated with the Bovie unit." All these years later, I find "bovied" still used a great deal—a useful term, succinct, and universally understood. Another such word is "saucerize," which refers to creation of a saucer-shaped excavation surgically.

I believe 20/20 hindsight might well be the determining factor in knowing what is a needed term, likely to survive and ultimately enter the language, and what is for the moment "flip," likely to have only narrow, local application, and short survival. My own criteria for using new words or slang would be (1) need for the word or term, (2) broad understanding of the term, and (3) potential for survival.

A new slang expression I have encountered only occasionally is "romied" and it may or may not last. Although it may fill a need, it is *not* commonly understood. I am not prepared to use it. It is a verb coined from an acronym, **r**ule **o**ut **m**yocardial **i**nfarction, and used thus: "The patient was admitted with severe precordial pain and cardiac arrhythmias, and was romied." My guess is that it is one of those terms that will not have wide circulation and will not survive because too few will know the acronym from which it is derived. It is an example of a sub-subspecies of an in-language, and may be known to some cardiologists (probably the newest of them only) and hence will not be a viable means of communication to a broader spectrum of the medical population.

It should also be remembered that our spoken language differs from our written (more formal) language, and that terms used in the operating room or on the ward are not necessarily what should be written in a report.

The following are other examples of acronyms that have become words: CABG (coronary artery bypass graft) and pronounced "cabbage," as in "The patient was given a CABG," or even "The patient was CABG'd." These evoke rather interesting images. (We have the option of using the acronyms or writing out the terms in full.) You may be astonished to hear a physician dictate, "Caloric testing produced COWS." "COWS" stands for "**c**old to the **o**pposite, **w**arm to the **s**ame" and is a mnemonic device used in otolaryngology to help remember the Hallpike caloric stimulation response.

It may be interesting to enter the arcane world of the operating room and discover the slang peculiar to it. For example, a "peanut" is a small gauze sponge used in surgery. This word is in widespread use, but some operating room personnel have their own terms for it. Cotton pledgets are small cotton balls (sponges) which are rolled so that they have somewhat pointed ends. They are used to absorb blood or other fluids from the operative site. In some parts of the country they are known as "pollywogs." The Chiba needle is often referred to as a "skinny needle." The term "stick-tie" means different things to different people in different operating rooms. In some operating rooms it refers to a suture ligature, or transfixion suture; in others it refers to a long strand of suture clamped on a hemostat. If a surgeon asks the scrub nurse for

''Mets'' (or ''Metz''), Metzenbaum scissors are wanted. It is understandable that under the time pressures in surgery, ''OR shorthand'' would be used, but in a formal document the word should be transcribed ''Metzenbaum scissors.''

In the dim, distant past, some words originated as medical slang and are now firmly rooted in our language. ''Gurney'' is one such. I do not know its origin; it may well have been a trade name. It may also have been the brainchild of someone in one hospital and traveled with surgeons or nurses to others across the country. None of the references I have consulted gives a derivation. It is, however, such a commonly used word that it would be absurd now to say, ''The patient was placed on a high wheeled cart for moving patients in a hospital and taken to the operating room.''

So you see, we are dealing with not only the present but also the past and the future. We can, to some degree, judge from the kinds of words that have been accepted and have survived over the years which ones will have currency in the future. A surgical word we hear all the time is ''prepped.'' Most attending surgeons with whose dictation I am familiar use ''prepared.'' ''Prepped'' is, however, universally understood, and my inclination is to type whatever the dictator says; if residents feel that they are being ''professional'' by using it, I won't argue the point. It seems a lost cause anyhow. Perhaps I am getting too old to fight for lost causes; perhaps my sense of proportion tells me it's not worth it, or perhaps I am saving my ammunition for more important issues.

The purpose in dictating all this material, and the purpose in transcribing it, is communication—with other physicians, with nurses, with other healthcare professionals and paraprofessionals; with quality assurance, billing, risk management people; with insurance companies; with lawyers. If we are not successful in this communication, if we are ''playing doctor'' by being exclusionary with our in-language, if we are obfuscating rather than clarifying, what then is the point in all this effort?

Actually, I have more questions than I have answers. But these are questions that must be raised. I do want to be clear, to be understandable. It is not, I repeat, not our role to *force* doctors to do anything *our* way. This is not in any way a crusade. Doctors like us to be right, but they do resent our being righteous!

Adapted from Vera Pyle, ''Medical Slang—Its Use and Abuse,'' *Journal of the American Association for Medical Transcription,* Fall 1983, pp. 38-39.

Key to Medical Specialties

To provide a context in which a term is likely to be encountered in medical transcription, one or more medical specialties may appear in parentheses in an entry.

Audiol	Audiology
Cardio	Cardiology; Cardiac Surgery
Dent	Dental; Oral Surgery
Derm	Dermatology
Emer Med	Emergency Medicine
ENT	Ear, Nose, and Throat
GI	Gastroenterology
Gyn	Gynecology
Hand Surg	Hand Surgery; Microsurgery
Hematol	Hematology
Lab	Laboratory Medicine
Neonat	Neonatology
Nephrol	Nephrology
Neuro	Neurology; Neurosurgery
Ob-Gyn	Obstetrics-Gynecology
Obs	Obstetrics
Oph	Ophthalmology
Oncol	Oncology
Oral Surg	Oral Surgery; Dental
Ortho	Orthopedics; Orthopedic Surgery
Path	Pathology
Peds	Pediatrics
Pharm	Pharmacology
Phys Ther	Physical Therapy
Plas Surg	Plastic Surgery
Pod	Podiatry
Psych	Psychiatry; Psychology
Pulm	Pulmonary Medicine
Radiol	Radiology
Rad Oncol	Radiation Oncology
Rehab	Rehabilitation; Physical Medicine
Resp Ther	Respiratory Therapy
Surg	Surgery
Thor Surg	Thoracic Surgery
Urol	Urology; Urological Surgery
Vasc Surg	Vascular Surgery

A, a

AAA (''triple A'')—medical slang for abdominal aortic aneurysm.

AAMT (American Association for Medical Transcription)—a professional association for medical transcriptionists. See *certified medical transcriptionist.*

Aaron's sign—pain on pressure over McBurney's point in a patient with appendicitis.

Aarskog syndrome—shawl scrotum, long philtrum, short stature, downward eye slant, pectus deformity.

ab, AB—abortion or miscarriage. AB 2 (or ab 2) means that the patient has had two abortions or miscarriages.

Abbe-Estlander flap (Plas Surg).

Abbe repair (Plas Surg).

Abbott-Rawson tube—a long gastrointestinal double-lumen tube.

Abbreviated Injury Scale (AIS).

ABC (airway, breathing, circulation) (Emer Med)—must be assessed immediately on trauma patients before anything else is done.

ABC (aspiration biopsy cytology).

ABCD (amphotericin B colloid dispersion)—a drug used to treat cryptococcal meningitis in AIDS patients.

abduct—to draw away from a position parallel to the median axis. Cf. *adduct.*

"a-b-duction"—dictated by a physician to clarify that *abduction,* not *adduction,* is intended.

aberrant—wandering or deviating from the normal; abnormal. Cf. *apparent.*

abetalipoproteinemia—see *Bassen-Kornzweig.*

ABGs (arterial blood gases)—refer to pO_2, pCO_2, and oxygen saturation. From these data and the serum pH, the bicarbonate (or base excess) can be calculated.

abirritant—a soothing agent.

ablation—separation, eradication, extirpation, as in cryo-ablation, radiofrequency ablation.

ABLC (amphotericin B lipid complex) —a drug used to treat cryptococcal meningitis in AIDS patients.

ABMT (autologous bone marrow transplant).

ABPP (bropirimine)—a drug used to treat AIDS.

ABR (auditory brain stem response)—an audiometric technique to test for sensorineural hearing loss.

Abramson catheter (Surg)—used for drainage.

abreaction (Psych)—the reliving of an experience in such a way that previously repressed emotions associated with it are released.

Abrodil (methiodal sodium) (Radiol)—used as a contrast medium in myelograms and in urinary tract studies.

abscess—a circumscribed, localized collection of pus, usually caused by infection, and by the decomposition of tissue. See *Brodie's abscess, collar button abscess.* Cf. *aphthous.*

Absolok—endoscopic clip applicator.

absolute neutrophil count (ANC) (Oncol).

absorbent—an agent or material that takes up or soaks up another material (usually a liquid). Cf. *adsorbent.*

ABVD (Oncol)—a standard chemotherapy protocol used to treat adult Hodgkin's disease. Consists of the drugs Adriamycin, bleomycin, vinblastine, and dacarbazine.

ABVE (Adriamycin, bleomycin, vincristine, etoposide)—chemotherapy protocol used to treat Hodgkin's lymphoma.

ACA (anticentromere antibody).

***Acanthamoeba* keratitis** (Oph)—an inflammation of the cornea caused by *Acanthamoeba.*

acanthosis—diffuse hyperplasia and thickening of the prickle-cell layer of the epidermis, as in psoriasis.

ACAT (automated computerized axial tomography).

Ac'cents—permanent lash liner applied by plastic surgeon.

access—admittance, as "This gave easy access to the abdominal cavity." Cf. *axis, excess.*

accommodation—adjustment, as of the eye for distance.

Accu-Chek II—a home blood glucose monitoring system.

Accu-Chek II Freedom—self-monitoring blood glucose system for visually impaired diabetics. It talks users through self blood-testing with clearly spoken cues.

Accucore II (Surg)—core biopsy needles with echo-enhanced tip for ultrasound guidance and precise depth markings.

Accu-Line knee instrumentation (Ortho)—to assist in total knee arthroplasty. Includes tibial resector, distal femoral resection instrument, dual pivot, chamfer resection guide, and patellar instruments.

AccuPoint hCG Pregnancy Test Disc for quick diagnosis (Obs).

Accupril (quinapril) (Cardio)—a once-a-day ACE inhibitor used to treat hypertension.

Accurate Surgical and Scientific Instruments (ASSI). A trade name, not a comment on quality.

AccuSpan tissue expander (Plas Surg). Cf. *expander, PMT AccuSpan.*

ACD (allergic contact dermatitis).

ACE (Adriamycin, Cytoxan, etoposide) —chemotherapy protocol used to treat small-cell lung carcinoma.

acebutolol (Sectral)—a beta adrenergic blocker used in treatment of mild to moderate hypertension; also used in treatment of ventricular arrhythmias; taken once a day.

acecainide (Napa) (Cardio)—an antiarrhythmic drug which is actually a metabolite of procainamide (Procan SR). The chemical name for this drug, N-acetylprocainamide, is abbreviated NAPA. Napa is the trade name.

Ace-Fischer fixator (Ortho).

ACE inhibitor (angiotensin converting enzyme)—to treat hypertension.
acemannan (Carrisyn)—a drug used in AIDS treatment.
acetylator—an agent capable of metabolic acetylation.
acetylcholine receptor antibody—see *AChRab.*
Ace Unifix (Ortho)—fixation device.
Achilles reflex. On percussion of the Achilles tendon just above the calcaneus, contraction of the muscles of the leg produces plantar flexion of the foot. Also, gastrocnemius reflex, ankle jerk.
Achilles tendon (*but* tendo Achill*is*).
achondroplastic dwarfism—a disorder of connective tissue metabolism; the patient is normal except for bone growth and development. Also, chondroplastic dwarfism.
AChRab (acetylcholine receptor antibody) (Neuro)—found in the sera of patients with myasthenia gravis.
Achromobacter lwoffi—see *Acinetobacter lwoffi.*
acid
- aminocaproic
- antiteichoic
- arachidonic
- chenodeoxycholic (CDA)
- eicosapentaenoic (EPA)
- ethacrynic
- 5-hydroxyindoleacetic (5-HIAA)
- hepatoiminodiacetic (HIDA)
- ibotenic
- isovaleric
- mefenamic (Ponstel)
- teichoic

acidemia, isovaleric.
acidic—having the characteristics of an acid. Cf. *ascitic.*
acidosis, renal tubular. See *Rector-Gordon-Healey-Mendoza-Spitzer type IV renal tubular acidosis.*
Acinetobacter lwoffi—normal flora of skin, mouth, and external genitalia; isolated from sputum and urine; associated with conjunctivitis, keratitis, and chronic ear infections. Also, *Achromobacter lwoffi, Mima polymorpha, Moraxella lwoffi.*
AC-IOL (anterior chamber intraocular lens) (Oph).
Ackrad H/S catheter (hysterosalpingography) (Gyn, Radiol).
aCL (anticardiolipin antibody).
Acland-Banis arteriotomy set (Surg)—used for end-to-side microvascular anastomosis.
Acland clip (Neuro).
ACL drill guide; repair (anterior cruciate ligament) (Ortho).
ACMI Martin endoscopy forceps.
ACOP (Adriamycin, Cytoxan, Oncovin, prednisone)—chemotherapy protocol used to treat non-Hodgkin's lymphoma.
acoustical shadowing (Radiol)—in ultrasonography. Reflection of large amounts of ultrasound from the surface of structures or materials that are physically incompressible (bone, gallstones), with blockage of further transmission.
acquired immunodeficiency syndrome (AIDS). See *AIDS.*
acquisition time—MRI term.
Acra-Cut cranial perforator (Neuro).
acrochordon (Path)—a skin tag.
A.C.S. (Alcon Closure System) (Oph) —a series of three ophthalmic needles and sutures—SC-1, PC-7, and Lewis Pair-Pak—used during intraocular surgery.
ACT (activated coagulation time).
Actigall (ursodiol) (GI)—given orally to dissolve small gallbladder stones without surgery. See *MTBE.*

activated charcoal—used as an antidote in some kinds of poisoning; it is an adsorbent, not an absorbent.

activated partial thromboplastin time (APTT).

active phase arrest (*not* of rest)—during labor, when the cervix stops dilating and no progress is being made toward delivery (Obs).

activities of daily living (ADLs) (Rehab).

Activitrax—brand name for a specialized heart pacemaker containing a microphone which senses muscle activity during exercise, and is programmable to increase the rate of a ventricle 5 to 10 beats per increment of sensed muscle tone. Manufactured by Medtronic.

actocardiotocograph (Ob-Gyn)—a fetal monitor that displays a tracing of the fetal heart rate and simultaneously records fetal movements and uterine contractions. Used to monitor pregnancies with multiple fetuses.

Acu-Derm I.V./TPN dressing (GI)—provides a moisture- and vapor-permeable covering that reduces the risk of catheter movement.

Acu-Dyne—an antiseptic (Ortho).

Acufex arthroscopic instruments, i.e., rotary punch, straight and curved basket forceps. (*Not* Acuflex.)

Acuson computed sonography—for Doppler and color Doppler imaging (Radiol).

acute abdomen—an abdomen showing signs of acute inflammation.

acute
graft-versus-host disease (GVHD)
intermittent porphyria (AIP)
lymphoblastic leukemia (ALL)
monoblastic leukemia (AMOL)
myeloblastic leukemia (AML)
nonlymphoid leukemia (ANLL)

acute *(cont.)*
renal failure (ARF)
respiratory failure (ARF)
tubular necrosis (ATN)

ACUTENS—transcutaneous nerve stimulator that includes elements of acupuncture or acupressure, for control of pain. It is typed in all capital letters, as in TENS unit.

Acuvue (etafilcon A)—disposable contact lens (Oph).

acycloguanosine—see *acyclovir.*

acyclovir (acycloguanosine, Zovirax)—an antiviral agent used in the treatment of herpes simplex, varicella-zoster virus infections, patients with AIDS and ARC, and CMV retininitis in AIDS patients. Used in treating chickenpox in otherwise healthy children, for faster healing of skin lesions with less scar formation.

A.D. (auris dextra)—right ear.

Adagen (pegademase bovine).

Adamkiewicz artery—supplying blood to the thoracolumbar spinal cord. Injury to this artery may be a cause of cauda equina syndrome (Neuro).

Adaptar (Oph)—a new "no-line" contact lens which can accommodate all stages of presbyopia.

ADD (attention deficit disorders) (formerly known as minimal brain dysfunction in children) (Peds). This is a group of developmentally inappropriate symptoms in children, such as moderate-to-severe distractibility, short attention span, hyperactivity, emotional lability, and impulsivity. Also called hyperkinetic child syndrome, minimal brain damage, minimal cerebral dysfunction, and minor cerebral dysfunction.

Addix needle and tier—for suturing the flap after submucous operation (ENT).

adduct—to draw toward a position near or parallel to the median axis. Cf. *abduct.*

"a-d-duction"—dictated by a physician to clarify that *adduction,* not *abduction,* is intended.

ADE (Ara-C, daunorubicin, etoposide) —chemotherapy protocol used to treat acute myeloid leukemia.

adenine arabinoside—antiviral drug, also known as *vidarabine, Ara-A,* and *Vira-A.*

adenocyst—adenocystoma (adenoma in which there is cyst formation). Cf. *adenosis.*

adenoma, aldosterone-producing (APA).

adenomyomatosis—a proliferation of the gallbladder's epithelium with glandlike formations and outpouchings of the mucosa into or through the hypertrophied muscular layer; these hyperplastic mucosal diverticula are also called Rokitansky-Aschoff sinuses (RAS).

adenosine echocardiography (Cardio). The antiarrhythmic agent adenosine (Adenocard) is given I.V. during echocardiography to assess patients with suspected coronary artery disease since it causes the coronary arteries to constrict, thus producing ischemic symptoms without a stress test. Even if the drug does produce coronary artery constriction and exacerbate patient symptoms, its effect is extremely brief for it has a half-life of only 10 seconds.

adenosis—disease of the glands or abnormal development of glandular tissue. Cf. *adenocyst.* Types:
blunt duct
florid
sclerosing

adhesion
banjo-string
filmy

adhesive (See also *bandage, dressing.)*
Aron Alpha
Biobrane
Coe-pak paste
Coverlet
Cover-Roll gauze
cyanoacrylate
fibrin glue
Histoacryl glue
hydroxyapatite
Implast bone cement
LPPS hydroxyapatite
methyl methacrylate cement
Palacos cement
Simplex cement
Superglue
Surfit
Surgical Simplex P radiopaque bone cement
Zimmer low viscosity

adiabatic fast passage—MRI term.

Adie's pupil (Oph).

adiposis dolorosa—a rare disorder of fat metabolism of unknown cause; fat accumulates in painful lumps over the body. Also, Dercum's disease.

Adjustable Leg and Ankle Repositioning Mechanism (ALARM).

adjuvant, see *Freund's complete adjuvant* and *Freund's incomplete adjuvant.*

adjuvant therapy—auxiliary therapy.

ADLs—activities of daily living (Rehab). "Plan: Improve the patient's ADLs."

adnexa (Gyn)—the uterine appendages including the ovary and fallopian tube on each side. *Adnexa* is plural and always takes a plural verb: "The adnexa were unremarkable." Also, ocular adnexa (Oph).

ADR-529 (Oncol)—used to prevent cardiotoxicity in cancer patients receiving Adriamycin.

ADR ultrasound—portable microprocessor based on electrocardiography system.

ADR Ultramark 4 ultrasound.

adrenergic antagonist (Pharm)—a drug which blocks the action of naturally produced neurotransmitters on adrenergic receptors of sympathetic nervous system.

Adson forceps; rongeur; suction tube.

Adson maneuver—to rule in or rule out scalenus anticus syndrome (Ortho).

adsorbent—an agent that attracts other molecules to, or maintains them on, a surface. Cf. *absorbent.*

adult respiratory distress syndrome (ARDS).

Advent flexible fluoropolymer contact lens (Oph).

Aebli corneal section scissors (Oph).

AE fold (aryepiglottic) (ENT).

Ae-H interval (anterograde conduction) (Cardio)—a term used in electrophysiologic studies of supraventricular tachycardia.

aeroallergens
- *Aspergillus*
- *Basidiomycetes* (a class of smut and rust fungi)
- *Chaetomium*
- *Curvularia*
- *Dermatophagoides* (mites)
- *Fusarium* (a slime mold)
- *Helminthosporium*
- *Phoma* (a slime mold)
- *Pullularia* (a slime mold)
- *Rhodotorula*
- *Saccharomyces*
- *Spondylocladium*
- *Stemphyllium*

AeroChamber—a face mask which attaches to a bronchial inhaler device. The metered-dose aerosol can be breathed over several seconds by patients who have difficulty using inhaler devices.

aerogenous (Lab)—descriptive term for bacteria which produce gas. Cf. *erogenous.*

Aeropent—trade name for aerosolized pentamidine, an inhaled agent used as prophylaxis against *Pneumocystis carinii* pneumonia.

aerosolized pentamidine—see *Aeropent.*

Aesculap forceps (Neuro).

Aesculap reciprocating saw.

aesthetic—artistic or beautiful in appearance. Cf. *asthenic.*

AFBG (aortofemoral bypass graft).

affect—(verb) to change; to produce an effect, as "This should not affect the outcome"; (noun) outward appearance of an inner emotion (Neuro, Psych), as "The patient demonstrated a flat affect" (or "flattened affect"). Cf. *effect.*

afferent—moving towards the center, as in an afferent defect in ophthalmology. Cf. *efferent.*

affinity chromatography.

AFIP (Armed Forces Institute of Pathology). Pathologists often send specimens to AFIP for consultation.

AFM (Adriamycin, fluorouracil, methotrexate)—chemotherapy protocol used to treat metastatic breast carcinoma.

AFO (ankle-foot orthosis) (Ortho).

AFP lab test (alpha-fetoprotein).

afterloading (Rad Oncol). Small plastic tubes are placed near the tumor in the operating room and later, in the patient's room, in isolation, the radioactive sources are loaded (to avoid putting hospital staff at risk for radiation).

Agar-IF (immunofixation in agar) of blood serum.

agarose gel electrophoresis (AGE) (Lab).

AGE (angle of greatest extension) (Ortho).

age-related macular degeneration (AMD) (Oph).

AGF (angle of greatest flexion) (Ortho).

aggregate—a mass or cluster of material, as aggregate measurements.

aggregated human IgG (AHuG).

Agnew tattooing needle (Oph).

agonist (Pharm)—a drug that stimulates activity of a receptor in the way it would be stimulated by naturally produced neurotransmitters. Cf. *antagonist.*

agranulocytosis, in *Kostmann's infantile agranulocytosis.*

Agricola lacrimal sac retractor (Oph).

Agrobacterium tumefaciens (Lab).

ahaustral—without haustra, the bands running circumferentially around the large bowel.

AHG (antihemophilic globulin)—can be administered via AV fistula for intravenous infusion control of intermittent bleeding in hemophilia.

AHI (apnea/hypopnea index).

AHIMA (American Health Information Management Association)—a professional association for health information management professionals who have credentials of the registered record administrator (RRA) or accredited record technician (ART). Formerly known as American Medical Record Association (AMRA).

AHuG (aggregated human IgG).

AICA (pronounced "I'-ka") (anterior inferior communicating artery).

AICD (automatic internal cardioverter defibrillator) (Cardio).

AID (artificial insemination–donor) (semen).

AID implantable defibrillator—manufactured by Medrac.

AIDS (acquired immunodeficiency syndrome)—a disease that attacks the immune system, leaving the body susceptible to such opportunistic infections as *Pneumocystis carinii* pneumonia, Kaposi's sarcoma, candidiasis, and others; these may also be accompanied by neurological manifestations. AIDS is caused by a retrovirus and transmitted by sexual contact or by contaminated hypodermic needles, blood or blood products (contaminated blood in blood transfusions, and occasionally by contamination by blood through an open wound in the skin), or by contact with the virus in semen. Related entries: AIDS drugs, AIDS virus, ARC, ARS, ARV, HIV, HTLV/III, Kaposi's sarcoma, and LAV.

AIDS drugs—see *medication* and alphabetic entries throughout the book. As of mid-1992 only three drugs had been approved by the FDA for treating AIDS: didanosine (ddI, Videx), dideoxycytidine (ddC, HIVID), and zidovudine (Retrovir). All other drugs are considered investigational for the treatment of AIDS symptoms. Some of the drugs are used only to treat patients with AIDS; others are used to treat HIV-positive patients, and patients with ARC (AIDS-related complex). Some drugs are used to treat Kaposi's sarcoma or other types of infections common to patients with AIDS. Other drugs are used to counteract the side effects of AIDS drugs.

AIDS vaccine—investigational vaccine consisting of purified protein derived from genetic material from the AIDS virus which is reproduced using recombinant DNA technology. This

AIDS vaccine *(cont.)* material stimulates the body to produce antibodies against the AIDS virus but, because it contains only pieces of HIV, the vaccine itself cannot cause AIDS. In mid-1992 at least six different AIDS vaccines were undergoing clinical trials: gp120, gp160, RG-83894, r-gp160, rp24, VaxSyn HIV-1.

AIDS virus—a retrovirus of the cytopathic lentivirus group that invades and inactivates helper/T-cells of the immune system. See *helper cells; HIV.*

AIH (artificial insemination-husband) (semen).

AIM CPM (continuous passive motion) for hand (Ortho).

AIP (acute intermittent porphyria).

air-bone gap (ENT)—in audiology testing. (*Not* "ear-bone gap" or "airborne gap").

air conduction (*not* ear conduction)—refers to the transmission of sound through the ear canal, tympanic membrane, and ossicular chain to the cochlea and auditory nerve. Air conduction is tested by holding an activated tuning fork near the external auditory meatus. Cf. *bone conduction, Rinne test.*

air-fluid level (Radiol)—a line representing the level of a collection of fluid seen in profile, with air or gas above it.

air hunger—in patients with chronic extreme anemia, uremia, and diabetic acidosis with great difficulty struggling to breathe; long, deep, slow or panting breathing.

air-space disease (Radiol)—as seen on chest x-ray, disease or abnormality of lung tissue that encroaches on space normally filled by air.

air splint (also inflatable splint) (Ortho). It is blown up like a balloon and usually used to immobilize the foot and ankle. There are other such splints used for the arm or the whole leg. Usage: "This is an acute ankle sprain, so she will be placed in an air splint and should keep her foot elevated."

air trousers—medical (or military) antishock trousers. See *MAST trousers.*

AIS (Abbreviated Injury Scale)—a system of scoring trauma injuries to each anatomic system.

AJ (ankle jerk) (Neuro). "He has preserved reflexes throughout, evaluated at 2+ AJs, 3+ KJs, trace brachioradialis, and 1+ biceps." (Note: KJ is knee jerk.)

akathisia—motor restlessness often localized in the muscles, resulting in inability to sit or lie quietly; a side effect of some antipsychotic drugs. Example: "A protracted akathisia-like dystonic-type reaction to this medication is very remote."

Aker pusher (Oph).

akinesia, Nadbath.

Akros extended care mattress for pressure relief.

alar flaring—flaring (dilatation) of the nostrils on inspiration, sometimes the only sign of dyspnea in a small child. Also called nasal flaring.

ALARM (Adjustable Leg and Ankle Repositioning Mechanism)—used in orthopedic surgery.

Alberts' Famous Faces Test—neurological test.

albumen—the white of the egg; it contains protein and not cholesterol. Cf. *albumin.*

albumin—the major plasma protein present in human serum. Cf. *albumen.*

albuminocytologic dissociation (cerebrospinal fluid elevation).

albuterol inhaler—for asthma.

Alcian blue—a stain used in testing for mucopolysaccharides.

alcohol, ethanol, EtOH—used interchangeably when referring to the consumption of alcohol.

Alcon intraocular lens (Oph).

aldosterone-producing adenoma (APA).

alfacalcidol (trade name, One-Alpha). Used in treating hypocalcemia and osteopenia resistant to vitamin D therapy. Used in Japan, Canada, and the United Kingdom in the same way as calciferol, Rocaltrol, and Calderol.

alfa interferon—see *interferon alfa.*

Alferon LDO—see *interferon alfa-n3.*

Alferon N—see *interferon alfa-n3.*

alglucerase (Ceredase)—treatment for Gaucher's disease, a rare hereditary metabolic disease. It is an enzyme which acts in the place of a deficit enzyme. The drug increases red blood cell and platelet counts, improves splenomegaly, and diminishes cachexia from Gaucher's disease.

algorithm—a problem-solving procedure, step-by-step, as with a computer; e.g., "We discussed the following: Should he not improve, there would be two more stools for ova and parasites and for culture. If these are normal, and should he still have symptomatology, he would have a barium enema. If this is normal, and symptomatology still persists, he would have flexible sigmoidoscopy, and finally, if his symptomatology still persists, then an upper GI with small bowel series. I told him that there is no urgency in approaching this algorithm."

ALHE (angiolymphoid hyperplasia with eosinophilia) (Path)—uncommon smooth-surfaced nodules, consisting of lymphocytes and eosinophils involving dermis and subcutaneous tissue.

alien hand sign (Neuro)—sequela of an extensive stroke in the medial frontal cortex. The hand opposite the affected side of the brain (the alien hand) instinctively grasps and does other purposeful behaviors which cannot be controlled by the patient. Often the patient must use his other (unaffected) hand to hold and restrain the alien hand.

aliquot ("al'-e-kwat")—an equal part of a whole, as in a solution. Used thus: "The patient was then given 5 mg of Valium in 2.5 mg aliquots to minimize the artifact in this EEG."

Alkeran—see *melphalan.*

alkylating, as in alkylating agent (*not* alkalating).

ALL (acute lymphoblastic leukemia); seen primarily in children.

Allen arm/hand surgery table.

Allen shoulder arthroscopy—traction system by Edgewater.

Allen's test for diagnosing certain circulatory problems.

Allergan 211—see *idoxuridine.*

allergen, *Rhizopus nigricans*.

allergic contact dermatitis (ACD).

allergic salute—repeated rubbing of the nose upward to scratch an itchy nose and open the obstructed airway (seen in patients with allergies).

allergic shiners—darkening of the skin around the eyes, resembling periorbital hematomas, as a symptom of allergic rhinitis.

Allevyn dressing (Surg)—nonadherent dressing material that is absorbent even under pressure.

Allis clamp, forceps.

Allis' sign (Ortho)—a sign of fracture of the femoral neck, when the fascia between the crest of the ilium and the greater trochanter relaxes.

allodynia—pain resulting from a non-noxious stimulus to normal skin.

allopurinol (Zyloprim)—commonly used as a treatment for gout. A solution of this drug is also used to preserve kidneys taken from cadavers prior to being transplanted.

allusion—an indirect reference to something, as "He made allusion to a history of some kind of tropical disease." Cf. *elusion, illusion.*

allylamines—class of antifungal drugs. Example: naftifine (Naftin).

Aloka color Doppler system—provides real-time, 2-dimensional blood flow imaging with Cine Memory (Radiol).

Aloka 650 ultrasound machine (Radiol)—made by Corometrics Medical Systems.

Aloka ultrasound diagnostic equipment (Radiol)—linear and sector scanners.

alopecia androgenetica—male pattern baldness (Derm).

Alpar intraocular lens implant (Oph).

Alpha Chymar (alpha-chymotrypsin).

alpha-chymotrypsin (Alpha Chymar) (Oph)—used for lysis of zonular fibers of the lens by enzymatic action.

alpha-fetoprotein lab test (AFP). Normal is less than 20; an elevated value (may go over 100,000) indicates the presence of an embryonal tumor, spina bifida, or Down's syndrome.

alpha interferon—see *interferon alfa.*

AlphaNine—a factor IX clotting agent, given by injection to patients with hemophilia B.

alpha$_1$-proteinase inhibitor—an intravenous drug for patients with emphysema due to alpha$_1$-antitrypsin deficiency.

alpha-TGI (alpha-triglycidyl isocyanurate)—see *teroxirone.*

Alredase (tolrestat)—a drug used to treat diabetic retinopathy.

AL-721—a drug used in treating AIDS.

Alström's disease (Oph, Nephrol)—the symptom complex includes pigmentary retinopathy, diabetes, obesity, with sensorineural deafness, and with severe visual loss in the first decade after diagnosis. There is also renal disease associated with this.

ALT (argon laser trabeculoplasty) (Oph).

Altace (ramipril).

Alternaria—an inhalant antigen.

Alteromonas putrefaciens—gram-negative organism.

ALT-RCC (autolymphocyte-based treatment for renal cell carcinoma)—a treatment in which a small number of the patient's WBCs are removed, activated in the laboratory, and then returned to the patient to combat the cancer cells. This procedure, done on an outpatient basis (two visits per month for six months), has been shown to increase survival time for these patients.

altretamine (Hexalen, Hexastat) (Oncol)—chemotherapy drug used to treat ovarian carcinoma. Known as hexamethylmelamine (HXM or HMM) while undergoing final testing before FDA approval.

ALVAD (abdominal left ventricular assist device) (Cardio).

alveolar ridge—the upper flattened surface of the mandible and the lower flattened surface of the maxilla, in the sockets of which the teeth are rooted (Oral Surg).

Alzate catheter.

ALZ-50 (Path)—a protein found in the central nervous system of patients with Alzheimer's disease. This may prove to be a good clinical marker in the diagnosis of this disease.

Alzheimer's disease—presenile dementia characterized by cortical atrophy and ventricular dilatation.

AMBI hip screw (Ortho).

amblyopia—dimness of vision not due to refractive error or organic lesion in the eye.

Ambu bag—a low-tech resuscitation tool in the emergency room.

AMD (age-related macular degeneration) (Oph).

AME bone growth stimulators (Ortho)—noninvasive; can be used over casted or noncasted fracture sites. For treatment of nonunion secondary to trauma. Requires minimum of 3-hour daily treatments. See *PEMF.*

AME PinSite Shields (Ortho)—for protection of the site (soft skin) into which are inserted halo pins, external fixation pins, Ilizarov fixation, and traction pins. Made by AME (American Medical Electronics).

American Association for Medical Transcription—see *AAMT.*

American Health Information Management Association—see *AHIMA.*

AMF (autocrine motility factor) (Urol).

amifostine—see *ethiofos.*

amiloride (Midamor)—commonly prescribed potassium-sparing diuretic. Administered via inhalation to treat cystic fibrosis.

amifostine—see *ethiofos.*

Amin-Aid—a special formula dietary supplement usually used by patients with chronic renal failure.

amine precursor uptake and decarboxylation (APUD).

aminoglutethimide (AGT, Cytadren, Elipten)—used to treat patients with advanced breast and prostatic carcinomas.

aminopyridine—see *4-aminopyridine.*

amiodipine (Norvasc) (Cardio)—a calcium channel blocking drug used to treat hypertension and angina.

Amipaque—brand name for a metrizamide radiopaque diagnostic agent. Used in intravenous digital arteriography.

Amko vaginal speculum.

AML (acute myeloblastic leukemia); seen at any age, but mostly in adults.

AMMOL (acute myelomonoblastic leukemia); seen at all ages but somewhat more often in adults.

AMOL (acute monoblastic leukemia)—seen at all ages, but a higher proportion of patients are adults.

amphotericin B colloid dispersion (ABCD)—a drug used to treat cryptococcal meningitis.

amphotericin B lipid complex (ABLC) —a reformulation of the common antifungal drug amphotericin B has made ABLC more effective in treating cryptococcal meningitis in AIDS patients.

Amplatz cardiac catheter; dilator.

Ampligen—mismatched double-stranded RNA used to treat AIDS patients. Also called polyribonucleotide.

amputation—see *Syme amputation.*

AMSA (methanesulfon-m-anisidide)—see *amsacrine.*

amsacrine (AMSA, Amsidyl)—chemotherapy drug used to treat adult acute leukemia.

Amsidyl—see *amsacrine.*

Amsler grid (Oph)—a grid with a small dot in the middle; it tests for irregularities in the central 20° of the visual field.

Amsterdam tube (Surg).

Amvisc (Oph)—trade name for sodium hyaluronate (Healon). It is used as a replacement for vitreous and to separate tissues to create a clear field for inspection and photocoagulation of the retina. Also used in cataract and intraocular lens implantation.

amyelia—congenital absence of spinal cord.

amygdala—general term for an almond-shaped structure; specifically a nucleus of the basal ganglia.

Anadrol-50—see *oxymetholone.*

Anafranil—see *clomipramine.*

anagen—the phase in which hair grows. See *telogen.*

anakmesis (Path)—arrest of maturation of leukocytes, resulting in smaller proportions of mature granular cells in the bone marrow, as observed in agranulocytosis. Leukanakmesis—arrest of maturation of white cell series.

anal reflex—see *anal wink.*

anal wink (or anal reflex)—contraction of the anal sphincter when the area around the anus is stroked. Loss of this response is indicative of a neurologic problem.

analog to digital converter—MRI term.

analogue—see *nucleoside analogue.*

analysis
- Diacyte DNA ploidy
- Dianon prostate profile and diagraph
- Fourier
- pentagastrin stimulated
- simkin

analyzer, sequential multiple (SMA).

anastomosis
- antecolic
- Baffe's
- Brackin ureterointestinal
- Coffey ureterointestinal
- end-to-end

anastomosis *(cont.)*
- end-to-side
- Fontan
- Furniss ureterointestinal
- Higgins ureterointestinal
- Ma and Griffith
- side-to-side

anatomical snuffbox—shallow depression between two tendons in the wrist, just proximal to the base of the thumb.

anchoring—see *Mitek.*

anchovy (No, you haven't strayed into the food department.) This is a term used in microsurgery and hand surgery and refers to a rolled-up piece of fascia lata (that looks like an anchovy) and is used thus: "Operation: Carpal/metacarpal joint arthroplasty, with tensor fasciae latae anchovy." Also: "The fascia lata was initially rolled into an anchovy and tied together with corner chromic sutures. This anchovy would not adequately fill the irregular joint cavity. The anchovy was then unraveled and the fascia lata divided into three strips. These were carefully inserted into the joint space with the joint opened and distracted."

Andrews SST-3000—spinal surgery table and frame for proper positioning during spinal surgery.

anechoic—in echocardiography, an area not generating echoes.

anesthesia—see *Bier block.*

Angelchik anti-reflux prosthesis—used in repair of sliding hiatal hernia and gastroesophageal reflux. The abdomen is entered and the stomach and a small portion of the esophagus pulled down below the diaphragm. The small C-shaped silicone prosthesis is placed around the esophagus and tied and the abdomen closed.

Angelchik prosthesis *(cont.)*
The prosthesis then lies around the esophagus, below the diaphragm, and above the stomach, reinforcing the esophageal sphincter.

angina
Ludwig's
Prinzmetal's

Angiocath PRN—a flexible catheter.

angiographically occult intracranial vascular malformation (AOIVM) (Neuro).

angiography, arteriography (Radiol)—the radiographic study of arteries into which radiopaque medium has been injected. Still pictures may be taken immediately after injection, or motion pictures may be made showing the flow of blood and contrast medium through vessels. See *digital subtraction angiography; fluorescein angiography.*

angiolymphoid hyperplasia with eosinophilia—see *ALHE.*

angioma—see *cherry angioma.*

angioplasty, laser-assisted balloon (LABA)

angioscope—see *Optiscope flexible fiberoptic angioscope.*

Angioskop-D—equipment used in digital subtraction angiography.

angiotensin converting enzyme (ACE) **inhibitor.** See *ACE inhibitor.*

angiotensin II—a vasoconstrictor associated with primary aldosteronism and secretion of large amounts of renin in the blood in some hypertensive patients.

angle
antegonial
Bauman's
Boehler's (Böhler's)
cerebellopontile
cerebellopontine

angle *(cont.)*
costosternal
gonial
Lovibond's

angular frequency; momentum—MRI terms.

anhedonia—loss of feelings of pleasure in things that usually give pleasure (Psych). Example: "The patient describes anhedonia and low energy."

anion gap ("an-eye-on")—referring to electrolytes.

Anis Staple implant cataract lens.

aniseikonia (Oph)—inequality in size and shape of an object, as seen by each eye. Cf. *anisoiconia.*

anisocoria (Oph)—condition of inequality of diameter of the pupils. Cf. *anisophoria.*

anisoiconia—rarely used spelling for preferred form, *aniseikonia.*

anisophoria (Oph)—condition in which the visual lines of the pupils are not on the same horizontal plane; caused by unequal pull on the muscles of the eyes. Cf. *anisocoria.*

anisoylated plasminogen streptokinase activator complex (APSAC)—see *anistreplase.*

anistreplase (Eminase) (Cardio)—also known as APSAC (anisoylated plasminogen streptokinase activator complex); used to break up thrombi obstructing the coronary arteries after a patient has a myocardial infarction. Similar in action to alteplase and streptokinase, anistreplase is given intravenously over just a few minutes, while the other two thrombolytic agents must be given intravenously over a few hours.

ankle air stirrup (Ortho).

ankle jerk—see *Achilles reflex* and *gastrocnemius reflex.*

ankle mortise (Radiol)—the normal articulation between the talus and the distal tibia and fibula.

anlage (pl., anlagen) (Ob-Gyn, Neonat)—a primordial structure in the developing embryo.

ANLL (acute nonlymphoid leukemia).

annuloplasty, De Vega tricuspid.

annulus of Zinn. Also *anulus.*

anomaly
- cor triatriatum
- cor triatriatum dexter
- Ebstein's cardiac
- Pelger-Huët
- Taussig-Bing

anorectoplasty, Laird-McMahon.

ansamycin (Mycobutin, rifabutin)—a drug used to prevent MAI infection in AIDS patients.

Anspach Cement Eater (Ortho). See *Cement Eater.*

Antabuse (Psych)—given to recovering alcoholics to thwart their consumption of alcohol. This drug is often misspelled as "Antiabuse" because it is "anti-alcohol."

antagonist (Pharm)—a drug that inhibits or counteracts the action of naturally produced neurotransmitters on a receptor. See *adrenergic antagonist, beta antagonist.* Cf. *agonist.*

antecolic—in front of the colon.

antecolic anastomosis.

antecolic gastrojejunostomy.

antegonial angle or notch—just in front of the gonion (the most inferior, posterior, and lateral point of the external angle of the mandible). A landmark in oral and plastic surgery.

anterior cruciate ligament (ACL).

anterior inferior communicating artery (AICA).

anterolisthesis—spondylolisthesis with anterior displacement of a vertebral body on the one below it (Ortho).

anthelix, antihelix—of the ear.

anthracenediones—a class of chemotherapy drugs; see *mitoxantrone.*

Anthron heparinized catheter—antithrombogenic catheter used in angiography (Radiol).

antibody
- acetylcholine receptor (AChRab)
- anticentromere (ACA)
- anticardiolipin (aCL)
- anti-EA
- antifibrin
- anti-HA
- anti-HAV
- anti-La
- antimelanoma
- antimitochondrial
- antinuclear
- anti-neutrophilic cytoplasmic
- anti-Ro
- anti-Sm
- CD5+
- cryptosporidiosis
- Duffy blood a. type
- E5
- HA-1A
- HBcAb
- HBeAb
- HBsAb
- IgM-RF (rheumatoid factor)
- islet cell (ICA)
- Kell blood a. type
- Kidd blood a. type
- Lewis blood a. type
- Lutheran blood a. type
- microsomal TRC
- monoclonal
- nuclear
- opsonizing

antibody molecules (immune globulins). They have heavy and light chains. There are five classes of heavy chains (G, A, M, D, and E)—IgG, IgA, IgM, etc., and two classes of light chains (kappa and lambda).

antibody, monoclonal. See *monoclonal antibody.*
anticardiolipin antibody (aCL).
anticentromere antibody (ACA)—appears in the majority of patients with CREST syndrome. See *CREST syndrome.*
anti-EA antibody—"EA" stands for "early antigen" of Epstein-Barr virus. Patients with chronic mononucleosis syndrome are thought to test positive to the antibody.
antiepilepsirine (Neuro)—used to treat generalized tonic-clonic seizures resistant to other drugs.
antifibrin antibody imaging (Radiol)—a method to diagnose deep vein thrombosis; it is thought to be a safer, faster, and more accurate way to detect blood clots than venography. In the procedure, a radiolabeled antifibrin antibody is injected into the patient. It then attaches itself to the fibrin in the clot; within an hour, imaging reveals the clot.
antigen
CEA (carcinoembryonic)
ENA (extractable nuclear)
Go[a] (Gonzales blood)
HbAg (or HBAg) (hepatitis B)
HB_eAg (hepatitis B "e")
HB_sAg (hepatitis B surface)
Histoplasma capsulatum (HPA)
HLA (human lymphocyte)
inhalant
PHA (phytohemagglutinin)
Rh (Rhesus) factor
SD
Sm
vWF (von Willebrand factor)
anti-HA, anti-HAV (antibody to hepatitis A virus).
antihelix, anthelix—of the ear.
antihemophilic globulin (AHG).
anti-La antibody—an unusual antibody found in patients with Sjögren's disease. Cf. *anti-Ro.*
antimesenteric border of ileum—a surgical landmark; the side of the small bowel away from the insertion of the mesentery.
antimicrobial catheter cuff (Surg). Placed subcutaneously where a central venous catheter exits from the skin, it slowly releases silver ions which prevent infection from microorganisms along the catheter exit site.
antimitochondrial antibody.
antimoniotungstate (HPA-23)—a drug used to treat AIDS. Also, antimonium tungstate.
antimonium tungstate (HPA-23).
antineutrophilic cytoplasmic antibody—the presence of this antibody is indicative of an acute necrotizing vasculitis.
antiperistaltic technique.
anti-RHO-D titer (Lab).
anti-Ro antibody—an unusual antibody found in patients with Sjögren's disease. Cf. *anti-La.*
Anti-Sept bactericidal scrub solution (Surg).
anti-Sm antibody—found in lupus erythematosus. The Sm is for Smith.
antiteichoic acid titer (Lab).
antithrombin III (ATnativ)—used to inhibit blood coagulation in patients with an antithrombin III deficiency. It is given I.V. prior to surgery or obstetrical procedures to prevent the formation of thrombi and emboli. Note the unique spelling of ATnativ, with two initial capital letters.
antithymocyte globulin (ATG).
antitussives—a class of drugs used as cough suppressants.

antiviral drugs—see *medications.*

Anton's symptom—cortical blindness, denied with confabulation.

anuresis (Urol)—inability of the kidneys to produce or excrete urine. Cf. *enuresis.*

anxiolytics—antianxiety drugs; minor tranquilizers.

AO indirect ophthalmoscope (American Optical).

AOA/CHICK—an ambulatory halo system, used for immobilization of the operative area in patients who have had surgery of the cervical spine (Neuro).

A-OK ShortCut knife (Oph)—an ophthalmic knife with a unique rounded tip and short length for intraocular incisions. Also called the ShortCut knife.

A_1 segment (Neuro).

aortofemoral bypass graft (AFBG).

A-O screws (Ortho).

AOIVM (angiographically occult intracranial vascular malformation).

AOPA (Ara-C, Oncovin, prednisone, asparaginase)—chemotherapy protocol.

AOPE (Adriamycin, Oncovin, prednisone, etoposide)—chemotherapy protocol.

aortic root *(not* route).

aortic valve prosthesis

Björk-Shiley—mechanical; tilting disk

Carpentier-Edwards—biological; pig aorta treated with glutaraldehyde

Ionescu-Shiley—biological; calf pericardium cut into three leaflets and attached to a frame

St. Jude Medical—mechanical; tilting disk

Starr-Edwards—mechanical; ball and cage

aortogram—see *flush aortogram.*

aortoplasty, subclavian flap (SFA).

APA (aldosterone-producing adenoma).

apallic syndrome—parasomniac conscious state.

A-pattern strabismus.

APACHE II—the second version of the Acute Physiology and Chronic Health Evaluation, a scoring system for severity of disease. Scores patients using 12 physiologic and biochemical measurements on a 0 to 4 scale; age and chronic health conditions also influence the final score.

APC (AMSA, prednisone, and chlorambucil)—chemotherapy protocol.

APE (Ara-C, Platinol, etoposide)—chemotherapy protocol used to treat children with advanced Hodgkin's disease.

APGAR—in Family APGAR Questionnaire, the acronym formed from the initial letters of *adaptability, partnership, growth, affection, resolve,* to match the name of Dr. Virginia Apgar, an anesthesiologist who devised a scoring system for the health status of neonates.

Apgar score (named for Dr. Virginia Apgar, an anesthesiologist)—rating of the condition of the newborn infant, performed at one and five minutes after birth. The criteria are color, heart rate, respiration, reflex response to nose catheter, and muscle tone. "The infant's Apgars were 8 and 9 at one and five minutes."

1. Color: If the infant is pale or blue, the score for color is 0; if the body is pink and the extremities are blue, the score is 1; if the body and extremities are pink, the score is 2.

2. Heart rate: If the heart rate

Apgar *(cont.)*
cannot be elicited, the score for heart rate is 0; if it is less than 100, the score is 1; if more than 100, the score is 2.

3. Respiration: If respirations cannot be elicited, the score for respiration is 0; if irregular or slow, the score is 1; if respirations are good, crying, the score for this is 2.

4. Reflex response: If there is no reflex response to the nose catheter, the score is 0; if the infant grimaces, the score is 1; if the infant sneezes or coughs, the score is 2.

5. Muscle tone: If the infant is limp, the score for muscle tone is 0; if there is some flexion of the extremities, the score is 1; if the infant is active, the score is 2.

All the sub-score totals are added together for the total score on a scale of 1 to 10 at one and five minutes.

apheresis (from Greek *aphairesis,* taking away)—removal of a component of the blood from the intravascular circulation. This process is used now as apheresis of plasma, erythrocytes, leukocyte fractions, platelets, and cold precipitable serum proteins in blood banking. It is used in treating babies who are Rh incompatible and is likely to be used in the future for selective apheresis of autoantibodies in the treatment of rheumatoid arthritis, systemic lupus erythematosus, and other autoimmune diseases. See *lymphapheresis, plasmapheresis. Cf. electrophoresis.*

aphtha (pl., aphthae), adj., aphthous (''af-thus'')—the small ulcers of the oral mucosa known colloquially as ''canker sores.'' Cf. *abscess.*

aphthous—see *aphtha.*

apical impulse (Cardio)—a thrust noted over the apex of the heart. May be referred to as PMI, point of maximal impulse.

APL (abductor pollicis longus) (Ortho).

Apley sign (Ortho).

apnea/hypopnea index (AHI).

APO (Adriamycin, prednisone, Oncovin)—chemotherapy protocol used to treat non-Hodgkin's lymphoma.

apocrine metaplasia—a change in the cells lining a breast duct so they appear similar to lactating breast. Frequently associated with mammary dysplasia.

apophysis—a projecting part of a bone; a bony outgrowth, such as a tubercle, process, or tuberosity, not separated from the main portion of the bone. Cf. *epiphysis, hypophysis.*

apparent—visible, obvious, evident. Cf. *aberrant.*

appendicular ataxia (Neuro)—ataxia of the extremities.

appendix
Morgagni's
vermiform

applanation—flattening of the cornea by pressure.

applanation tonometry—measures intraocular pressure (Oph). See *Schiötz tonometry.*

applanometer—an instrument used to determine the intraocular pressure in testing for glaucoma. See *tonometry.*

Appolionio implant cataract lens.

Appose disposable skin stapler.

apposition—the placing or bringing together of two adjacent parts, e.g., drawing together the cut edges of an incision on closure of a wound: ''The wound edges were placed in apposition and sutured in place.'' Cf. *opposition.*

apprehension test (Ortho)—"There is a positive mild to moderate apprehension test."

apron—excessive subcutaneous fat that hangs from the abdominal wall like an apron; also called *hanging panniculus.*

APR total hip system (Ortho)—porous, coated cement fixation.

APSAC (anisoylated plasminogen streptokinase activator complex). See *anistreplase.*

APSGN (acute poststreptococcal glomerulonephritis).

APTT (activated partial thromboplastin time).

APUD (amine precursor uptake and decarboxylation).

apudoma—tumor composed of APUD cells; potentially malignant or overtly malignant gastrin-secreting tumor; the most frequent cause of the Zollinger-Ellison syndrome. See *APUD.*

Aquaphor gauze (Ortho)—non-adhering dressing.

Aquaplast splint (Ortho).

Aquaspirillum itersonii—a gram-negative organism.

Aquatech cast padding.

aqueous flare (Oph)—scattering of slit-lamp light beam when the light is directed into the anterior chamber. This is found with increased protein in the aqueous and is an indication of iritis. See *cell and flare; Tyndall effect.*

Ara-A (adenine arabinoside)—antiviral drug, also known as vidarabine and Vira-A.

arachidonic acid—an unsaturated fatty acid that occurs in certain fats and in animal phosphatides.

arachnoid (Greek *arachne,* spider)—the membrane between dura and pia mater; the web-like strands between it and the pia give rise to the name.

araldehyde-tanned bovine carotid artery graft (heterograft or xenograft).

Arani catheter.

arbovirus (**ar**thropod-**bo**rne virus)—any one of a group of viruses carried by mosquitoes and ticks. Arboviruses are the cause of some febrile diseases, such as yellow fever, and of types of viral meningitis. See *togavirus.*

ARC (AIDS-related complex)—an incompletely understood syndrome resulting from infection with the HIV virus, but not full-blown AIDS. It is not known yet if people can recover from ARC or how many cases will progress to AIDS. The older term for ARC was "pre-AIDS," which was dropped for lack of precision because of these unknowns. See *ARS.*

arc, precipitin.

arcade, temporal (Oph).

Arcelin's view. See *views.*

arch bar (Oral Surg)—a wire or bar support, shaped to fit the arch of the teeth, used to splint a fractured jaw or loosened teeth. See *Winters arch bar.*

Arco pacemaker (Cardio).

ARDS (adult respiratory distress syndrome).

Aredia (pamidronate disodium).

Arenberg-Denver implant (ENT)—a pressure-sensitive unidirectional inner-ear valve implant. For use in patients with Mondini's dysplasia, and to control endolymphatic hypertension and hydrops in Ménière's disease, congenital hydrops, and large vestibular aqueduct syndrome.

ARF (acute renal failure)—a critical condition characterized by rapid deterioration in renal function, and oliguria.

ARF (acute respiratory failure).

argentaffin carcinoma.

arginine tolerance test (ATT) for growth hormone.
argon/krypton laser (Oph)—a vitreoretinal laser used for iridotomies and trabeculoplasties, for management of glaucoma, and in macular procedures.
argon laser (Oph)—is used for photocoagulation in diabetic retinopathy and detached retina. Cf. *laser, CO_2 laser, Nd:YAG laser.*
Argyle CPAP nasal cannula.
Argyle-Salem sump tube.
Arias-Stella phenomenon.
ariboflavinosis—a vitamin deficiency state, indicated by flattening of the papillae of the tongue.
Aries-Pitanguy correction of mammary ptosis (Plas Surg).
arm, Utah artificial (Ortho).
arm board, in *Flexisplint flexed arm board.*
Army-Navy retractor.
Arneth's grouping of polymorphonuclear neutrophils—according to the number of lobes in their nuclei, e.g., one lobe, class I; two lobes, class II; three lobes, class III, etc.
Arnold's nerve—the auricular branch of the vagus nerve.
Aron Alpha adhesive (Neuro).
array (MRI terms)
convex linear
high-density linear
phased
processor
symmetrical phased
arrest of labor—stopping of progress in labor *(not* "a rest of labor").
Arrowgard Blue Line catheter (Cardio)—a central venous catheter that contains chlorhexidine and silver sulfadiazine antiseptics bonded onto the outer surface to reduce the risk of catheter-induced bacteremia. From the manufacturer: ARROWg+ard.
Arrow-Howes multilumen catheter—provides multiple apertures with the use of only one venipuncture site, thus permitting hyperalimentation, central venous pressure monitoring, intravenous administration of medications, and blood sampling without the necessity of multiple needle punctures.
Arrow pneumothorax kit (Radiol)—for nonsurgical treatment of pneumothorax, using percutaneous catheter-over-needle technique.
Arrow Twin Cath—multilumen peripheral catheter.
Arruga lacrimal trephine (Oph).
ARS (AIDS-related syndrome)—a term used less than *ARC* for the same syndrome. In either case, if one of these terms appears in a diagnosis, the whole phrase should be written as *acquired immunodeficiency syndrome-related complex.*
arterial—referring to an artery. Cf. *arteriole.*
arterial blood gases (ABGs).
arterial line (A-line).
arterial oxygen saturation (SaO_2).
arteriole—a tiny arterial branch. Cf. *arterial.*
arteriovenous oxygen difference (AVD O_2).
arteritis—inflammation of an artery or arteries. Examples: giant cell arteritis (GCA); Takayasu's arteritis. Cf. *arthritis.*
artery of Adamkiewicz—the great anterior radicular artery.
arthritides ("ar-thrit-ih-dees")—plural form of arthritis.
arthritis—inflammation of a joint. Cf. *arteritis.*
Arthro-Flo system (Ortho)—provides powered irrigation for arthroscopic procedures.

Arthro-Lok system (Ortho)—Beaver blades for arthroscopic surgery and all types of meniscal tears. Blades include banana, rosette, retrograde.

arthroplasty
Aufranc-Turner
Crawford-Adams
Gustilo-Kyle
Keller
Koenig metatarsophalangeal joint
laser image custom (LICA)
McKee-Farrar total hip
Mumford-Gurd
Neer hemiarthroplasty
New England Baptist
Putti-Platt
Schlein-type elbow
Stanmore shoulder
Swanson PIP joint

Arthropor cup prosthesis (Ortho).

ArthroProbe laser system (Ortho)—a laser system for arthroscopic surgery, which provides both resection and hemostasis. Used through an arthroscopic cannula.

Arthus reaction—immune complex deposition in dermal walls; it can cause gangrene at the site of injection of an allergen. Named for a French bacteriologist (d. 1945).

artificial blood
pyridoxylated stroma-free hemoglobin (SFHb)
recombinant hemoglobin (rHb1.1)

artificial heart
Symbion J-7-70-mL-ventricle
University of Akron

artificial insemination–donor (semen) (AID).

artificial insemination–husband (semen) (AIH).

artificial lung—see *IVOX* (intravascular oxygenator).

ARV (AIDS-related virus)—the term given to the AIDS virus by the group of scientists working at U.C. San Francisco under Dr. Jay Levy. The virus is now officially known as *HIV.* See *HIV.*

Arvin (Cardio)—a drug used to dissolve blood clots following a stroke. Obtained from snake venom.

aryepiglottic fold (AE fold) (ENT).

A.S. (auris sinistra)—left ear.

ASA (acetylsalicylic acid, aspirin). The trade name of the drug marketed by Lilly is A.S.A. (with periods).

Asacol (mesalamine).

A-scan (Oph)—an ultrasound device used to differentiate abnormal from normal tissues in the eye.

Asch septal forceps.

Aschoff-Tawara node—atrioventricular node.

ascitic—characterized by ascites or an accumulation of fluid in the peritoneal cavity. Cf. *acidic.*

ascribe—to attribute; e.g., "The patient ascribes occasional shortness of breath to the fact that she has put on a great deal of weight in the past four months, although she still smokes more than a pack a day." Cf. *describe.*

AS-800 (Urol, Gyn)—artificial sphincter for surgically treating urinary incontinence in women.

Asendin (amoxapine) (Psych)—an antidepressant drug which helps patients *ascend* from the depths of depression. Note that the *c* in *ascend* does not appear in the drug name.

ASH (asymmetric septal hypertrophy) (Cardio)—the newer term for what was formerly called IHSS (idiopathic hypertrophic subaortic stenosis).

A-SHAP (Adriamycin, Solu-Medrol, high-dose Ara-C, Platinol)—chemotherapy protocol used to treat advanced lymphoma.

ash leaf spots in the eye, seen in cases of tuberous sclerosis.

ASIS (anterior superior iliac spine) (Ortho).

AS–101—a drug used in treating AIDS patients.

A68 (Path)—a protein found in the brains of patients with Alzheimer's disease. Cf. *ALZ-50.*

Aspen electrocautery (Ortho)—used in arthroscopic procedures.

Aspen laparoscopy electrode—electrosurgical device used in laparoscopic surgical procedures.

Aspergillus—the fungus causing aspergillosis, which is seen in disseminated form in AIDS. See *Penicillium.*

aspheric (Oph)—refers to the reflecting surface of a lens.

aspirating curet, Laufe (Gyn).

aspiration biopsy cytology (ABC).

assay
CA15-3 RIA
cell
C1q
C-terminal
enzyme-linked immunoassay (EIA)
enzyme-linked immunosorbent (ELISA)
Factor III multimer
glycosylated hemoglobin
Heprofile ELISA
Pylori Fiax
Pylori Stat
Raji cell a. test
thyroxine radioisotope

ASSI (Accurate [a brand name, not a comment on quality] Surgical and Scientific Instruments Corporation) bipolar coagulating forceps and disposable cranio blades (no hyphen and no period after "cranio") and wire pass drills for use in neurosurgery and other surgical specialties.

AST (antistreptolysin titer).

astasia–abasia (Neuro)—inability to stand or to walk, although the legs are otherwise under control.

astemizole (Hismanal)—an antihistamine, for nasal congestion (ENT).

asthenic—lacking in strength and energy, or pertaining to an individual with an ectomorphic body build. Cf. *aesthetic.*

asthenopia (Oph)—eye discomfort that feels like eyestrain, may also be accompanied by headache.

asthma, synonym for *reversible obstructive airway disease.*

astigmatism—an eye condition in which there is unequal curvature of one of the refractive surfaces of the eye, causing lack of sharpness in focus of a ray of light on the retina.

Astler-Coller modification of Dukes' C classification of carcinoma; it provides a subscript for the C (C_1 and C_2).

ASTRA profiles (Lab)—blood chemistry analyzers.

Astrup blood gas values.

asymmetric septal hypertrophy (ASH) —new term for what was formerly called IHSS (idiopathic subaortic septal stenosis).

ataxia
appendicular
equilibratory
Marie's
telangiectasia

ATFL (anterior talofibular ligament).

ATG (antithymocyte globulin)—used to prevent rejection of transplanted kidney.

atherectomy catheter (Cardio)—catheter which is used to retrieve cholesterol plaque from diseased arteries.

AtheroCath (Radiol)—see *Simpson atherectomy catheter* (used in interventional radiology).

Atkinson endoprosthesis—a silicone rubber tube with a preformed distal shoulder. Also, Atkinson tube.

Atkinson-type lid block—local eye anesthesia.

ATL syndrome (acute tumor lysis).

ATL real-time Neurosector scanner—used in ultrasonography (Neuro). ATL stands for Advanced Technology Laboratories, Inc.

ATLS examination (advanced trauma life support) (Emer Med).

ATN (acute tubular necrosis).

ATnativ—see *antithrombin III.*

ATNR (asymmetric tonic neck reflex).

AT-125—see *acivicin.*

Atraloc needle—double-pointed needle used for blood vessel anastomoses; the double point allows the needle to be passed in either direction without reversing it on the needle holder, thus saving time.

Atraloc surgical needle.

Atrauclip hemostatic clip (Cardio).

atrio-His tract or pathway in the heart, as in bundle of His (Cardio). Pronounced "atrio-hiss."

atrophy—see *Sudeck's atrophy.*

ATT (arginine tolerance test)—a test for growth hormone.

attention deficit disorder (ADD) (Peds). Also, hyperkinetic child syndrome, minimal brain damage, minimal cerebral dysfunction, minor cerebral dysfunction. See *ADD.*

AuBMT (autologous bone marrow transplantation) (Oncol).

Auchincloss modified radical mastectomy (Surg).

audiometer, Maico-MA 20.

AudioScope, Welch Allyn—an instrument for screening hearing loss in children; it is combined with an otoscope in a single device.

auditory brain stem response (ABR).

Auer body; rod—found only in myelogenous and monocytic leukemia.

Aufranc-Turner
acetabular cup
arthroplasty
prosthesis

Aufrecht's sign of tracheal stenosis—faint breath sounds heard about the jugular notch.

Aufricht elevator; retractor.

augenblick diagnosis (literally "eyeblink").

aural (ENT)—pertaining to the ear, or to the sense of hearing, as *aural acuity* or *aural surgery.* Cf. *oral.*

auramine-rhodamine stain (Path).

auris dextra (A.D.)—right ear.

auris sinistra (A.S.)—left ear.

Austin Flint murmur of relative mitral stenosis. This differs from the murmur of true mitral stenosis by having no audible opening snap.

Austin Moore hip prosthesis (named for Dr. Thomas Austin Moore). No hyphen.

Auth atherectomy catheter (Cardio).

Autima II dual-chamber cardiac pacemaker.

Autoclix—see *fingerstick devices for blood glucose testing.*

autoclot (Surg)—a preformed clot of the patient's blood, reinjected to stop bleeding.

autocrine motility factor (AMF) (Urol)—a protein secreted by cancerous cells which can be detected in the urine. The test for AMF aids in early detection of bladder cancer.

Autoflex II (Ortho)—continuous passive motion (CPM) units.

Autolet—see *fingerstick devices for blood glucose testing.*

autologous bone marrow transplant (ABMT).

autologous clot—used for control of hemorrhage. Some of the patient's blood is mixed with epsilon aminocaproic acid, and clot forms. This is then cut in small fragments. Gelatin sponge is then soaked in 50% diatrizoate sodium, and the clot alternated with strips of the gelatin sponge is injected into the bleeding vessels until hemorrhage stops.

autologous fat graft—use of the patient's own fat (to fill a cavity, such as that left by removal of a tumor or cyst).

autologous transfusion—transfusion of one's own blood or blood components, thereby eliminating risks (e.g., hepatitis and alloimmunization) associated with homologous blood transfusion.

autolymphocyte-based treatment for renal cell carcinoma (ALT-RCC).

Automator device (Ortho)—a computerized device which attaches to the telescopic rods used in the Ilizarov leg lengthening procedure, it is programmed to automatically adjust the hardware four times per day to increase bone distraction. In the recent past, this adjustment had to be done manually by the patient.

Autophor femoral prosthesis.

Autoplex—Factor VIII inhibitor bypass product (anti-anti Factor VIII) (yes, anti-anti).

Auto Suture Multifire Endo GIA 30 stapler (GI)—for laparoscopic use in appendectomy, bowel resection, blebectomies, wedge resections, etc.

Auto Suture Premium CEEA stapler (GI)—used for circular anastomosis requiring double and triple stapling technique in intestinal procedures.

Auto Suture surgical stapler.

Autosyringe insulin pump.

autotransfusion system—see *Cell Saver Haemolite.*

AV bundle in heart (atrioventricular). See *Kent bundle.* Terms used in electrophysiologic studies of supraventricular tachycardia.

AVD O_2 (arteriovenous oxygen difference).

aversion therapy (Psych)—a type of therapy used to change behavior patterns by associating them with unpleasant stimuli.

Avitene—microfibrillar collagen hemostatic material; used like Gelfoam; applied topically for hemostasis in localized oozing, in areas inaccessible for suturing, and in procedures involving friable organs or vessels.

avium-intracellulare, Mycobacterium —see *MAI infection.*

Avlosulfon (dapsone)—previously used for treatment of leprosy, and now used to treat *Pneumocystis carinii* pneumonia in AIDS patients.

AVM (arteriovenous malformation).

AVM (atrioventricular malformation).

axial images—MRI term (Radiol).

axillofemoral bypass (Vasc Surg)—used only in high risk patients.

Axiom DG balloon angioplasty catheter.

Axiom double sump tube (Surg).

axis—a real or imaginary straight line going through a structure, around which it revolves, or would revolve if it could. Cf. *access, excess.*

axis, HPA (hypothalamic-pituitary-adrenal).

Axostim nerve stimulator.

aywl, ayw2, ayw3, ayw4, ayr—these are hepatitis B surface antigen (HBsAg) subdeterminants.

azacytidine (AZC, 5-azacytidine) (Oncol)—a chemotherapy drug used to treat acute myelogenous leukemia. Note the different spelling of azacitidine and 5-azacytidine.

azalides—a new class of antibiotics. The first drug in this group is azithromycin (Zithromax) which is similar to erythromycin.

Azar Tripod implant cataract lens.

azathioprine (AZTP) (Urol)—a derivative of the chemotherapy drug mercaptopurine. Used to prevent rejection of renal transplants.

AZC (azacitidine).

AzdU (azidouridine)—a drug reported to be much less toxic than AZT to human bone marrow cells in in vitro studies. Used to treat patients who are HIV-patients who are HIV-positive or have ARC or AIDS.

azidothymidine (AZT)—see *zidovudine.*

azidouridine (AzdU).

azithromycin (Zithromax)—antibiotic for treating AIDS patients with MAC infection; also for strep pharyngitis, chlamydial infections, urethritis, toxoplasmosis, and cryptosporidiosis.

Azmacort (Pulm)—a drug used to treat asthma. Easy to misspell because it does not follow the spelling of *asthma.*

AZQ (aziridinylbenzoquinone, diaziquone)—a chemotherapy drug used in treatment of brain tumors, lymphoma, and acute leukemias.

AZT (azidothymidine)—see *zidovudine.*

AZTP (azathioprine).

Azulfidine—trade name for a sulfasalazine preparation; used in treatment of Crohn's disease. *Not* Asulfidine or Asulfadine.

azygos lobe; vein—unpaired. (*Not* azygous or azygus.)

B, b

babesiosis—infection with the tick-borne parasite *Babesia.*

Babinski sign (Neuro, Ortho)—upward deviation of the great toe on stroking the sole of the foot, an indication of brain stem injury. A positive Babinski is an extensor plantar response: "The toes are upgoing"; a negative Babinski is a flexor plantar response: "The toes are downgoing."

BABYbird respirator *(BABY,* all caps) —a time-cycled infant ventilator. Also, Bird respirator.

Bachman, anterior internodal tract of, in the heart.

Bacillus coagulans (Lab).

bacillus

Döderlein's

Ducrey's

Friedländer's

bacitracin—an antibacterial polypeptide, active against many pathogenic gram-positive bacteria, and used topically rather than systemically because of toxicity. Extracted from cultures of a particular strain of *Bacillus subtilis* first isolated in 1945 from wound drainage of a patient named Margaret Tracy.

BackBiter (Ortho)—grooved orthopedic instrument which cuts from the rear to allow easier access to the anterior horn of the meniscus.

backward failure (Cardio). When all the blood returned to the heart cannot be pumped out, venous pressure rises and the lungs and viscera congest.

Bacon–Babcock (Gyn)—operation for correction of rectovaginal fistula.

BACT (BCNU, Ara-C, Cytoxan, 6-thioguanine)—chemotherapy protocol.

bactericidal—see *cidal.*

Bacteroides corrodens—genus of anaerobic gram-negative rods; found normally in the oropharynx; has been isolated from infected tonsils, in pharyngitis, pneumonia, and postoperative wound infections. Also, *Eikenella corrodens.*

Bactrim (sulfamethoxazole and trimethoprim)—see *TMP-SMZ.*

BAEP (brain stem auditory evoked potential) (Neuro).

BAER (brain stem auditory evoked response). Pronounced "bear."

Baffe's anastomosis (Cardio)—between the inferior vena cava and the left atrium.

baffle
intra-atrial
pericardial
Senning intra-atrial

bagassosis—extrinsic allergic alveolitis caused by exposure to moldy sugar cane.

BAGF (brachioaxillary bridge graft fistula).

bagged—ventilated by hand using an Ambu bag, as "The patient was being bagged via endotracheal tube in the emergency room."

Baggish hysteroscope (Gyn)—an operative sheath used in both Nd:YAG laser and conventional surgery in the uterine cavity as well as aspiration from the uterine cavity. Also, Baggish contact panoramic hysteroscope systems.

Bagolini lens—used in testing and assessing retinal correspondence in eye deviations (Oph).

bagpipe sign—a continuous wheeze at the end of expiration.

Bailliart's ophthalmodynamometer.

Bair Hugger—a plastic warming body cover.

Bakanjian flap (ENT)—a deltopectoral flap turned in a radical neck dissection.

Bakelite (Urol)—a strong, lightweight material used to make cystoscopy sheaths.

Bakes dilator (no apostrophe)—a common duct dilator.

BAL (British antilewisite)—therapy for lead poisoning. Lewisite was a poison gas used during World War I.

BAL (bronchoalveolar lavage).

balanced electrolyte solution (BES).

balanced salt solution (BSS) (Oph).

Balb/c mice—a strain of mice used in laboratories.

bald gastric fundus—absence of rugal folds when the gastric fundus is distended by gas or by the presence of barium from an (immediately previous) upper GI study.

Baldy-Webster operation—for retrodisplacement of the uterus.

Balke protocol (Cardio)—for exercise stress testing.

Ball operation for treatment of pruritus ani (GI).

Ballantine forceps.

Ballard gestational assessment (Peds).

ballism (Neuro)—intense and violent flailing movements. Also, ballismus, hemiballism, hemiballismus.

balloon
Epistat double
Fogarty
Grüntzig
Honan
Hunter-Sessions
Microvasive Rigiflex
Microvasive Rigiflex TTS
Rand microballoon

balloon biliary catheter. See *Fogarty balloon biliary catheter.*

balloon tuboplasty—opens blocked fallopian tubes without surgery. Technique is similar to that used in the Grüntzig balloon catheter angioplasty. In the tuboplasty, a guide wire is passed up through the uterus and eased through the fallopian tube to the point of blockage, which is then perforated. The balloon catheter is inserted and inflated to further enlarge the opening.

Baloser hysteroscope (Gyn).

banana blade—a Beaver blade used in arthroscopic surgery.

band, bands
BB
Ladd's

band *(cont.)*
MB
MM
oligoclonal
Parham
spiral band of Gosset

bandage (See also *dressing.)*
Ace
Champ elastic
Comperm tubular elastic
E Cotton
Elastic Foam
Elastomull
Esmarch
Fractura Flex
Flexilite conforming elastic
Hydron Burn Bandage
Kerlix
POP (plaster of Paris)
spica
Velpeau

bandeau (Plas Surg)—a narrow band or fillet; bandlike. A type of defect.

Bang's horseshoe-crab blood test—see *LAL.*

banjo-string adhesion.

Bankart procedure (Ortho)—operation of the shoulder girdle to treat recurrent shoulder dislocation.

Bankart shoulder prosthesis by Kirwan Surgical Products (Ortho).

BAR (biofragmentable anastomotic ring). See *Valtrac BAR.*

Bárány's symptom (ENT)—see *caloric testing.*

barbotage ("bar-bow-tahzh")—alternate injection and withdrawal of fluid.

Bard cardiopulmonary support system—a new portable heart-lung machine that does not require opening the patient's chest. The patient's blood is shunted to an external machine via a narrow catheter inserted into the femoral vein up to the heart. The blood is oxygenated, warmed, and pumped back into the body via a second catheter threaded through the femoral artery.

Bardach's modification—Obwegeser's mandibular osteotomy (Plas Surg).

Bard's sign—on cardiac palpation, a prominent and broad thrust sustained throughout ventricular systole in left ventricular hypertrophy.

Bardex catheter.

Barkan goniotomy knife (Oph).

Barlow test (Ortho)—for dysplasia of the hip.

Barnes-Crile forceps.

Baron implant cataract lens (Oph).

Baron suction tubes.

barotrauma—tissue injury caused by abnormally high or low atmospheric pressure, e.g., in flying, scuba diving; also, from high respirator pressures.

Barraquer-Krumeich-Swinger refractive set (Oph). See *BKS-1000.*

Barr body—see *buccal smear.*

Barrett's esophagus—a condition in which the esophagus is lined with columnar epithelium (as seen in the stomach); it is uncertain whether this is congenital or the result of reflux esophagitis; often seen with hiatal hernia.

Barron pump—four-speed pump used to control delivery of chemotherapeutic agents through an arterial line.

Bartley anastomosis clamp.

Bartter's syndrome—hypokalemic alkalosis, hyperaldosteronism secondary to adrenal cortical hyperplasia, hypertrophy and hyperplasia of the juxtaglomerular apparatus of the kidneys, and normal blood pressures associated with subnormal reactivity of blood pressures to angiotensin II.

basal ganglia—gray masses in the cerebrum involved in motor coordination.

base excess—one of the measurements on a blood gas study related to bicarbonate. "The arterial blood gases showed pH 7.35, pO_2 110, pCO_2 40 with a base excess of -3 and saturation of 95%."

bas-fond ("bah-fawn'")—bladder fundus.

Basidiomycetes—class of smut and rust fungi causing allergic problems in allergic individuals who work around wheat and granaries.

basis pontis—the ventral portion of the pons; part of the brain stem.

basket (Urol)
Dormia stone
Ellik kidney stone
Pfister stone

Bassen-Kornzweig abetalipoproteinemia.

Bassini inguinal hernia repair.

Bateman UPF II bipolar endoprosthesis (universal proximal femur)—hip replacement system by Kirschner.

Batten disease—a form of cerebral macular degeneration (Oph).

Battey-avium complex. See *MAC infection.*

Battle's sign—discoloration (ecchymosis) over the mastoid process, a sign of basilar skull fracture (Neuro).

Bauhin, valve of—ileocecal valve.

Bauman's angle (Ortho).

Baumgartner holder.

Bayley Scales of Infant Development—from manual by Nancy Bayley.

bayonet-type incision (Surg)—a basically rectilinear incision with a jog near the middle, giving it a configuration like that of a rifle with a bayonet attached.

Baypress (nitrendipine) (Cardio)—vasodilator and calcium channel blocker, used to treat hypertension.

Bazex syndrome (Oncol)—palmoplantar keratoderma with features similar to psoriasis on the hands, associated with carcinoma of the upper respiratory tract; this is a cutaneous marker to an internal malignancy.

BB shot—small, 0.46 cm in diameter round pellet used in air rifles or BB guns. "There was a small BB-sized cystic lesion on the lateral thigh."

BBVP-M (BCNU, bleomycin, VePesid, prednisone, methotrexate)—protocol used to treat advanced non-Hodgkin's lymphoma resistant to CHOP chemotherapy protocol.

BCD (bleomycin, Cytoxan, dactinomycin)—chemotherapy protocol.

B-cell (also called B-lymphocyte)—part of the immune system; some mature B-cells become plasma cells, which secrete antibodies, but not without help from T-cells, one variety of which is attacked by the AIDS virus. See *T-4 cell, helper cell.*

Bdellovibrio ("del'-o-vib'-re-o)—a genus of parasitic gram-negative organisms that live on certain other gram-negative bacteria.

B-D spinal needle (Becton-Dickinson).

BEAC (BCNU, etoposide, Ara-C, Cytoxan)—chemotherapy protocol used to treat advanced non-Hodgkin's lymphoma.

beads of methyl methacrylate—see *methyl methacrylate, beads of.*

Beale intraocular implant lens (Oph).

Beall Surgitool mitral valve (Cardio).

BEAM (brain electrical activity map, or mapping)—a computerized EEG that maps different areas of the brain (Neuro, Radiol).

beam splitter—used with an operating microscope to permit use of attachments that will enable a second person to look through the microscope with the surgeon; makes it possible to take photographs through the microscope and to videotape what is seen.

beaten silver appearance—increase in the convolutional markings on x-rays of the skull (Neuro).

Beau's line—seen in fingernails, a transverse groove in the nail; can result from severe emotional or physical shock. Cf. *Mee's line.*

Beaver blade
arachnoid shape
banana
cataract knife
discission knife
keratome
retrograde
rosette
sickle-shape

Beaver DeBakey blades—for hip surgery (Ortho).

BEB (blind esophageal brushing).

Bebax (Ortho, Peds)—advertised as "the plaster cast disguised as a shoe" for treatment of forefoot deformities.

Bechert nucleus rotator (Oph).

Bechtol hip prosthesis.

Beck Depression Inventory (Psych).

Becker accelerator cannula—a liposuction cannula (Plas Surg).

Becker probe.

Becker tissue expander/breast prosthesis (Plas Surg)—an inflatable tissue expander used to reconstruct the breast following mastectomy. Also serves as a permanent breast implant. Only the access port and tubing have to be removed in a brief outpatient procedure under local anesthesia with I.V. sedation.

Beckwith-Wiedemann syndrome.

becquerel (Bq)—the unit of measurement in the International System of Measurement (SI) that is the absorbed dose equivalent in radioactivity. See *International System.*

bedewing of cornea ("bee-doing")—swelling and superficial clouding of the cornea, caused by increased intraocular pressure for an extended period of time. The surface of the cornea becomes "grainy" in appearance, thus interfering with the transmission of light rays. May also be referred to as *Sattler veil.*

Bedge antireflux mattress (GI)—egg-crate foam wedge used to elevate the upper body to prevent gastroesophageal reflux.

Behçet's syndrome ("ba'-sets")—severe uveitis and retinal vasculitis, optic atrophy.

Belcher clamp.

Belganyl (suramin)—an anti-infective agent, used in the treatment of AIDS.

Bell's phenomenon—the eye rolls upward and outward on attempting to close the eye.

belly of muscle—the center of the muscle where its area of greatest mass lies. The site where an I.M. injection may be given in certain large muscles in the arms, legs, and buttocks.

Belsey Mark IV fundoplication (Surg).

BEMP (bleomycin, Eldisine, mitomycin, Platinol)—chemotherapy protocol used to treat squamous cell carcinoma of the uterine cervix.

benazepril (Lotensin) (Cardio)—ACE inhibitor used to treat hypertension.

bench method (Lab)—refers to manual performance of a laboratory test (at a workbench, hence the name) rather than by automated machinery.

bench method *(cont.)*
"Calcium determinations were 10.3 and 9.7 on the SMA, and 9.7 by bench method."

Bender Gestalt test (Psych)—mental status examination.

Benedikt's ipsilateral oculomotor paralysis (Neuro).

benign—normal, not showing evidence of disease or abnormality; a benign tumor is one that is not malignant.

Benjamin binocular slimline laryngoscope (ENT).

Benjamin–Havas fiberoptic light clip—used as light source in laryngoscopes (ENT).

Benjamin pediatric laryngoscope.

Benjamin proverbs (Psych).

Bennett PR-2 ventilator—a time-cycled ventilator, used mainly in treating children.

bentonite flocculation test—to diagnose trichinosis.

benzalkonium chloride patch test—for allergies.

benzodiazepines (Psych)—a class of drugs that includes antianxiety agents and sedatives.

BEP (bleomycin, etoposide, Platinol)—a standard chemotherapy protocol used to treat testicular carcinoma, ovarian carcinoma, and chronic myelogenous leukemia.

bepridil (Vascor) (Cardio)—a calcium channel blocker that relaxes the smooth muscle of the coronary arteries and relieves angina. Because it can cause arrhythmia and blood disorders, it is reserved for use in patients who have not responded to other antianginal medications.

beractant (Survanta).

Berci-Shore choledochoscope.

Berens lid everter (Oph).

Berens muscle clamp (Oph).

Berens 3-character test—eye test used in small children who do not know the letters of the alphabet.

Berger's disease—appears to be a variant of Henoch-Schönlein nephritis, but without the rash. Cf. *Buerger's disease.*

Berkeley-Bonney retractor—a self-retaining three-blade abdominal retractor. See *Goligher modification.*

Berke ptosis forceps (Oph).

Berkow formula—a method of assessing the percentage of body surface that has been burned. This is an adaptation of the Rule of Nines, but makes allowance for the age of the patient. In a one-year-old child, for example, the head is larger in proportion to body size; therefore, the head is rated at 19, while the head of an adult would be rated at 7. See *Rule of Nines.*

Berkson-Gage calculation—for determining breast cancer survival rates.

Berman locator (Oph)—a magnetic device used in locating intraocular foreign bodies.

Berotec (fenoterol) (Resp)—a drug used to prevent bronchial asthma attacks.

berry aneurysm—abnormal berry-like dilatation of an artery.

Bertel's position (Radiol)—used to visualize the floor of the orbits and the orbital fissures.

Berwick's dye (Gyn).

BES (balanced electrolyte solution).

Bessey-Lowry units—measure alkaline phosphatase. See also *Bodansky unit, King-Armstrong unit.*

Best right-angle colon clamp. (Best is a proper noun.)

beta antagonist—see *antagonist.* Also known as beta blockers.

Betadine Helafoam solution—an antibacterial agent.

beta-endorphin—an opiate-like peptide that acts on the central nervous system; it is of anterior pituitary origin. See *endorphins*.

beta-lactamase—an enzyme produced by certain bacteria which is able to split the beta-lactam chemical ring structure of penicillins and cephalosporins. Beta-lactamase positive bacteria are resistant to the antibiotic effect of penicillins and cephalosporins.

Betapace (sotalol).

Betaseron (recombinant human interferon beta)—used to treat CMV retinitis in AIDS patients.

Betatron I.V. insulin infusion pump, battery powered.

bethanidine (Cardio)—used to treat ventricular fibrillation.

Betz cells—large pyramidal cells forming layer of the gray matter of the brain. Vladimir Betz, Russian anatomist.

Bevan incision—vertical elliptical skin incision in the abdomen.

Beyer rongeur (Ortho).

bG (blood glucose).

Biaxin (clarithromycin)—an antibiotic belonging to the macrolide class. Similar in effectiveness to penicillin and erythromycin but with fewer side effects. Particularly effective against *Mycoplasma pneumoniae*, MAC infection, and resistant strains of *Haemophilus influenzae.*

bibasally (Radiol)—at the bases of both lungs (on chest x-ray).

Bible printer's lung—extrinsic allergic alveolitis caused by exposure to moldy paper.

BICAP cautery.

Bicarbolyte (Nephrol)—a bacteriostatic solution, premixed liquid bicarbonate dialysate. Used for hemodialysis.

Biceps bipolar coagulator (Surg).

biceps jerk (BJ) (Neuro).

Bielschowsky's head tilt—a test of oblique ocular muscle paralysis.

Bier block anesthesia (''beer'')—used in surgery of the extremities.

Bietti implant cataract lens.

biferious pulse (or bisferious)—see *bisferious pulse* (pulsus bisferiens, or biferiens).

BiLAP—bipolar cautery unit with cutting and coagulation functions.

bilharziasis—another name for schistosomiasis. Infection with flukes of the genus *Schistosoma.*

Biliblanket Phototherapy System—an alternative to phototherapy light used to treat jaundice in newborn babies, this device consists of a small jacket that gives off high intensity, fiberoptic light.

Bili mask—an eye shield used on infants undergoing phototherapy for bilirubinemia.

Billroth gastroenterostomy (GI, Surg). Billroth I is a partial resection of the stomach (65–75%), and anastomosis of the end of the stomach to the duodenum. (The stomach is first tapered to the size, or caliber, of the duodenum.) The Billroth II is used for duodenal ulcer; a gastrojejunostomy is performed, bringing the jejunal loop up to the remnant of the stomach posteriorly through a hole in the transverse mesocolon, or anterior to the transverse colon. The antecolic anastomosis is used more frequently because it is a simpler procedure. Dr. Theodor Billroth lived in Vienna

Billroth *(cont.)*
in the second half of the 19th century and was one of the foremost surgeons of his time. He was a music lover, an excellent amateur musician, and a friend of Brahms, Schumann, and other composers.

Bing auditory acuity test (ENT). A vibrating tuning fork is placed at the mastoid process and the acoustic meatus is closed off and opened. If the patient hears a decrease and increase in sound (a positive Bing), hearing is normal or the hearing loss is sensorineural. If the patient does not notice any difference in sound (a negative Bing), there is a deficit in conductive hearing.

bingeing or binging—overindulging in excessive amounts of food (as in bulimia) or alcohol.

Binkhorst iridocapsular implant cataract lens (Oph).

Binkhorst-McIntyre irrigation cannula (hydrodissection cannula) (Oph).

Biobrane (Surg)—a temporary biosynthetic skin substitute (for relatively short-term use). See *Biobrane adhesive, Biobrane glove.*

Biobrane adhesive—a biosynthetic skin substitute. The adhesive is used to protect clean superficial abrasions and burns. It maintains a clean wound until healing takes place, or is removed when autografting is necessary and possible.

Biobrane glove—a glove-like wrapping made of a biosynthetic skin substitute. It is used to protect clean excised burn wounds of the hand until healing occurs, or is removed when autografting is possible.

Biocell RTV implant (Plas Surg)—a saline-filled breast implant.

Biocept-5—a blood test for pregnancy (Obs).

Biocept-G—pregnancy test.

Bioclusive transparent dressing (Surg)—a clear, waterproof sterile dressing that protects the wound, permits continuous monitoring of the wound, is vapor permeable (thus preventing skin maceration), and prevents dehydration of the wound.

Biocoral (Neuro)—trade name for processed madreporic coral; manufactured by Inoteb Cy, a French company. See *madreporic coral.*

Biodel (Oncol, Ortho)—a new biodegradable polymer formed into wafers or beads impregnated with a chemotherapy drug or antibiotic. Used to treat osteomyelitis and malignant gliomas. See *Gliadel, Septacin.*

Biofix system—bioabsorbable fixation rod by Acufex made of Dexon sutures.

biofragmentable anastomotic ring (BAR).

Biograft
AV fistula
bovine heterograft
Dardik

Biomatrix ocular implant (Oph)—an implant made of hydroxyapatite and used in patients who have had enucleation or evisceration of an eye. About six to eight weeks after surgery, the blood vessels and tissues have grown into the implant, and the artificial eye is then attached to the implant. This lets the artificial eye move naturally with the other eye, for very good cosmetic effect. See *enucleation, evisceration, hydroxyapatite.*

Biomet plug.

biomicroscope—a microscope used to visualize living tissue in the body. Used synonymously with slit lamp in ophthalmology. It permits study of the structures of the eye, with the intense beam of light permitting visualization *through* the tissues of these structures. See *slit-lamp microscopy.*

Bioplus dispersive electrode (Cardio).

BioPolyMeric graft for femoropopliteal bypass.

Bioport collection and transport system(Path)—a sterile, self-contained device to preserve the viability of aerobic microbial specimens.

biopsy
Kushner-Tandatnick endometrial
mirror image breast
stereotaxic fine-needle aspiration
Tru-Cut needle

Biopty cut needle (Gyn, Urol)—a needle used in breast biopsy and in prostate biopsy. *Not* biop*s*y.

Biopty gun; Bard Biopty gun (Gyn, Urol)—a device used in needle core breast biopsy and prostate biopsy. *Not* biop*s*y.

Biotrack coagulation monitor (Cardio). Using only one drop of blood, this monitor can calculate the APTT value to assess heparin levels while a cardiac catheterization is being performed.

Biotropin—human growth hormone used to treat HIV-positive patients.

Biot's breathing—an irregular breathing commonly found in meningitis.

BIP (bleomycin, ifosfamide, Platinol)—chemotherapy protocol used to treat cervical carcinoma.

biplane sector probe (Urol)—used with Bard Biopty gun to perform transrectal prostatic ultrasonographic biopsy.

bipolar affective illness (also manic-depressive; bipolar disorder)—alternating attacks of mania and depression (Psych).

bipolar coagulation—electrosurgery that utilizes a pair of electrodes, and tissue between them is coagulated by flow of current from one to the other. Also, bipolar forceps.

bipolar disorder—see *bipolar affective illness* (Psych).

bipolar esophageal recording.

Birbeck granule—identification of this part of a Langerhans' cell is diagnostic of histiocytosis X. Also, X-body.

Bird respirator. See also *BABYbird respirator.*

birdcage splint (Ortho)—descriptive term for a splint used on a digit with a crush injury: "The wound was dressed and a birdcage splint was applied to the index finger."

Birkhauser eye testing chart (Oph).

bisferious pulse (or biferious) (pulsus bisferiens, or biferiens)—a pulse with two beats, sometimes palpable in combined aortic stenosis and aortic regurgitation.

Bishop-Harman (Oph)
anterior chamber irrigator
forceps
irrigating cannula

bishop's nod—rhythmic nodding of the head, synchronous with the pulse, in aortic regurgitation (Cardio).

bite line—a horizontal line of whitened, thickened buccal mucosa caused by habitual biting or chewing of the surface.

Bizzari-Giuffrida laryngoscope.

BJ (biceps jerk) (Neuro).

Bjerrum's scotoma—further development of Seidel's scotoma.

Björk-Shiley aortic valve prosthesis.

BKS-1000 refractive set (Barraquer-Krumeich-Swinger)—used to section and reshape the cornea (Oph).

Black and Decker drill—neurosurgical battery-operated drill.

Blackfan-Diamond syndrome—a rare hypoplastic anemia seen in infants and young children; caused by defective erythropoiesis and lack of adequate nucleated erythrocytes in the bone marrow, but with normal platelet and leukocyte counts. Also known as Josephs-Diamond-Blackfan syndrome. See *Kaznelson's syndrome.*

black hairy tongue—discoloration and alteration of the surface texture of the tongue by fungal infection.

blackout—loss of consciousness; syncope.

black patch delirium (Oph)—hallucinations caused in some patients with both eyes patched.

bladder carcinoma classification—see *Jewett's classification.*

BladderScan (Urol)—measures postvoid residuals and bladder distention by ultrasound to avoid catheterization.

blade
- arachnoid-shape
- banana
- Bard-Parker
- Beaver cataract knife
- Beaver DeBakey
- Beaver discission knife
- Beaver keratome
- Curdy
- Hebra
- K
- MVR
- Paufique
- sickle-shape
- Superblade
- Swann-Morton surgical

bladebreaker knife (Oph)—Oertli razor bladebreaker knife.

Blair head drape (Oph).

Blair silicone drain. See *J-Vac closed wound drainage system.*

Blakemore-Sengstaken tube—a triple-lumen tube. It is useful in stopping hemorrhage from gastric and esophageal varices, to suction gastric contents, and in differentiating between bleeding from esophageal varices and other causes of upper gastrointestinal bleeding. This tube has a gastric balloon (always inflated), an esophageal balloon, and a gastric tip that permits suction.

Blalock-Hanlon procedure (Cardio).

Blalock-Taussig procedure (Cardio)—for "blue baby" syndrome.

Blaydes corneal forceps (Oph).

bleb, filtering (Oph).

Bledsoe brace for knee and lower extremity fractures (Ortho).

bleed (noun)—a hemorrhage, usually gastrointestinal. Intracranial bleeds are common in very premature infants.

bleeding time—see *Duke; Ivy.*

Bleier clip for tubal sterilization (Gyn).

Blenoxane (sterile bleomycin sulfate)—for palliative treatment of head and neck cancer and in some lymphomas and testicular carcinomas.

bleomycin sulfate (Blenoxane).

blepharitis—inflammation of the eyelid margin.

blepharostatsee *McNeill-Goldmann.*

blind esophageal brushing (BEB) (GI)—a method of diagnosing infectious esophageal disease in patients with AIDS. This technique protects the endoscopist from exposure to HIV better than the standard procedure of esophagogastroduodenoscopy.

BlisterFilm—transparent dressing.
Bloch, clear cells of.
Bloch equation—MRI term.
block
 Atkinson lid
 dorsal penile nerve (DPNB)
 Mobitz I and II AV heart
 paraffin
 shock
blocker
 calcium channel
 calcium entry
Blom-Singer valve (ENT)—a prosthetic device used to improve esophageal speech in patients after laryngectomy. See also *Panje voice button.*
blood, artificial—see *artificial blood.*
blood-brain barrier (Neuro)—barrier by which many substances that pass easily through vessel walls in other parts of the body are chemically prevented from passing through blood vessel walls into central nervous system tissue.
blood coagulation factors—see *coagulation factors, blood.*
blood glucose (bG).
blood patch (Neuro)—a method of stopping postspinal tap headaches. The patient's own blood is injected into the epidural space and seals the hole in the dura made by the spinal tap needle which prevents leakage of cerebrospinal fluid, the cause of the headache pain. Also called postspinal headache.
blood perfusion monitor (BPM), Laserflo. See *Laserflo.*
blood pool (Radiol)—the circulating blood, into which radionuclides are injected for various types of circulatory scans.
blot test—see *Western blot electrotransfer test.*
blow-by oxygen—a tube with humidified flowing oxygen is positioned near the patient's nose and allowed to blow by. FiO_2 (forced inspiratory oxygen) is not precise.
blow-in fracture.
blown pupil—slang for a dilated pupil unresponsive to light in a brain-damaged patient.
blow-out fracture (Neuro)—a result of blunt impact to the orbit. It usually involves the floor of the orbit.
blue bloater—a patient with severe respiratory failure, showing dyspnea, cyanosis, and peripheral edema due to right ventricular failure. Cf. *pink puffer.*
blue diaper syndrome—tryptophan malabsorption.
blue-dot sign (Urol)—when, in testicular torsion, the infarcted appendix epididymidis can be seen through the scrotal skin.
Blue FlexTip catheter (Cardio)—a cardiac catheterization catheter with a special blue flexible tip to decrease the risk of vessel perforation.
blue rubber-bleb nevus syndrome (BRBNS).
blue toe syndrome—multiple emboli of atheromatous material in small arteries, causing cyanosis and pain in the toes.
Blumberg's sign—rebound tenderness over the site of a suspected abdominal lesion, a sign of possible peritonitis.
Blumenthal irrigating cystitome (Oph)—used during cataract surgery.
Blumer's shelf—in anorectum.
blunt dissection (also, blunt finger dissection and finger dissection) (Surg)—separating tissues with the fingers or a sponge.

blunted costophrenic angle (Radiol)—on chest x-ray, a costophrenic angle that is flattened or distorted by scarring or pleural fluid.

B-lymphocyte—see *B-cell.*

BMI (body mass indices)—used to identify and monitor obesity in children.

B-mode—see *B-scan.*

BNMSE (Brief Neuropsychological Mental Status Examination).

boat hook (Oph)—a combination of a Sinskey hook and an iris hook, the boat hook is used to manipulate an intraocular lens. It was so named because it is similar in shape (a C curve going in one direction with a straight short tip going in the opposite direction) to boating hooks used by sailors.

Bochdalek's hernia—congenital hernia through a hiatus in the posterolateral part of the diaphragm because of the persistence of the pleuroperitoneal canal in an infant.

Bodansky unit—unit of measurement of alkaline phosphatase. Very high levels (over 100 Bodansky units) are seen in primary biliary cirrhosis. Alcoholic liver disease, cholestatic hepatitis, and drug-induced cholestasis also produce high alkaline phosphatase levels. Other units of measurement in alkaline phosphatase are King-Armstrong and Bessey-Lowry.

body
- Auer
- Barr
- Councilman
- creola
- cytomegalic inclusion
- cytoplasmic inclusion
- Gamna-Gandy
- Heinz
- Hirano
- inclusion

body *(cont.)*
- Lafora inclusion
- Lewy inclusion
- lyssa inclusion
- Negri inclusion
- Pick inclusion
- psammoma
- vitreous
- X-body

body mass indices (BMI)—used to identify and monitor obese children.

body of Luys—subthalamic nucleus—an important "way-station" in the extrapyramidal system. Also called corpus Luysii and nucleus of Luys.

body surface Laplacian mapping (BSLM) (Cardio)—noninvasive way to map out the heart's electrical activity in patients with arrhythmias. This technique utilizes Laplacian electrodes to translate the three-dimensional heart into a two-dimensional picture.

Boehler's angle (or Böhler's) (Radiol)—view of the two superior surfaces of the calcaneus.

Boerhaave's syndrome—a spontaneous rupture of the esophagus.

boggy uterus (Obs)—undesirable soft spongy uterus felt on abdominal palpation following delivery, rather than firm uterus which is needed to stop hemorrhaging.

Boies nasal fracture elevator.

Böhler's angle—see *Boehler's angle.*

Boltzmann distribution—MRI term.

bolus—a single dose of a drug given intravenously over a few minutes, usually by the I.V. push method. A bolus produces immediate therapeutic levels of the drug and is used in emergency situations. See also *I.V. push.*

bombé, iris (Oph)—curved or swelling outward.

Bonaccolto forceps (Oph).

bone age according to Greulich and Pyle (Radiol).

bone cement—see *adhesive.*

bone conduction—refers to the transmission of sound through the bones of the skull to the cochlea and auditory nerve. Bone conduction is tested by holding an activated tuning fork against the mastoid bone. Normally the sound is heard twice as long by air conduction as by bone conduction. See *Weber test, air conduction, Rinne test.*

bone-cutting forceps (Pod)—used in podiatric surgery.

Bonefos (Oncol)—a drug used to treat increased bone resorption (loss of bony substance) in patients with carcinoma.

bone replacement material (See *graft.)*
- Bonfiglio
- Calcitite
- hydroxyapatite
- Durapatite
- Interpore
- Nicoll
- Unilab Surgibone

bone scan—see *TSPP rectilinear bone scan.*

bone wax—a sticky material prepared from beeswax and used to control bleeding on bony surfaces.

Bonfiglio bone graft (Ortho).

bonito fish insulin.

Bonn micro iris hook (Oph).

bony island (Radiol)—benign developmental abnormality consisting of a localized zone of increased density in a long bone.

Bookwalter retractor—used in colorectal, vaginal, Ob-Gyn, and small-incision surgery.

Bookwalter retractor system (Surg)—a metal circular frame on a post to which many retractors are clamped to expose the surgical field from all directions.

Boorman gastric cancer typing system (types I-IV):
- I polypoid carcinoma
- II ulcerocancer
- III ulcerating and infiltrating carcinoma
- IV diffusely infiltrating carcinoma

boot
- Bunny
- gelatin compression
- Unna

BOP (bleomycin, Oncovin, Platinol)—chemotherapy protocol used to treat metastatic testicular carcinoma, malignant germ cell tumor of ovary and teratoma of the ovary.

Bordetella—genus of small gram-negative coccobacilli, or rods, of the family *Brucellaceae,* formerly *Haemophilus.* The organism causing whooping cough is *B. pertussis* (formerly *Haemophilus pertussis*).

Bores forceps.

Borrelia burgdorferi—the tick-borne spirochete which causes Lyme disease.

Bosker TMI system (Oral Surg)—mandibular fixation device using an osseointegrated rigid box-frame structure which can induce bone growth in the mandible.

boss (noun), **bosselated** (adj.)—a rounded eminence, as on the surface of a bone or tumor; for example, bosselated surface.

Bosworth procedure (Ortho)—to repair acromioclavicular separation, using screw fixation of the clavicle to the coracoid.

Bosworth screw (Ortho).

bottle operation (Urol).

botulinum toxin type A (Oculinum, Ortholinum) (Oph, Ortho)—a drug derived from a culture of *Clostridium botulinum.* Oculinum is injected into certain muscles of the eye to correct strabismus and blepharospasm. As a treatment for strabismus, it permanently affects muscle fibers and allows them to lengthen. As a treatment for blepharospasm, it temporarily paralyzes the muscle in spasm, thus providing relief. Ortholinum is used to treat torticollis. See also *Clostridium botulinum toxin type A.*

Bouchard's nodes (Hand Surg).

bouche de tapir ("boosh duh tahpeer") (Fr., "tapir's mouth")—elongation of the face, so that it resembles that of a tapir, caused by extreme weakness of the muscles about the mouth.

Bouin's solution (Path)—a fixative for gastrointestinal biopsy specimens (and other tissue specimens).

Bourns-Bear ventilator—a volume-cycled ventilator which delivers a preset volume of air.

Bourns infant ventilator.

boutonnière deformity—of the finger.

bovied (lowercase)—verb form denoting the use of the Bovie electrocautery.

bovine heterograft (Vasc Surg).

bow-tie sign (Ortho)—an abnormality seen on x-ray which is associated with a cervical facet fracture. The body and facet of the cervical vertebra rotate and overlap, causing a shadow in the shape of a bow tie to appear.

boxcarring (Oph).

boxer's fracture (Ortho, Hand Surg)—caused by striking close-fisted hand on hard object, as in boxing. "Preliminary interpretation of x-rays of the left hand is of a boxer's-type fracture of the distal aspect of the second metacarpal."

Boyd intraocular implant lens.

Bozeman dilator.

BPD (biparietal diameter) (Ob-Gyn).

BPD (bronchopulmonary dysplasia).

BPM^2 (blood perfusion monitor)—incorporates laser and fiberoptic technology to provide continuous tissue perfusion data. See *Laserflo.*

Bq (becquerel).

Braasch bulb catheter.

brace

Bledsoe
clam-shell
CRS
C.Ti.
DonJoy Goldpoint knee
49er knee
Galveston metacarpal
Jewett
Kydex
Lenox Hill
LSU reciprocation-gait orthosis
Nextep knee
OS-5/Plus 2 knee
OS-5/Plus knee
Palumbo knee
Rolyan tibial fracture
Seton hip
Swede-O
Townsend
UBC (Univ. of British Columbia)

brachial—refers to the arm, as in brachial plexus—a network of nerves located partly in the neck and partly in the axilla. Cf. *branchial, bronchial.*

brachioaxillary bridge graft fistula (BAGF) (Urol)—used for patients on chronic hemodialysis when sites for direct arteriovenous anastomosis are no longer usable.

brachiosubclavian bridge graft fistula (BSGF) (Urol)—used for patients on chronic hemodialysis when sites for direct arteriovenous anastomosis are no longer usable.

brachytherapy (Rad Oncol)—interstitial implantation of radioactive isotopes, permitting the localized delivery of high doses of radiation to a tumor mass. See *remote afterloading brachytherapy.*

Bracken iris forceps (Oph).

Brackin ureterointestinal anastomosis (Surg).

bradyarrhythmia—slow, irregular heartbeat.

bradykinin—endogenous peptide that causes vasodilation, induces contraction of smooth muscle, and induces hypotension.

bradyphemic (Neuro)—afflicted with slow speech.

Brailler, Perkins.

brain death—irreversible coma.

brain death syndrome (Neuro)—state in which brain function, including autonomic control, is totally and permanently absent.

brain electrical activity map (BEAM).

brain stem (two words, as a noun and an adjective).

brain stem auditory evoked potential (BAEP).

brain stem auditory evoked response (BAER).

brain tests, noninvasive (Neuro). Cf. also *EP* (evoked potential).
- BAEP—brain stem auditory evoked potential
- BAER—brain stem auditory evoked response
- EP—evoked potential
- ER—evoked response
- MEP—multimodality evoked potential (a combination of visual, somatosensory, and brain stem auditory evoked potential)
- SEP—somatosensory evoked potential
- SER—somatosensory evoked response
- VEP—visual evoked potential
- VER—visual evoked response

branch retinal vein occlusion (BRVO). Said to be second only to diabetic retinopathy as the most common form of retinal vascular disease (Oph).

branched calculus—staghorn calculus (Urol, Radiol).

branchial cleft. Cf. *brachial, bronchial.*

Branham's sign. Compression over an arteriovenous fistula causes slowing of the pulse, giving a positive sign.

Branhamella catarrhalis (new genus—formerly *Neisseria*).

brash—a burning sensation in the stomach. Cf. *water brash.*

BRAT diet (Peds)—for children who, after having been on intravenous fluids, are started on **b**ananas, **r**ice cereal, **a**pplesauce, and **t**oast.

Braun-Yasargil right-angle clip (Neuro).

brawny edema *or* **brawny induration.**

Braxton Hicks contractions—sometimes called *false labor* (Obs). Light, irregular contractions, usually painless; may become more intense, frequent, and regular later in pregnancy.

Brazelton Neonatal Assessment Scale.

BRBNS (blue rubber-bleb nevus syndrome).

breast fibrocystic disease, stages of:
- mazoplasia—in patients in late teens and early 20s.
- adenosis—early 30s and 40s.
- cystic disease—late 30s through 40s and early 50s.

breath hydrogen excretion test—a screening test in premature infants to detect necrotizing enterocolitis.

breathing, Biot's.

Brecher and Cronkite technique—for platelet counting.

Bremmer halo (Neuro).

Brent pressure earring—used for treating earlobe keloids.

Brescio-Cimino AV fistula—arteriovenous fistula, used as hemodialysis access.

Breslow classification system (Oncol, Path)—pathologic classification of melanoma.

Breuerton view—a special x-ray view of the hand, to permit visualization of early changes of the joints from rheumatoid arthritis (Radiol, Ortho).

Brevibacterium linens.

Bricker procedure (Urol)—ureteroileostomy.

bridge flap, Cutler-Beard.

bridging osteophytes—osteophytes on adjacent vertebrae that meet and fuse, forming a "bridge" across the joint space.

bridle suture (*not* bridal)—used in eye surgery.

Brief Neuropsychological Mental Status Examination (BNMSE).

brim sign (Radiol)—in Paget's disease, a thickened pelvic brim.

bris—the Jewish circumcision rite, from the Hebrew *berith.* Also, briss.

Bristow procedure—for recurrent anterior dislocation of the shoulder. Stabilizes the shoulder by coracoid process transfer.

British antilewisite (BAL). See *BAL.*

brittle bone disease (osteogenesis imperfecta)—marked by a china blue discoloration of the sclerae.

broach (Surg)—an elongated, tapered, and serrated cutting tool for shaping and enlarging holes. See *ELP; Harris; Mittlemeir.*

Broca's motor speech area of the brain (Neuro).

Brockenbrough needle (Cardio)—used in diagnostic cardiovascular procedures such as with a Mullins sheath in transseptal catheterization.

Broders' index (devised by A. C. Broders, an American pathologist)—a classification of the malignancy of tumors, based on the degree of differentiation, and therefore the aggressiveness, of the tumor; graded from 1 to 4, grade 1 representing the most differentiation and the best prognosis, and grade 4 the least differentiation and the poorest prognosis.

Brodie's abscess (Ortho, Radiol)—centrally placed lucency in the metaphysis adjacent to the growth plate, usually in adolescents and associated with subacute or chronic hematogenous osteomyelitis. Named for Benjamin Brodie in 1832.

bromodeoxyuridine (BUdR, broxuridine). See *BUdR.*

Brompton solution (from the Brompton Hospital in London), used for analgesia in terminal cancer patients. Contains cocaine, morphine sulfate, Compazine, ethyl alcohol, and syrup. Also, Brompton mixture.

bronchial—refers to the bronchi and bronchial tubes. Cf. *bronchiole, brachial, branchial.*

bronchial washings cytology.

bronchiole—one of the smaller branches into which the segmental bronchi divide. Cf. *bronchial.*

bronchoalveolar lavage (BAL).

bronchogram, tantalum—using powdered tantalum.

Bronkaid (Pulm)—used to treat bronchial asthma. Easy to misspell because it does not follow the spelling of *bronchial.*

Bronkosol (Pulm)—used to treat bronchial asthma. Easy to misspell because it does not follow the spelling of *bronchial.*

Bronson-Turtz iris retractor (Oph).

bronze diabetes—diabetes with accompanying pancreatic damage. Also called iron storage disease.

bronze disease—same as Addison's disease; called "bronze" because one of the symptoms of this hypofunction of the adrenal glands is a bronze or brownish color of the skin.

Brooke ileostomy.

bropirimine (ABPP)—a drug used to treat AIDS.

Brostrom procedure (Ortho)—repair of ankle ligament injuries using direct suturing to reconstruct a ligament with available tissue and reimplant into the bone.

Broviac atrial catheter.

Brown dermatome—oscillating blade-type dermatome (Plas Surg).

Browne—see *Denis Browne clubfoot splint.*

Brown-McHardy pneumatic dilator—used in treatment of dysphagia associated with achalasia. The unit of measure used in procedures with this dilator is p.s.i. ("sigh"), pounds per square inch.

Brown-Roberts-Wells (BRW) **stereotactic system** (Neuro)—consisting of an arc system, frame, stereotactic adapter used in performing stereotactic procedures on the brain.

Brown-Séquard lesion (Neuro).

Brown's syndrome (Oph).

Brown's tendon sheath syndrome—the superior oblique tendon is short, causing strabismus (Oph).

Bruce protocol, staging on treadmill test (Cardiol). Scored in mets—1 met equals 3.5 ml O_2/kg/min. There are six stages, I through VI.

Bruch's membrane (Oph)—the glassy-appearing membrane of the choroid of the eye. (K.W.L. Bruch, Swiss anatomist.)

Brudzinski's sign—a positive sign in meningitis. Bending a patient's neck (pressing the chin toward the sternum) produces flexion of the knees and hips.

Bruel-Kjaer transvaginal ultrasound probe (Gyn).

Bruel-Kjaer ultrasound scanner (Urol)—used in intracavitary prostate ultrasound procedure. "Incremental multiplane scanning of the prostate and seminal vesicles in real-time mode was performed using the Bruel-Kjaer ultrasound scanner, type 1846, and a 7 MHz 112° rectal multiplane transducer, type 8551."

Bruhat maneuver—CO_2 laser surgery neosalpingostomy.

bruit ("broo'ee"), pl., bruits—a sound or murmur heard on vascular auscultation, especially an abnormal one. Example: aneurysmal bruit.

Bruner modified incision (Hand Surg).

brunescent—dark brown, as in brunescent cataract.

Brun plastic shears.

Bruser's skin incision (knee surgery).

brushing, blind esophageal (BEB).

brux, bruxism—to grind the teeth spasmodically (Oral Surg). "She complained of a weak chin and malocclusion, and desired a normal bite and profile. She bruxes and clenches,

brux *(cont.)*
but denied any TMJ [temporomandibular joint] pain or dysfunction."

BRVO (branch retinal vein occlusion).

BRW CT stereotaxic guide (Brown-Roberts-Wells). May also be used with MRI and PET scan techniques.

Bryant's traction (Ortho)—used on small children for the correction of congenital hip dislocation, or for stabilization of femur fractures. Overhead suspension is used, so that the hips are flexed to 90°.

B-scan (also called B-mode)—an ultrasound technique which permits visualization of structures by delineating echoes from these structures in various shades of gray. It can differentiate between the lumen of an artery and the arterial wall, to determine the thickness of the wall.

BSGF (brachiosubclavian bridge graft fistula).

BSS (balanced salt solution) (Oph).

BSS Plus (Oph)—balanced salt solution with added bicarbonate, dextrose, and glutathione, used as a sterile intraocular irrigating solution. It is better than plain BSS in preserving the integrity of the corneal epithelium following surgery .

bubble ventriculography—used in diagnosing hydrocephalus.

buccal mucosa *(not* buckle)—the mucosa lining the inside of the cheek.

buccal smear—test used in X-chromosome determinations; made from cells scraped from the buccal mucosa, placed on a slide, and stained; demonstrates the Barr bodies (sex chromatin) seen in normal females.

Bucholz prosthesis (Ortho).

Buck's traction (Ortho)—used on the leg and in knee injuries. Also used as a temporary measure to help reduce muscle spasm, while the patient is awaiting surgical repair for fracture of the hip.

Bucrylate—a liquid acrylic monomer made by Ethicon which polymerizes on contact with blood, forming a plug for a vessel. Used to stop bleeding in life-threatening situations.

Budd-Chiari syndrome, acute parenchymatous jaundice. Related terms:
Budd's disease
Budd's jaundice
Chiari's disease
Rokitansky's disease
von Rokitansky's disease

buddy splint (Ortho)—used in dislocation of fingers; the dislocated finger is taped to an adjacent finger (its "buddy") which acts as a splint.

Budin toe splint (Pod)—treats overlapping toes and hammertoes.

BUdR (bromodeoxyuridine, broxuridine)—a clinical radiosensitizer, used in tumors that are poorly radio-responsive to enhance radiotherapy response. Used concurrently with irradiation. Cf. *FUdR, IUdR.*

Buec uterine elevator.

Buerger's disease (Cardio)—an inflammatory disease of the blood vessels which can lead to ischemia and gangrene. Cf. *Berger's disease.*

Buerhenne technique for stone basket.

buffalo hump—a zone of focal edema over the upper mid back, seen especially in Cushing's syndrome and in prolonged adrenal steroid therapy.

buffy coat—layer of white blood cells found on centrifugation of anticoagulated blood between the plasma and the red cells. You may hear of a test being "buffy coat positive." See *buffy coat smear.*

buffy coat smear—used in diagnosis of lupus erythematosus, in determining the presence of certain protozoa and fungi in the peripheral blood, and for some bone marrow exams.

bulimia nervosa—binge eating followed by self-induced vomiting or purging.

bulimorexia—an eating disorder including features of both anorexia nervosa (severe caloric restriction due to distortion of body image, with dangerous nutritional deficiency) and bulimia nervosa (binge eating followed by self-induced vomiting or purging).

bull's eye lesion—a skin lesion consisting of concentric rings of erythema.

bunching suture.

bundle
- AV (atrioventricular)
- His
- Keith's
- Kent
- Mahaim
- Thorel's

Bunge evisceration spoon (Oph).

bunion, tailor's.

bunionectomy, tricorrectional (Pod)—bunion repair procedure also used to repair juvenile hallux valgus deformity. The bunion deformity is corrected in all three planes with a distal metatarsal osteotomy involving a transverse V-osteotomy with a long plantar hinge using cannulated bone screws for fixation. Does not interfere with the epiphyseal growth center of the first metatarsal.

Bunker intraocular implant lens.

Bunnell active hand and finger splints (Hand Surg).

Bunnell tendon transfer.

Bunny boot (Ortho).

bur, Rotablator rotating.

Burch iliopectineal ligament urethrovesical suspension (Urol).

Buretrol—a volume control device for the administration of intravenous infusions.

Burford rib retractor (Thor Surg).

buried bumper syndrome (GI)—complication which begins to cause symptoms several months after percutaneous endoscopic gastrostomy (PEG), done to insert a permanent feeding tube. The internal "bumper" of the gastrostomy tube burrows into the gastric mucosa and becomes permanently embedded. It must be freed surgically and a new gastrostomy tube inserted.

Burkitt's lymphoma—one of the cancers to which AIDS patients are particularly susceptible.

burn diagram—see *Lund Browder.*

burns classification
- first degree—erythema, involving only epidermis. Only superficial destruction of tissue and no blistering.
- second degree—entire epidermis and some of the dermis involved. There are blisters, mottling of the surface, and pain. In deeper burns, hair follicles and sebaceous glands may be destroyed.
- third degree—full thickness of skin injury.
- fourth degree—extends to subcutaneous tissue, muscle, or bone. There may be charring.

Burow's solution (*not* Burrow's, but pronounced the same).

bursitis—see *Tornwaldt's.*

BUS (Bartholin's, urethra, Skene's) **glands** (Ob-Gyn).

BuSpar (buspirone)—antianxiety drug.

busulfan (Myleran)—alkylating agent used in treatment of adult-type chronic myeloid leukemia.

butorphanol tartrate—see *Stadol NS.*

butterfly drain—a soft tissue drain consisting of a butterfly needle connected to a Vacutainer; used after surgery.

butterfly flap—technique used in hand surgery for correction of incomplete syndactyly.

butterfly needle—a fine-gauge needle with color-coded plastic tabs on each side (like wings of a butterfly) for gripping while inserting. Useful for drawing blood from a hand vein or used for scalp vein I.V. in premature infants.

butterfly rash—a rash that has a shape roughly like that of a butterfly; it is seen over the malar area and bridge of the nose in systemic lupus erythematosus.

butterfly shadow—on x-ray (Cardio).

butyl-DNJ (deoxynojirmycin).

butyrocholinesterase level.

BVAT (Oph). Mentor BVAT is a computer screen chart used in testing visual acuity.

BVM device (bag-valve-mask) (Pulm)—a resuscitating device consisting of a ventilating bag with a valve, attached to a mask.

Byers flap (Urol).

bypass circuit (Cardio).

Byron intraocular implant lens.

C, c

CA (cardiac-apnea)—see *CA monitor.*
"CA"—slang for *carcinoma.*
CABG (''cab-bage'')—coronary artery bypass graft. ''The patient underwent a CABG,'' or ''The patient was given a CABG.''
cable
Dwyer
FlexStrand
CAC (cisplatin, Ara-C, caffeine)—chemotherapy protocol.
CAD (coronary artery disease).
CAD (Cytoxan, Adriamycin, dacarbazine)—chemotherapy protocol used to treat metastatic sarcoma.
CADD-PLUS—an intravenous infusion pump which can be used on an outpatient basis to give drugs through a central line.
Cade, oil of.
Cadence AICD (automatic implantable cardioverter/defibrillator).
CAE (Oncol)—a chemotherapy protocol used to treat refractory non-Hodgkin's lymphoma. It consists of the drugs Cytoxan, Adriamycin, and etoposide.
CAF (Oncol)—a chemotherapy protocol used to treat advanced breast cancer. It consists of the drugs Cytoxan, Adriamycin, and fluorouracil.
caffeine (Neonat)—given to premature infants to prevent episodes of apnea.
Caffinière prosthesis (Hand Surg)—a cemented prosthesis used in replacement of the trapeziometacarpal joint.
CA15-3 RIA—a serum assay for monitoring breast cancer, based on two monoclonal antibodies which react with circulating antigen expressed by human breast carcinoma cells. This monitors a breast cancer patient's response to therapy. Used in the manner of carcinoembryonic antigen (CEA).
CAFTH (Cytoxan, Adriamycin, fluorouracil, tamoxifen, Halotestin)—chemotherapy protocol used to treat hormone-sensitive metastatic breast carcinoma.
CAGEIN (catheter-guided endoscopic intubation) (GI)—used at the start of endoscopy as a method to intubate the esophagus in patients who have constricted anatomy, such as from a Zenker diverticulum.
caisson disease—decompression sickness (called ''the bends''), seen in

caisson disease *(cont.)* workers and divers who work for long periods of time under water, breathing air at higher than atmospheric pressure, and then come up too quickly. The name is from the watertight structures in which underwater construction is performed, as in building bridges or tunnels.

calamus scriptorius (Neuro)—the lowest portion of the floor of the fourth ventricle, shaped like a writing pen (hence its name). Used in surgical correction of syringomyelia.

Calandruccio compression apparatus (Ortho).

Calandruccio triangular compression fixation device (Ortho)—used for fixation of the distal tibia.

calcarine fissure—sulcus on medial surface of the occipital lobe; the visual cortex is around this fissure.

Calcitite (Ortho, Plas Surg)—alloplastic material used as bone replacement. It is a solid hydroxyapatite, similar to cortical bone. See *hydroxyapatite.*

calcium acetate (PhosLo) (Urol)—used to bind with phosphate in the blood and decrease the high levels seen in end-stage renal failure.

calcium channel blockers (Oncol)—a class of drugs commonly used to treat angina, hypertension, and arrhythmias, and now a part of some chemotherapy protocols. Certain types of cancer are resistant to the effects of chemotherapy agents, but this resistance can be overcome with the use of calcium channnel blockers such as nifedipine and verapamil. See also *P-glycoprotein.*

calcium entry blockers—alternative name for calcium channel blockers.

calcium—see *fenoprofen calcium.*

calcium pyrophosphate deposition (or disease) (CPPD).

calculation—see *Berkson-Gage.*

calculus
- branched
- jackstone

Caldwell view (Radiol)—occipitofrontal view for x-raying the ethmoid and frontal sinuses.

CALF (Cytoxan, Adriamycin, leucovorin calcium, fluorouracil)—chemotherapy protocol.

CALF-E (Cytoxan, Adriamycin, leucovorin calcium, fluorouracil, ethinyl estradiol)—chemotherapy protocol used to treat breast carcinoma.

caliber—the internal diameter of a needle; also known as the bore. Cf. *calipers.*

calipers (cf. *caliber*)—instrument with two curved legs used to hold a thickness of skin and measure the subcutaneous fat underneath to assess overall nutritional status. Examples:
- Jameson
- Lange skin-fold
- Machemer
- Oscher
- Stahl
- Tenzel
- Vernier

Calleja exercises (Ortho).

callous (adjective)—hard, as "There is a callous area on the heel of the left foot." Cf. *callus.*

callus (noun)—localized growth of a hard, horny epidermal material, as "There is a callus on the palm of the hand, near the ring he is wearing on his ring finger." Cf. *callous.*

Calnan-Nicolle synthetic joint prosthesis (Ortho)—used to lengthen a shortened metatarsal.

caloric testing of vestibular function (ENT)—stimulates the labyrinth by

caloric testing *(cont.)* syringing fluid into the ear (either above or below body temperature). Resulting nystagmus lasting more than two minutes indicates hyperirritability of the labyrinth. Absence of response indicates eighth nerve damage. Also, *cold water calorics.* See *Bárány's symptom.*

Caluso PEG tube (GI)—a percutaneous endoscopic gastrostomy tube.

calusterone—an androgen used experimentally in treatment of carcinoma.

camera—see *Circon video camera for arthroscopy; Newvicon; Saticon; Vidicon.*

cameral fistula—a very rare condition of the coronary arteries, with an arteriovenous fistula betwen the artery and one of the cardiac chambers. Also called coronary artery cameral fistula.

Camey ileocystoplasty (Urol)—see *LeDuc-Camey ileocystoplasty.*

Camey reservoir (Urol)—a continent supravesical bowel urinary diversion, performed for bladder reconstruction to treat invasive bladder cancer. Also, Camey ileocystoplasty.

Camino intracranial catheter (Neuro). Inserted into the lateral ventricle, subarachnoid space, or subdural space, this catheter uses a transducer to monitor intracranial pressure.

CA monitor (cardiac-apnea)—for newborns (Peds).

Campbell de Morgan spots—see *cherry angioma.*

Campylobacter fetus—a gram-negative organism causing enteritis in AIDS patients.

Campylobacter jejuni—enteric pathogen in humans, probably transmitted by infected animals, or from consumption of contaminated water or foods of animal origin.

CAM tent (Peds).

canal
Dorello's
Guyon's
haversian
Hunter's
Schlemm's
Sondermann

canaliculus —a small canal; generally refers to the one that leads from the lacrimal punctum to the lacrimal sac of the eye. Cf. *colliculus.*

canals of Sondermann (or canaliculi)—blind outpouchings from the canal of Schlemm.

cancellous—of a reticular, spongy, or lattice-like structure, mainly of bony tissue.

cancellus—any structure arranged like a lattice.

cancer classifications—see *classification* and *staging.*

Candida albicans—a fungus which can disseminate in AIDS, but is also an exceedingly common cause of dermatitis, vaginitis, and thrush in persons with intact immune systems. Also, esophageal candidiasis is seen in AIDS patients.

C&S, C and S (culture and sensitivity). Do not confuse with *CNS* (central nervous system). See *CNS.*

CA 19-9 (Oncol)—tumor marker which is a sialylated Lewis A antigen expressed by many adenocarcinomas of the digestive tract.

Cannon waves (Cardio). The two chambers of the heart may contract at the same time, when the heart loses coordination of the atria and ventricles. Blood then flows upward across the mitral and tricuspid valves, and a venous wave is seen in the neck. Named for a physician named Cannon, who first observed this phenomenon.

cannula
Argyle CPAP nasal
Becker accelerator liposuction
Binkhorst-McIntyre irrigation
Bishop-Harman irrigating
Concorde suction
Elsberg
Flexicath silicone subclavian
Fluoro Tip
Gottschalk Nasostat
Kanavel brain-exploring
Kellan
Kellan hydrodissection
Lifemed
Mercedes tip
Packo pars plana
Padgett Concorde suction
Padgett shark-mouth
Polystan perfusion
Portnoy ventricular
Sarns aortic arch
Scheie anterior chamber
Trocan disposable CO_2
Tulevech lacrimal
USCI
Veirs
Visitec

Canthobacter (Lab).

Cantor tube (GI).

CA 125 (Gyn)—an ovarian tumor-associated antigen marker; found in serum assays for the presence of gynecological malignancies.

CAP (Cytoxan, Adriamycin, Platinol) —chemotherapy protocol used to treat ovarian carcinoma.

capacity, functional residual (or reserve) (FRC).

CAPD (continuous ambulatory peritoneal dialysis).

Capetown aortic prosthetic valve.

capillary blood sugar (CBS).

capillary leak syndrome.

capnograph (Pulm). An infrared spectrometer is used to analyze samples of expired air for various values of carbon dioxide. The results are displayed on a graph (capnograph, as *capno-* pertains to carbon dioxide) as CO_2 wave forms, and as numbers denoting values for P_ECO_2 (partial pressure of end-tidal CO_2) and F_ECO_2 (fraction of expired CO_2).

CaPPi (calcium pyrophosphate)—one of the salts of which bone is composed.

CAPPr (Cytoxan, Adriamycin, Platinol, prednisone)—chemotherapy protocol.

CAPS-free diet
C caffeine
A alcohol
P pepper
S spicy foods

capsule
Crosby-Kugler pediatric
Glisson's

capsulorhexis (Oph)—circular anterior capsulotomy. (Note that there is only one *r* in capsulorhexis, unlike capsulorrhaphy.)

capsulorhexis, continuous curvilinear (CCC). See *capsulorhexis.*

Capulets—a multivitamin preparation (not related to Juliet).

caput—the head; also used in reference to the expanded part of an organ or muscle. See also *caput medusae.*

caput medusae—dilated veins around the umbilicus. So named because of the resemblance to the snakes which formed the hair of Medusa in Greek mythology. Seen in patients with cirrhosis of the liver, and in some newborns. Cf. *caput.*

carbacephems—a new class of antibiotics similar to cephalosporins. Example: loracarbef (Lorabid).

carbolfuchsin stain, Tilden's method, to study mouth organisms.

carbonaceous material—debris from smoke inhalation deposited in the nose and upper respiratory tract of victim.

carbonate-apatite (Lab).

carboplatin (Paraplatin)—used for advanced ovarian cancer, this drug is related to cisplatin but causes fewer side effects.

carbovir—a drug used to treat AIDS.

carboxyhemoglobin (Lab). Levels are measured in patients exposed to fires and in attempted suicides using automobile exhaust. Carbon monoxide binds competitively with hemoglobin molecules, excluding oxygen.

carcinoembryonic antigen (CEA).

carcinoma, argentaffin.

carcinoma in situ (CIS).

carcinoma of bladder classification. See *Jewett's classification.*

cardiac retraction clip (Cardio)—used to retract the fatty layer over the heart during coronary artery anastomosis.

cardiac risk factors—elevated blood lipids, obesity, habitual dietary excesses, lack of exercise, hypertension, cigarette smoking, and stress.

cardiac sling (Cardio)—used to support the heart and expose the circumflex branch of the coronary artery during surgery.

cardiokymographic test (CKG)—for measuring interference in pacemaker function. Cardiokymography is used clinically at some institutions for detecting segmental wall motion abnormalities of the heart. It may interfere with cardiac pacemaker function and can cause the pacemaker to operate at its upper rate limit.

Cardiolite scan (Radiol)—a cardiac scan showing areas of myocardial infarction, using the radioactive imaging agent ^{99m}Tc sestamibi (trade name: Cardiolite).

cardiomyoplasty (Cardio)—a surgical treatment for weakened heart muscle leading to congestive heart failure. In cardiomyoplasty, the latissimus dorsi muscle is surgically excised except for a pedicle which contains its blood and nerve supply. It is then inserted into the chest cavity through an opening created by excision of the second rib on the anterior chest. Two pacing electrode leads are placed in the muscle flap, and two sensing leads are placed on the heart itself. These leads are connected to a programmable pulse pacemaker which is placed surgically beneath the rectus abdominis muscle. The pacemaker synchronizes the contraction of the muscle flap to the R wave of the heart's own electrical rhythm. The number of bursts from the pacemaker is gradually increased after surgery until, after a few months, the skeletal muscle contracts with every heartbeat or every other heartbeat. After exposure to burst stimulation from the pacemaker, the skeletal muscle gradually changes its muscle fibers at the cellular level until they resemble those of heart muscle which can contract repeatedly without fatigue.

cardioplegic solution—an iced solution injected into the coronary arteries during open-heart surgery to produce cardiac arrest. Composed of calcium, magnesium, potassium, chloride, and sodium bicarbonate in solution, it produces cardiac standstill, and protects the myocardium from damage due to intracellular ion im-

cardioplegic solution *(cont.)* balance and acidosis. Types:
ECS—extracellular-like, calcium-free solution
ICS—intracellular-like, calcium-bearing, crystalloid solution

cardiopulmonary support system (CPS).

Cardio Tactilaze peripheral angioplasty laser catheter (Cardio)—a catheter containing an Nd:YAG laser to vaporize atheromatous plaques.

CardioTek scan (Radiol)—a cardiac scan showing areas of myocardial infarction, using the radioactive imaging agent ^{99}Tc teboroxime (trade name: CardioTek). Used for emergency scans, it clears rapidly from the blood to allow subsequent scans, if necessary.

cardiothoracic ratio (CTR).

Cardizem CD (Cardio)—another form of diltiazem, not to be confused with Cardizem SR. Cardizem CD is an extended release capsule, given once per day, and is available in 180 mg, 240 mg, and 300 mg strengths. Cardizem SR is a sustained release capsule, given twice per day, and is available in 60 mg, 90 mg, and 120 mg strengths. *Not* Cardiazem.

Cardona corneal prosthesis trephine (Oph).

Cardura—see *doxazosin mesylate.*

Carlens' fiberoptic mediastinoscope.

C-arm fluoroscopy—image intensifier, portable x-ray unit used in the operating room.

Carolina rocker—a wheelchair on a rocker platform, used in physical therapy for patients with stroke, and also for tardive dyskinesia.

carotene—the yellow or red coloring found in egg yolk, carrots, and sweet potatoes. Cf. *creatine, creatinine, keratin.*

carpal tunnel syndrome (CTS) (Ortho)—caused by repetitive hand motions, such as prolonged keyboard use, or hammering, filing, or writing, resulting in compression of the rather soft median nerve against the volar carpal ligament by the nine comparatively harder tendons that are in the tunnel with it. Depending on the degree of pressure, symptoms range from aching and numbness over the median nerve distribution (but sparing the little finger), to constant hypesthesia and paralysis of the abductor pollicis brevis. Also, repetitive strain injury (RSI).

Carpentier-Edwards valve (Cardio).

carphology (Psych)—purposeless plucking at clothing or bedclothes; sometimes seen in dementia or terminal illness.

carprofen (Rimadyl) (Ortho)—a nonsteroidal anti-inflammatory drug.

Carrel patch (Surg).

Carrisyn (acemannan)—a drug used in treating AIDS.

Carroll bone-holding forceps.

Carr-Purcell sequence—MRI term.

Carr-Purcell-Meiboom-Gill sequence—MRI term.

Carswell's grapes—clusters of tubercles around the smaller bronchioles, looking like a bunch of grapes; seen in pulmonary tuberculosis.

Carter pillow (Ortho, Plas Surg)—a foam cushion which immobilizes and elevates simultaneously; often used in replantation procedures.

caseation—necrosed tissue resembling cheesy material.

CA 72-4 (Oncol)—a cancer antigen serum tumor marker to monitor metastatic gastric cancer.

Casey pelvic clamp.

Caspar alligator forceps (Oph).

C-asparaginase (Crasnitin).

cast, casting material (Ortho)
Fractura Flex
Gypsona
Hexcelite
hip spica
MaxCast
Risser localizer
Sarmiento
spica

Castaneda anastomosis clamp (Vasc Surg) (Aldo Castaneda, b. 1930).

Castaneda bottle—used in the culture of certain organisms from blood.

Castaneda suture tag forceps.

Castelli tube (ENT).

Castroviejo
bladebreaker knife
cyclodialysis spatula
forceps
scissors
trephine

CAT (''cat'') (computerized, or computed, axial tomography) (Radiol)—a radiologic technique producing a two-dimensional image in cross-sections or ''slices'' of tissue, in a transverse plane. This is done by means of several x-ray sources positioned around the patient, a scanner, and a computer. Also called ACAT, CT, and CAT scan.

cat cry syndrome—a chromosome abnormality including multiple heart and eye abnormalities, mental retardation, microcephaly, and a mewing cry from which the syndrome gets its name. Also, cri du chat syndrome.

cat's eye pupil (also cat's eye reflex) (Oph)—an unusual appearance of the pupil resembling that of a light shining into a cat's eye. It is seen in retinoblastoma.

cat's eye reflex—sign of retinoblastoma.

Catapres (clonidine).

cataract—opacity of the lens of the eye, or its capsule, or both. Types:
brunescent
capsular
congenital
cortical
diabetic
infantile
lamellar
mature
morgagnian
nuclear
polar
posterior subcapsular (PSC)
senile
traumatic

catch—term for a sharp, localized pain, usually in the chest, and provoked or aggravated by drawing a breath (inspiration).

catgut—see *surgical gut.*

cathepsin D (Oncol)—lysozomal enzyme used to label fibroblasts, macrophages, sweat ducts and glands, smooth muscle and stratum granulosum in normal tissue and now being used as a prognostic marker in breast tumors.

catheter
Abramson
Ackrad H/S (hysterosalpingography)
Alzate
Amplatz cardiac
Angiocath PRN
Anthron heparinized
Arani
Arrowgard Blue Line
Arrow-Howes multilumen central venous
Arrow Twin Cath
atherectomy
AtheroCath
Auth atherectomy
Axiom DG balloon angioplasty

catheter *(cont.)*
balloon biliary
Bardex
Blue FlexTip
Braasch bulb
Broviac atrial
Buerhenne
Camino intracranial
Cardio Tactilaze peripheral angioplasty laser
Cath-Finder
Cathlon I.V.
central venous (CVC)
Chemo-Port
Comfort Cath I
Comfort Cath II
Cook TPN
coudé
Critikon balloon thermodilution
cutdown
Datascope
Double-J stent
EAC
EchoMark
Endotak C
Ependorf angiocatheter
Erythroflex
Evermed
expandable access
Express PTCA coronary angioplasty
Flexxicon Blue dialysis
Flexxicon dialysis
Fogarty
Fogarty balloon biliary
Foltz
Grollman
Groshong
Groshong double-lumen
Grüntzig balloon
Hickman
Hieshima coaxial
ICP (intracranial pressure)
ILUS (intraluminal ultrasound)
Ingram
Intracath

catheter *(cont.)*
Intran disposable intrauterine pressure measurement
intrepid PTCA angioplasty
Jackson-Pratt
Jelco
JL4 (Judkins left 4 cm curve)
JL5 (Judkins left 5 cm curve)
KDF-2.3
Kifa
Kinsey atherectomy
KISS (Kidney Internal Splint/Stent)
Konton
LAP-13
Lifecath
Mahurkar dialysis
Malecot
Manu
Marathon guiding
Max Force
McGoon coronary perfusion
McIntosh double-lumen
Medina ileostomy
Med-Tech
Mixtner
Multi-Med triple-lumen infusion
nephrostomy-type
NoProfile balloon
Nutricath
Olbert balloon dilatation
ORC-B
Oreopoulos-Zellerman
Orion balloon dilatation
P.A.S. Port
P.A.S. Port Fluoro-Free
Passage
PIC (peripherally inserted)
PICC (peripherally inserted central)
pigtail
Pipelle endometrial suction
Polystan venous return
ProFlex5 balloon
Pruitt irrigation
Pruitt occlusion
Quinton Mahurkar dual-lumen

catheter *(cont.)*
Raaf Cath
Raimondi ventricular
Ranfac cholangiographic
Reddick cystic duct cholangiogram
Redifurl TaperSeal IAB
Rigiflex TTS
Royal Flush angiographic flush
SCOOP 1
SCOOP 2
Seroma-Cath
Simpson atherectomy
Simpson peripheral AtheroCath
Skinny dilatation
Slinky
Speedy balloon
split sheath
Suction Buster
Swan-Ganz
Tactilaze angioplasty laser
Tenckhoff
Tenckhoff peritoneal
Tennis Racquet
thermodilution
Tis-u-trap endometrial suction
Torcon NB selective angiographic
Tracker-18
Tracker-18 Soft Stream
transtracheal oxygen
TTS (through the scope)
twist drill
umbilical artery (UAC)
vanSonnenberg-Wittich
Von Andel
whistletip ureteral
Wills-Oglesby locking
Witzel enterostomy
Wurd
XL-11

catheter cuff, antimicrobial.

catheterization, endoscopic transpapillary, of the gallbladder (ETCG)

catheter vitrector, Verbatim balloon probe.

Cath-Finder—catheter tracking system, part of the P.A.S. Port system that tracks the catheter tip during placement, without fluoroscopy.

Cattell Infant Intelligence Scale.

cauda—tail, or structure resembling a tail. See *tail.*

caudate, adj., having a tail, as in "caudate lobe." Cf. *chordate, cordate.*

cauliflower ear—slang term for an external ear deformed by repeated or severe trauma, as in boxers and wrestlers.

cautery
BICAP
BiLAP bipolar
bipolar
Concept hand-held
electrocautery
Mira
NeoKnife
Op-Temp
Scheie ophthalmic
wet field

CAV (Cytoxan, Adriamycin, vincristine)—chemotherapy protocol used to treat neuroblastoma.

CAVH (continuous arteriovenous hemofiltration) (Nephrol). This procedure filters toxins from the blood of patients in renal failure. It has a lower risk of side effects than hemodialysis because the equipment is simpler and blood is removed from the patient's body at a much slower rate.

Cavitron dissector (Neuro).

Cavitron ultrasonic aspirator (CUSA)—used in tumor decompression.

CAVP16 (Cytoxan, Adriamycin, VP-16)—chemotherapy protocol.

CBS (capillary blood sugar)—a test for hypoglycemia. It enables a patient to take a blood sugar reading by a fingerstick.

CBV (Cytoxan, BCNU, VP-16)—chemotherapy protocol used to treat Hodgkin's lymphoma.

CBWO—see *closing base wedge osteotomy.*

C Cap (compliance cap)—a new device on containers of medications for glaucoma, to help patients track medication compliance.

CCE (clubbing, cyanosis, or edema) or (clubbing, cyanosis, and edema).

CCUP (colpocystourethropexy).

CDA (chenodeoxycholic acid)—a drug used to dissolve gallstones in carefully selected patients: those at higher surgical risk, who are slender, who have noncalcium gallstones, and who tend to have higher serum cholesterol levels. Cf. *2-CdA.*

CDC—the Centers for Disease Control (*not* Center) in Atlanta, Georgia, the federal clearinghouse for information on epidemic diseases. In addition to being a pool of information for researchers and practicing physicians, they sometimes have investigational drugs available.

CDE (Cytoxan, doxorubicin, etoposide)—chemotherapy protocol used to treat small-cell lung carcinoma.

CD4, recombinant soluble human (Receptin, rsCD4)—a drug used in the treatment of AIDS.

CD4-IgG—a drug used to treat HIV-positive mothers and babies.

CD5+ monoclonal antibody—used in treatment of graft-versus-host disease.

CD5-T lymphocyte immunotoxin—see *XomaZyme-H65.*

CDH (congenital dysplasia of the hip) (Ortho, Peds). Also, dislocation.

cDNA (complementary DNA).

CE (capillary electrophoresis) (Lab)—a technique for rapid separation and analysis of peptides and proteins.

CEA (carcinoembryonic antigen).

CEAker (Radiol)—an anti-CEA monoclonal antibody labeled with indium-111 and used to detect recurrent colorectal carcinoma.

CEA-Tc 99m (Radiol)—carcinoembryonic antigen (a monoclonal antibody) plus ^{99m}Tc (a technetium isotope). See *RAID* and *ImmuRAID.*

CEB (carboplatin, etoposide, bleomycin)—chemotherapy protocol used to treat metastatic testicular carcinoma.

Cebotome (Ortho)—made by Zimmer. Also, Neurairtome, Surgairtome.

CECA (cisplatin, etoposide, Cytoxan, Adriamycin)—chemotherapy protocol.

CEF (Cytoxan, epirubicin, fluorouracil)—chemotherapy protocol used to treat breast carcinoma.

cefmetazole (Zefazone)—a second-generation cephalosporin similar in action to that of cefoxitin (Mefoxin). Used for treating infections by susceptible gram-positive and gram-negative bacteria, and is given prophylactically in abdominal surgery.

cefprozil (Cefzil)—a cephalosporin antibiotic used to treat ENT, pulmonary, and skin infections.

ceftazidime (Ceptaz, Fortaz, Tazidime)—an antibacterial agent.

Cefzil (cefprozil).

Celestin latex rubber tube—used in dilation of the esophagus in treatment for peptic stricture.

celiacography (Radiol)—used to diagnose hemangiomata.

celiprolol (Selecor) (Cardio)—a cardioselective beta blocker drug used to treat hypertension and angina.

cell
Betz
Bloch clear
clue
eating (phagocyte)
foam
glitter
ground-glass
HeLa
helper
helper/inducer T-cell
inducer
irreversible sickled (red) (ISC)
islet
koilocytotic
Kulchitsky
Kupffer
LAK (lymphokine-activated killer)
Leydig
large unstained (LUC)
mast
NK (natural killer)
null
oxyphil
Pelger-Huët
phagocytic
prickle
Purkinje's
Sézary
suppressor
Tart
T-cell (thymus)
T-8 suppressor
T-4
theca
thymus dependent
TRC
umbrella
Warthin's
zymogen

cell and flare (*not* flair) (Oph)—an accumulation of white blood cells and an increase of protein in the aqueous which can be seen on slit-lamp examination of the anterior chamber of the eye. A sign of iritis or ciliary body inflammation.

cell assay test. See *Raji cell assay test.*

Cellano phenotype (Kell blood group).

cell-mediated immunity (CMI).

Cellolite—a form of patty material (see *cottonoid patty)* produced as an alternative to cottonoid; made of polyvinyl alcohol foam cross-linked with formaldehyde, and impregnated with particles of barium sulfate.

cell ratiosee *helper/suppressor.*

cell saver—see *Solcotrans Plus.*

Cell Saver Haemolite—trade name for a washed red cell autotransfusion system for use in low-volume blood loss procedures. Can be used intraoperatively and postoperatively.

cell sorter, Fluorescence activated.

celltrifuge—a coined word for a device to remove white blood cells from blood of patients with leukemia.

CEM (cytosine arabinoside, etoposide, methotrexate)—chemotherapy protocol.

cement—see *adhesive.*

Cement Eater, Anspach—trade name for a drill used in re-doing arthroplasties; it drills out the hard, old cement holding the prosthesis in place.

cementophyte (Ortho). In contrast to osteophyte, which is a bony excrescence or osseous outgrowth, a cementophyte is an excrescence of cement (such as methyl methacrylate), the result of a previous arthrotomy.

Cenflex central monitoring system.

Centers for Disease Control (CDC).

centigray (cGy) (Radiol)—a unit of absorbed radiation dose equal to 1 rad. See *gray.*

centimeter (cm)—often pronounced "sonometer").

centistoke—a unit of measurement of plasma viscosity and serum viscosity.

Centovir—a drug used to treat cytomegalovirus infection. Also known as monoclonal antibody C-58.

Centoxin—the HA-1a monoclonal antibody which acts as an immunostimulant.

central venous catheter (CVC)—an intravenous catheter is inserted into the subclavian vein (occasionally into the internal jugular vein) and advanced so that the tip is just above the right atrium. Used to administer fluids, drugs, or total parenteral nutrition on a long-term basis.

Centry ("sen-tree") **bicarbonate dialysis control unit** (Nephrol).

CEP (Cytoxan, etoposide, Platinol)—chemotherapy protocol used to treat nonsmall-cell lung carcinoma and metastatic solid tumors.

cephalopelvic disproportion (CPD)—a condition in pregnancy in which the mother's pelvis is too small to accommodate the fetal head.

cephalosporins—a group of antibiotics with a broad spectrum of antibacterial activity. They are divided into first-, second-, and third-generation cephalosporins. This designation has nothing to do with when these antibiotics were discovered or first marketed, but instead divides them by their therapeutic antibiotic properties. First-generation cephalosporins, such as cefazolin (Ancef) and cephalexin (Keflex), are generally inactivated by bacteria that produce penicillinase. Third-generation cephalosporins, such as cefixime (Suprax) and ceftazidime (Fortaz, Tazidime), show the greatest activity against gram-negative bacteria and against resistant strains of bacteria.

Ceptaz (ceftazidime).

cerclage—encircling, hooping, banding. See *Dall-Miles cerclage.*

cerebellopontile angle—the area between the cerebellum and the pons. See *cerebellopontile angle tumor.*

cerebellopontile angle tumor—a brain tumor located between the cerebellum and the pons. It involves cranial nerves V, VI, VII, and VIII. Spasms of eyelid muscles, oscillating eye movements, loss of corneal sensation, and impaired hearing are characteristic symptoms.

cerebrovascular accident (CVA)—stroke.

Ceredase (alglucerase).

certified medical transcriptionist (abbreviated CMT)—an individual who has satisfied the requirements for voluntary certification (by examination or experience) by the American Association for Medical Transcription (AAMT).

Cerubidine (daunorubicin HCl)—medication for use in nonlymphocytic leukemia (myelogenous, monocytic, erythroid) in adults; administered intravenously.

Cervex-Brush (Gyn)—used to simultaneously obtain ectocervical and endocervical cells for cytologic exam.

cervical intraepithelial neoplasia (abbreviated CIN)—a phrase used to describe preinvasive lesions of the cervix. The degree of abnormal cytology is expressed as grades 1-3. CIN-2 would be severe dysplasia.

cervical support
AOA halo traction
Bremmer halo
Georgiade visor
Houston halo traction
Miami acute collar
Miami J collar

cervical *(cont.)*
Philadelphia collar

cesium chloride (Radiol)—used in myocardial scanning.

cetiedil citrate—a drug used to treat sickle cell crisis.

cetirizine (Reactine) (ENT)—a nonsedating antihistamine, given orally.

Cetus trial—You may hear this in reference to tumor necrosis factor in conjunction with interleukin-2. Cetus is the corporation that manufactures tumor necrosis factor, and the physician is talking about a trial of this agent in the treatment of cancers that have been unresponsive to other therapy. See *tumor necrosis factor.*

cf. (L., *confer,* ''compare'').

C-fiber—small unmyelinated nerve fiber. See *fiber of Remak.*

CFIDS (chronic fatigue immune dysfunction syndrome).

CFL (calcaneofibular ligament).

CGL (chronic granulocytic leukemia).

C'H$_{50}$—total hemolytic complement.

Chadwick's sign—purplish or bluish discoloration of the cervix and vaginal mucosa, a normal finding in pregnancy early in gestation. Also *Jacquemier's sign.*

Chaffin-Pratt drain.

chair-back brace (Ortho).

chair, Gardner.

chalazion—chronic inflammatory granulomatous process of a meibomian gland. See *meibomian cyst, tarsal cyst.*

chamfer reamer (lowercase *c*) (Ortho).

Champ elastic bandage.

Champion Trauma Score (CTS)—a scoring system used to evaluate multiple trauma injuries.

Chance fracture (Ortho)—a fracture of the lumbar vertebrae caused by extreme forward flexion of the spine above and below a seat belt during an automobile accident. Named for Dr. C. Q. Chance, who first described this type of traumatic spinal fracture in 1948. Also known as a seat belt fracture and a fulcrum fracture because the seat belt acts as the point of a fulcrum which separates the upper and lower segments of the spinal column.

chandelier sign (Gyn)—extreme tenderness of the uterine adnexa, elicited on pelvic examination. (The term fancifully implies that the pain causes the patient to leap into the air and cling to the chandelier.)

Chan wrist rest—a device used by ophthalmic surgeons to stabilize their hands, particularly when performing vitrectomies.

charcoal, activated.

Charcot-Bouchard aneurysm—aneurysmal formation in small arteries within the neural parenchyma.

Charcot-Leyden crystals—found in sputa of patients with bronchial asthma.

Chardack-Greatbatch Implantable Cardiac Pulse Generator (Cardio).

Charles intraocular lens.

Charles vacuuming needle.

charley horse—a painful spasm in a lower extremity, generally due to injury or strain.

Charnley-Mueller hip prosthesis.

Charnley total hip system (Ortho).

Charriere bone saw (Ortho).

CHART (continuous hyperfractionated accelerated radiotherapy).

Chausse's view.

Cheatle-Henry hernia.

Cheatle slit (for takedown of colostomy).

Check-Flo introducer—used to introduce balloon, electrode, closed end,

Check-Flo *(cont.)*
and other catheters; the seal on this prevents blood reflux and air aspiration.

checking (Neuro)—fine control of voluntary movement; the act of stopping a motion when its goal or purpose has been attained.

cheese worker's lung disease—extrinsic allergic alveolitis caused by exposure to moldy cheese.

cheilectomy ("ky-lék-to-me")—(1) excision of a lip (Plas Surg); (2) an operative procedure in which bone edges that impede joint motion are removed, e.g., in hallux rigidus (Ortho).

Chemet (succimer).

chemical shift—MRI term.

ChemoCap—see *Kold Kap.*

chemoembolization (Oncol)—the use of degradable starch microspheres (DSM) administered simultaneously with a chemotherapy drug. These microspheres temporarily block the blood flow at the capillary level. The chemotherapy drug is then concentrated in the region of the cancer and achieves high tissue uptake. See *DSM.*

Chemo-Port catheter—for administration of chemotherapeutic agents or for the delivery of nutritional fluids.

chemosis—edema of the conjunctiva of the eye.

chemosurgery, Mohs.

chemotherapy code for evaluating progress:
−2 definitely worse
−1 probably worse
0 no change since last scan
+1 probably better
+2 definitely better

chemotherapy drugs—see *medication.*

chemotherapy protocol—see individual main entries alphabetically throughout the book. Also listed under *medication,* for quick reference.

Chemstrip bG (lowercase b, capital G). Trade name of a plastic strip used in checking blood glucose. Cf. *Dextrostix,* used in a similar manner. The blood spot on the treated strip is wiped off and rinsed with water, and then the resulting color is compared with a color chart, which gives the blood glucose value.

Chemstrip MatchMaker blood glucose meter—for self-testing by diabetics.

chemstrip, Micral.

Chenix (chenodiol) (GI)—a drug given orally to dissolve small gallbladder stones in patients without surgery. See *MTBE.*

chenodiol (Chenix).

Cherney incision—lower transverse abdominal incision.

cherry angiomas (Derm)—benign hemangiomas that are round, cherry-red, dome-shaped papules; usually seen in the elderly. Called Campbell de Morgan spots, or De Morgan's spots.

Cherry-Crandall test—of serum lipase.

chest, flail—see *flail chest.*

chest PT (physiotherapy) (Pulm)—the use of positioning (postural drainage) and clapping with a cupped hand over the patient's chest and back (frappage) to loosen pulmonary secretions. The patient may cough up the secretions, or they may be suctioned out.

chevron incision—the name derives from the V shape of the incision.

CHF (congestive heart failure).

C'H_{50}—total hemolytic complement.

Chiari—see *Budd-Chiari syndrome.*
Chiba needle (also, *skinny needle)*—used in percutaneous transhepatic cholangiography.
Chibroxin (norfloxacin).
CHICK fracture table (Ortho).
Chilaiditi's syndrome ("ky-la-dee-tees")—interposition of the colon (sometimes the small intestine) between the liver and the diaphragm. This is a result of a congenital anomaly of the diaphragm or the falciform ligament, which is a fold of peritoneum from the diaphragm to the surface of the liver. Usually seen in adults but also found in children.
Child's classification of hepatic risk criteria, class A, class B, and class C. Relates to operative risk.
chimney, Roux-Y—see *Roux-Y chimney.*
CHIP (iproplatin) (Oncol)—a chemotherapy drug for children with neuroblastoma; a single agent, not a protocol.
ChlVPP (chlorambucil, vinblastine, procarbazine, prednisone)—chemotherapy protocol used to treat Hodgkin's disease.
Chlamydia trachomatis—a gram-negative organism.
chloracetate esterase (Leder stain).
chlorotrianisene (TACE)—estrogen.
CHOD (Cytoxan, hydroxydaunomycin, Oncovin, dexamethasone)—chemotherapy protocol used to treat CNS lymphoma.
choked disk (Oph)—edema of the optic nerve head, as seen on funduscopic examination.
cholecystectomy
endoscopic laser
laparoscopic laser
video-laseroscopy
cholecystoduodenostomy, Jenckel.
cholecystokinin (CCK)—thought to be one of the important hormones regulating gallbladder contraction. See *noncholecystokinin substance.*
choledochoscope—see *Berci-Shore.*
cholescintography, radionuclide test (Radiol). ^{99m}Tc PIPIDA is injected intravenously, giving prompt visualization of the liver, bile ducts, and gallbladder. Absence of dye in the gastrointestinal tract indicates obstruction of the common duct. If the gallbladder is not visualized, this is an indication of acute cholecystitis or of obstruction of the cystic duct or hepatic duct. See *PIPIDA.*
chondromalacia patellae *(not* patella, even though only one knee is involved); patellae is (Latin) genitive case, meaning *of the patella* (Ortho).
CHOP (Cytoxan, Halotestin, Oncovin, prednisone)—chemotherapy protocol used to treat non-Hodgkin's lymphoma and CNS lymphoma.
Chopart ankle dislocation of navicula and cuboid across talus and calcaneus (Ortho).
CHOP-BLEO (Cytoxan, Halotestin, Oncovin, prednisone)—chemotherapy protocol used to treat non-Hodgkin's lymphoma.
CHOPE (Cytoxan, Halotestin, Oncovin, prednisone, etoposide)—chemotherapy protocol used to treat Hodgkin's and other lymphomas.
chordate—having a notochord (primitive backbone). See *caudate, cordate.*
chordee—a congenital defect that involves stricture of the fibrous tissue of the penis and that causes the penis to bow. This condition is often associated with a hypospadias.

chordoma (*not* cordoma)—a malignant tumor arising from the embryonic remains of the notochord (primitive backbone).

chordotomy—see *cordotomy.*

chorionic villi biopsy (CVB).

choristoma—a benign tumor containing tissues foreign to the tissue in which the tumor is found, e.g., bone found in muscle tissue.

choroidal neovascular membrane (CNVM).

Chorus DDD pacemaker (Cardio)—uses atrial sensing.

Choyce anterior chamber lens (Oph).

Choyce implant cataract lens (Oph).

Chrisman and Snook procedure (Ortho)—modification of the Elmslie procedure using half of the peroneus brevis tendon to correct lateral ankle instability.

Christmas disease (Hematol)—factor IX deficiency (hemophilia B). See *hemophilia A.* Named for the child in whom it was first identified.

Christmas tree appearance of pancreas (Radiol).

Christmas tree pattern (Derm)—seen in the skin eruption of pityriasis rosea.

Christopher-Williams overtube—tube used with the Fujinon colonoscope.

chromatography
affinity
gas

chromohydrotubation (Gyn)—test used in the evaluation of infertility. Dye is injected into the cervix through the vagina; a laparoscopic incision permits visualization of where the dye goes, to determine if the fallopian tubes are patent. Also called *chromopertubation.*

chromopertubation—see *chromohydrotubation.*

chromosome
mitotic
Philadelphia
polytene

chronic—persistent or prolonged, as in chronic bronchitis, chronic steroid therapy.

chronic fatigue immune dysfunction syndrome (CFIDS)—newer name by the Centers for Disease Control for what is usually called chronic fatigue syndrome.

chronic fatigue syndrome (CFS) (also known as chronic fatigue immune dysfunction syndrome, myalgic encephalomyelitis, postviral fatigue syndrome, and yuppie flu)—characterized by fatigue, irritability, sleep loss, forgetfulness, and muscle pain. Many of the patients are also depressed, and whether this is one of the symptoms of the disease or relates to the isolation, exhaustion, pain, and the fact that many physicians do not recognize this as a disease entity is not known. Symptoms last for months or even years, and seem to affect more women than men.

chronic granulocytic leukemia (CGL).

chronic lunger—a patient who has had chronic long-term lung disease, particularly tuberculosis or chronic obstructive pulmonary disease. A pejorative term not used in the patient's hearing. "The patient is a chronic lunger who no longer smokes."

Chrysosporium pruinosum.

CHRYS CO_2 laser—a portable carbon dioxide laser as small as a desktop computer. Intended for use in physician offices and outpatient surgery centers.

chymonucleolysis—use of chymopapain for removal of nucleus pulposus.

Cibis ski needle—a flat needle used as an aid in placing an encircling band in retinal surgery.

cidal level (serumcidal; bactericidal): the amount of an antibiotic needed in the blood to kill an organism.

CIE (countercurrent immunoelectrophoresis)—test for amebic antigen.

cifenline succinate (Cipralan) (Cardio)—an antiarrhythmic drug with a chemical structure unlike any other antiarrhythmic currently in use.

Cilastin tube.

cilazapril (Inhibace) (Cardio)—an ACE inhibitor used to treat hypertension and congestive heart failure.

Cilco intraocular lens—Binkhorst-type (Oph).

Cilco MonoFlex PMMA lenses (Oph).

Cilco Slant lens (Oph)—a single-piece intraocular lens with a design that incorporates slanted haptics and a low profile for easy insertion through the longer scleral tunnel and more acute angle of entry now used in intraocular lens surgery. Slant is a trade name. Also called Slant lens.

Ciloxan (ciprofloxacin)—an ophthalmic antibiotic solution.

cimetidine (Tagamet) (GI)—a drug used in treatment of Crohn's disease, duodenal ulcer, and other GI diseases.

CIN (cervical intraepithelial neoplasia)—a designation to describe preinvasive lesions of the cervix. The degree of abnormal cytology is expressed in grades 1-3. CIN-2 would be severe dysplasia.

cinchonism (''sin-koh-nism'') (from cinchona, the plant from which quinine is obtained)—the manifestations of quinine toxicity: tinnitus, blurred vision, nausea, headache, and possibly thrombocytopenia.

cinctured—encircled.

cine CT (computed tomography) (Radiol, Cardio). Compare motion pictures and still photographs and you will get the picture. The cine CT scanner can visualize contractions of the heart wall and the blood flow in the brain, as well as evaluate coronary artery bypass graft function, detect regional thickening of the myocardium, or abnormalities in wall motion, and can also estimate cardiac output. Also called ultrafast CT.

cine view (cinematograph) (in multiple gated acquisition scan, or MUGA) (Radiol, Cardio)—a moving picture of the cardiac cycle, constructed from individual frames, of which each is a composite image of one point in the cardiac cycle obtained by cardiac gating.

cingulate gyrus (''sing-gyu-late'')—one of the elevations of the brain surface, just above the corpus callosum.

Cintor knee prosthesis (Ortho).

Cipralansee *cifenline succinate.*

ciprofloxacin (Ciloxan, Cipro) (Oph)—a fluoroquinolone antibiotic.

circinate (''sur-sin-ate'')—ringlike or circular.

circinate retinopathy (Oph)—condition marked by white spots encircling the macular area, which results in complete foveal blindness.

CircOlectric bed.

Circon-ACMI electrohydraulic lithotriptor probe (Urol).

Circon video camera—for arthroscopy. This camera is connected to the arthroscope and provides color reproduction reported almost identical to that perceived by the human eye. Also, Saticon and Newvicon. Cf. *Vidicon vacuum chamber pickup tube for camera.*

circulation—see *extracorporeal circulation.*

circumduction ("sur-kum-duk-shun") —the rotational movement, active or passive, of an eye, or of an extremity. Cf. *sursumduction.*

circumference, occipitofrontal (OFC).

circumferential fracture (Neuro)—extends completely around the skull, leaving the skull essentially in two pieces.

circus-movement tachycardia (CMT).

circus senilis—often used interchangeably with *arcus senilis*—a hazy gray ring around the periphery of the cornea, composed of lipid droplets.

cirsodesis ("sur-sod-ee-sis")—ligation of varicose veins.

CIS (carcinoma in situ).

CISCA (cisplatin, Cytoxan, Adriamycin)—chemotherapy protocol.

cisplatin (cis-platinum, Platinol)—an antineoplastic drug.

cis-retinoic acid—see *isotretinoin.*

cisternogram, metrizamide CT.

cisternography, oxygen.

cite—to bring forward, as for illustration; to quote, as proof or by way of authority; to summon to appear. "It may be necessary to cite an example." Cf. *site.*

Citelli rongeur (Oph).

Citelli-Meltzer atticus punch (ENT).

citrate phosphate dextrose (CPD).

Citrobacter amalonaticus (formerly *C. freundii*)—associated with enteritis, septicemia, urinary tract infections, pneumonia, and burn and wound infections.

citrovorum rescue (Oncol)—see *leucovorin rescue.*

citta ("sit'-ah")—the craving for unusual foods during pregnancy (strawberries, pickles, etc.) (Obs).

CIWA-A scale—see *Clinical Institute Withdrawal Assessment-Alcohol.*

CK (creatine kinase).

CK_1, CK_2, CK_3 —isoenzymes of creatine kinase.

CK/AST ratio (creatine kinase/aspartate aminotransferase).

Cladosporium—an inhalant antigen.

Clagett-Barrett esophagogastrostomy.

clamp

- Allis
- Bartley anastomosis
- Belcher
- Berens muscle
- Best right-angle colon
- Casey pelvic
- Castaneda anastomosis
- Cooley-Derra
- Cope crushing
- Cope modification of Martel intestinal
- Crafoord
- Crafoord coarctation
- DeBakey-Semb
- Edna towel
- Eisenstein
- Fogarty Hydrogrip
- Foss
- Garcia aorta
- Glassman
- Gregory bulldog
- Gusberg hysterectomy
- Harken auricle
- Harrah lung
- Henley vascular
- Jahnke anastomosis
- Kay aorta
- Kiefer
- Lambert-Kay aorta
- Leland Jones
- Liddle aorta
- Locke
- Masters intestinal
- Masters-Schwartz intestinal

clamp *(cont.)*
Mattox aorta
modified Collier
Morris aorta
mosquito
Niedner anastomosis
Noon AV fistula
Omed bulldog vascular
Parker-Kerr intestinal
Pennington
Sarot bronchus
Selverstone
side-biting
Wertheim

clam-shell brace (Ortho).

clarithromycin (Biaxin)—an antibiotic belonging to the macrolide class of drugs, similar in effectiveness to penicillin and erythromycin but with fewer side effects. Particularly effective against *Mycoplasma pneumoniae,* resistant strains of *Haemophilus influenzae,* and MAC infection.

Claritin (loratadine) (ENT)—a long-acting antihistamine.

Clark classification of malignant melanoma, levels I–IV. Named for the pathologist who devised it, Wallace H. Clark, Jr., M.D.

Clark perineorrhaphy (Gyn).

classification; staging
Astler-Coller modification of Dukes' c.
Breslow c. for malignant melanoma
Broders' tumor index
burns
Child's c. of hepatic risk
Clark malignant melanoma
diabetes
diabetes mellitus, c. in pregnancy
Duane's
Dukes' c. of carcinoma
FAB (French/American/British)
FIGO
Frykman c. of hand fractures

classification *(cont.)*
Hunt and Hess neurological
Jewett's c. of bladder carcinoma
Karnofsky status
Keith-Wagener c. of retinopathy
Kiel c. of non-Hodgkin's lymphoma
leukemia
Lukes-Collins c. of non-Hodgkin's lymphoma
Neer (shoulder fractures I, II, III)
NYHA (New York Heart Association) c. of congestive heart failure
Reese-Ellsworth c. of retinoblastoma
Rye histopathologic c. of Hodgkin's disease
Singh-Vaughn-Williams arrhythmia
TNM malignant tumor
van Heuven's anatomic c. of diabetic retinopathy
Wiberg c. of patellar types

claustrum—thin layer of gray matter lateral to the external capsule of the brain. Cf. *colostrum, clostridium.*

clavus (pl., clavi) (Pod)—a corn on the foot or toe.

Clayman-Kelman intraocular lens forceps.

clean-catch urine specimen—an uncontaminated urine specimen obtained by first thoroughly washing the genitalia. The urine stream is started and then, midstream, the specimen is caught without the urine stream or container touching the genitalia or perineum.

ClearSite transparent wound dressing.

ClearView CO_2 laser (GI, Gyn)—includes a device to continually evacuate smoke generated by laser use.

Cleasby iris spatula.

cleft
branchial
Sondergaard's

Cleland's ligament—in the hand; it keeps the skin sleeve from twisting

Cleland's ligament *(cont.)* around the bone of the digit. You may hear reference to this ligament in operative procedures for Dupuytren's contracture. See also *Grayson's ligament;* they are not, however, synonymous.

Clindamycin—antibiotic combined with primaquine, an antimalarial drug, to treat *Pneumocystis carinii* pneumonia in AIDS patients.

Clinical Institute Withdrawal Assessment–Alcohol scale (CIWA-A)—a psychological/physiological scale used to assess the degree of alcohol withdrawal that a patient is experiencing. For a score above 10, the patient is given a drug such as chlordiazepoxide (Librium) or diazepam (Valium) to produce sedation and prevent seizures.

Clinitron bed.

clip
- Acland
- Atrauclip hemostatic
- Benjamin-Havas fiberoptic light
- Bleier
- Braun-Yasargil right-angle
- cardiac retraction
- Drake
- fenestrated Drake
- Heifitz
- Hem-o-lok
- Hem-o-lok polymer ligating
- Hulka
- Khodadad
- LeRoy
- Ligaclip
- Liga surgical
- McFadden
- Michel
- Multiclip
- Phynox cobalt alloy
- Raney
- Secu

clip *(cont.)*
- Sugita
- Sundt
- Sundt-Kees
- Weck

clip applicator, Absolok.

CLL (chronic lymphocytic leukemia); seen primarily in late adulthood (usually after age 50).

clobazam (Frisium) (Psych)—an antianxiety drug.

clofazimine ("klo-fa'-zih-meen) (Lamprene)—for use in treatment of Hansen's disease (leprosy) and now to treat MAC infection in AIDS patients.

clomipramine (Anafranil) (Psych)—an oral tricyclic antidepressant for treatment of obsessive-compulsive disorders.

clonidine (Catapres) (Cardio, Oncol)—commonly used to treat hypertension, and also used to relieve pain in cancer patients via the epidural route.

clonogenic technique—a technique for growing tumor cells in test tubes and testing sensitivity to various chemotherapeutic agents.

Clonorchis sinensis—liver fluke.

clonus—see *drawn ankle clonus.*

C-loop of duodenum (Radiol).

closed fracture (Ortho)—in which there is no break in the skin. Formerly called simple fracture.

closing base wedge osteotomy (CBWO) (Pod).

***Clostridium botulinum* toxin type A** (Dysport, Oculinum) (Oph)—injected into eye muscles to treat blepharospasm. See *botulinum toxin type A.*

Clostridium difficile—an organism isolated from meconium and feces of infants, from wounds, and from the urogenital tract of asymptomatic people.

closure
mucosa-to-mucosa
Smead-Jones-type
Tom Jones

clot, autologous. See *autologous clot.*

Clot Stop drain (Plas Surg)—a drain with an antithrombogenic covering, used in cosmetic surgery.

clotting agent, AlphaNine.

clove hitch—a sailor's knot; also used in surgery.

cloverleaf skull (Ger., *Kleeblattschädel).*

Cloward back fusion (Ortho).

clozapine (Clozaril) (Psych)—indicated for the treatment of schizophrenia in patients who have not responded to other antipsychotic medications or who have undesirable side effects on those medications. Patients receiving this drug must have their WBC counts monitored, as the drug causes the severe side effect of agranulocytosis.

Clozaril (clozapine).

clubbing of the fingers and toes—thickening and bulbous enlargement of the tissue at the base of the nail; often seen in patients with cystic fibrosis, ulcerative colitis, cirrhosis of the liver, and cardiopulmonary disease.

clubbing, cyanosis, or edema (CCE).

clubfoot splint—see *Denis Browne.*

clue cells—You may hear of these in reference to a Pap smear. They are so-called because their presence is a clue to possible infection with *Gardnerella vaginalis* (formerly *Haemophilus vaginalis*).

clumping, RPE (retinal pigment epithelium).

CME (cystoid macular edema) (Oph).

CMF (Oncol)—a standard chemotherapy protocol used to treat breast cancer. Consists of the drugs Cytoxan, methotrexate, and fluorouracil.

CMFP (Oncol)—a standard chemotherapy protocol used to treat breast cancer. Consists of Cytoxan, methotrexate, fluorouracil, and prednisone.

CMFPT (Cytoxan, methotrexate, fluorouracil, prednisone, tamoxifen)—chemotherapy protocol used to treat inflammatory breast carcinoma.

CMFPTH (Cytoxan, methotrexate, fluorouracil, prednisone, tamoxifen, Halotestin)—chemotherapy protocol.

CMFVP (Cytoxan, methotrexate, fluorouracil, vincristine, and prednisone)—chemotherapy protocol used to treat advanced breast cancer.

CMH (Cytoxan, m-AMSA, hydroxyurea)—chemotherapy protocol.

CMI (cell-mediated immunity).

CML (chronic myelocytic leukemia)—seen mostly in young adults (age 20 to 50).

CMOPP (Oncol)—a standard chemotherapy protocol used to treat adult non-Hodgkin's lymphoma. Consists of the drugs Cytoxan, mechlorethamine, Oncovin, procarbazine, and prednisone.

CMT (circus-movement tachycardia).

CMT—see *certified medical transcriptionist.*

CMV (cisplatin, methotrexate, vinblastine)—chemotherapy protocol used to treat transitional cell carcinoma of the bladder.

CMV (cytomegalovirus).

CNOP (Cytoxan, Novantrone, Oncovin, prednisone)—chemotherapy protocol used to treat non-Hodgkin's lymphoma.

C/N ratio (contrast-to-noise)—a term used in MRI scans.

CNS (central nervous system). Not to be confused with C&S. See *C&S.*

CNVM (choroidal neovascular membrane) (Oph).

CO_2 laser (carbon dioxide laser). See *argon laser, laser, Nd:YAG laser.*

coagulation factors, blood

I fibrinogen
II prothrombin
III thromboplastin
IV calcium ions
V proaccelerin (or accelerator globulin [AcG])
VI Factor VI (which is rapidly destroyed by thrombin; hence, cannot be identified by its activity in the serum) is assumed to be the active form
VII proconvertin (or serum prothrombin conversion accelerator [SPCA])
VIII antihemophilic factor (or von Willebrand's factor)
IX plasma thromboplastin component (Christmas factor)
X Stuart factor (or Stuart-Prower factor)
XI plasma thromboplastin antecedent
XII Hageman factor
XIII fibrin stabilizing factor

coagulator

Biceps bipolar
Concept bipolar
Fabry

coagulum pyelolithotomy (Urol)—a procedure for removal of kidney stones. Coagulum is introduced through two Intracaths, and cryoprecipitate and calcium chloride mixture are instilled simultaneously. After seven minutes an incision is made in the pelvis of the kidney, and the stones, now surrounded by the gel that has formed, are easily scooped out without rough edges traumatizing the renal tissues.

coal tar, crude. *Not* cold tar.

COAP (Cytoxan, Oncovin, Ara-C, prednisone)—chemotherapy protocol used to treat acute lymphoblastic leukemia.

coaxial sheath cut-biopsy needle—see PercuCut cut-biopsy needles (Radiol).

Cobacter luendi.

Coban dressing or wrapping (Ortho, Plas Surg)—an elastic dressing.

cobblestoning—coarsely lumpy appearance of a mucosal surface, such as the tongue, nasal mucosa, or conjunctiva, caused by inflammation.

Cobb-Ragde needle (Urol)—double-prong ligature carrier used for bladder neck suspension.

Cobb's syndrome—characterized by the presence of spinal and vertebral angiomas (Neuro).

Cobe gun (Surg)—a staple gun.

Coburn equiconvex lens (Oph)—an intraocular lens with an equal curvature from anterior to posterior.

Coburn intraocular lens (Oph).

Coburn Mark IX eye implant.

coccygodynia—pain in the coccyx and neighboring region.

cochlear implant (ENT)—electronic device that provides direct electrical stimulation to the auditory fibers in the inner ear.

cochleosacculotomy, Schuknecht.

Codman exercises—to increase range of motion in a stiff shoulder. The patient bends over at a 90° angle at the waist and, with a weight held in each hand, moves the arms in arcs.

Cody tack operation (ENT)—for treatment of progressive endolymphatic hydrops (Ménière's disease). Similar to the Fick sacculotomy.

Coe-pak (Dental)—hard- and fast-set periodontal paste.

COF/COM (Oncol)—a chemotherapy protocol to treat nonmetastatic breast carcinoma. Consists of Cytoxan, Oncovin, fluorouracil + Cytoxan, Oncovin, methotrexate.

coffee-grounds material; vomitus. "She has vomited twice. This was productive of stomach contents and bile, no hemoptysis, hematemesis, or coffee-grounds material." The appearance of the vomitus is similar to that of the grounds left over after roasting coffee. Coffee-grounds emesis is indicative of the presence of blood in the gastric contents. Note: Coffee grounds, *not* coffee ground.

Coffey ureterointestinal anastomosis.

Cognex (tacrine) (Psych, Neuro)—drug used to treat Alzheimer's disease.

cogwheel breathing—jerkiness or intermittency of breath sounds on inspiration, due to sudden expansion of previously collapsed air sacs.

cogwheel gait—muscle jerkiness due to spasticity in patients with Parkinson's disease.

cogwheel rigidity—seen in Parkinson's disease.

Cohen uterine incision.

Coherent CO_2 (carbon dioxide) **surgical laser**. Coherent—brand name.

coil (MRI terms)
crossed
Gianturco wool-tufted wire
Golay
gradient
Helmholtz
radiofrequency
receiver

coil *(cont.)*
saddle
shim
solenoid
surface

coil dialyzer—see *hemodialyzer.*

coin test of pneumothorax. One coin is pressed against the anterior chest and tapped with another, while the posterior chest is auscultated. A characteristic sound is diagnostic of pneumothorax.

Colbenemid (probenecid-colchicine)—used to treat chronic gouty arthritis.

colchicine (Neuro)—commonly used to treat gout. Also helpful in decreasing the progression of neurological symptoms in patients with multiple sclerosis.

cold water calorics (ENT, Neuro)—a test for vertigo, nystagmus, and vestibular function, with cold water gently injected by syringe into the ear canal. Also, *ice water calorics test.*

colfosceril palmitate (Exosurf Pediatric). See also *RDS, Survanta.*

Colibri forceps (Oph).

CollaCote (Oral Surg)—collagen wound dressing.

collagen
Zyclast
Zyderm I or II

collagen suture—an absorbable suture made of beef tendon.

CollaPlug (Oral Surg)—wound dressing.

collar
Miami Acute (MAC)
Miami J
Plastizote

collar-button abscess of the palm.

collar-button appearance in colon (Radiol).

CollaTape (Oral Surg)—tape used with wound dressing.

collateralization—formation of collateral vessels.

collateral vessels—vascular channels that are newly formed from existing ones to maintain the circulation of a tissue or organ whose normal blood supply has been impaired by disease or injury. Cf. *collateralization.*

collecting system (Radiol)—on an intravenous pyelogram (IVP), the nonexcretory portions of the kidney, which collect newly formed urine and conduct it to the ureter; the minor and major calices and the renal pelvis.

colliculus—a small protuberance. Cf. *canaliculus.*

Collier's sign—when the upper lid is elevated, showing more sclera above the iris than is usually seen, producing the so-called thyroid stare; a sign of thyroid disease.

collimation—used in scanning (Neuro).

Collimator, Multileaf.

Collin-Beard procedure (Oph)—resection of the levator muscle, with advancement onto the tarsal plate.

Collins' solution—used for preservation of a liver which is to be transplanted; the liver may be kept in this solution for about six hours before implantation. Ringer's solution may be used for this purpose if the liver is to be kept for a shorter period.

Collis–Nissen fundoplication (GI)—used in association with transthoracic parietal cell vagotomy to manage advanced gastroesophageal reflux with peptic stricture and Barrett metaplasia.

collodion—a topical protectant used often on infants and small children to keep a surgical wound dry.

colloid oncotic pressure—see *COP.*

colloid shift on liver-spleen scan.

colloid, technetium-sulfur.

colloids—as blood replacement: dextrose, hetastarch, plasma protein fraction, and serum albumin. See *crystalloid.*

Collostat—a collagen hemostatic agent in the form of a soft sponge. Pieces of this material are placed over bleeding sites and pressure applied.

colocolponeopoiesis (Ob-Gyn)—new term for a technique used to create a new vagina in females with congenital vaginal aplasia or in males having a sex change operation. A portion of the sigmoid colon is resected, but its blood supply is preserved. Using sutures or a stapler, the colonic segment is formed into a conduit for use as a vagina. Also called modified Kun colocolpopoiesis.

Colorgene DNA Hybridization Test—a DNA probe test to detect herpes simplex virus in two hours rather than waiting days for culture results.

colostomy appliance, Gentle Touch.

colostrum—a thin, milky fluid which is secreted by the mammary glands around the time of parturition. It contains antibodies which provide the baby with passive immunization. Cf. *claustrum.*

colpocystourethropexy (CCUP).

Colyte—a bowel preparation used before colonoscopy or barium enema x-ray examination (Radiol).

Comfeel Ulcus—a synthetic (hydrocolloid) occlusive dressing for lower extremity ulcers (Ortho).

Comfort Cath I or II (Urol)—male external catheter.

comitant ("accompanying, following") (Oph)—related to deviation of the eye. Here is the definition supplied by an ophthalmologist: *Comitant* refers to the eye's deviation in the same

comitant *(cont.)* amount in all positions of gaze. Let's say it's an inturning eye and it deviates 10 diopters of inward deviation, and that deviation is the same in upgaze, downgaze, right gaze, and left gaze; we call that comitant deviation or comitant esotropia. If the deviation varies in different gaze positions, we call it noncomitant; it is more likely to be paralytic. Cf. *concomitant.*

Command PS pacemaker (Cardio).

commissure of Gudden—located within the optic chiasm.

compensated—corrected or mitigated; said of a defect or disability, as in *compensated congestive heart failure; compensated hearing loss,* hearing loss improved with a hearing aid; *edentulous and compensated,* toothless but fitted with dentures.

Compere fixation wires (Ortho).

Comperm tubular elastic bandage (Ortho)—provides 360° compression and support for sports injuries, postcast support, postburn scarring, sprains, and strains.

complementary DNA (cDNA).

complement fixation (Lab)—a type of serologic test in which the consumption of a serum protein, called *complement,* is taken as evidence that the expected antigen-antibody reaction has occurred. Cf. *compliment.*

complementation—a process by which inactive genes in a defective virus can be replaced with active genes from another virus, inside a cell, such that a functioning virus results.

complex
- AIDS-related (ARC)
- anisoylated plasminogen streptokinase activator (APSAC)
- Battey-avium

complex *(cont.)*
- Eisenmenger's
- Ghon
- Golgi
- MAC (*Mycobacterium avium*)
- MAI (*Mycobacterium avium-intracellulare*)
- Ranke

compliance—a patient's following physician's directions and advice regarding diet or medicinal treatment. Cf. *noncompliance,* when the patient is not cooperative.

compliment—an expression of admiration or praise. Cf. *complement.*

compound Q (trichosanthin)—a drug used in treating AIDS. Made from a Chinese cucumber plant. See *GLQ223.*

compound S (azidothymidine, AZT).

Comprecin (enoxacin)—an antibiotic effective against gram-negative bacteria.

compromise—impairment or damage to a normal structure or function, as in neural compromise, circulatory compromise, and compromise of the immune system.

Compuscan Hittman computerized electrocardioscanner, as in "Tapes were analyzed with a Compuscan Hittman computerized electrocardioscanner and graded according to the method of Lown and Woolf." Used in studies of ventricular septal defect, pulmonary stenosis, and Ebstein's anomaly of the atrioventricular valve.

computed tomography (CT) **scan** (also called computerized axial tomography, or CAT scan) (Radiol)—an application of computer technology to diagnostic radiology. Instead of exposing a film after passing through the patient, x-rays are detected and

computed tomography *(cont.)* recorded by a scintillation counter. The x-ray tube moves around the patient on a frame called a gantry, rotating through an arc and "cutting" across one plane of the patient. A series of scintillation counters are so placed that each detects the rays passing through the patient at a different angle. (Alternatively a single counter may rotate in perfect alignment with the x-ray source.) Data on the amount of x-ray that penetrates the patient at each angle are collected from the counters, digitized, stored, and analyzed by a minicomputer programmed to generate a cross-sectional image of the patient corresponding to the plane cut by the moving x-ray beam. Contrast medium may be injected into the circulation immediately before CT scanning. Intravenous contrast enhances the sensitivity of CT scanning of certain structures and body regions and improves the visibility of some tumors.

concealed straight leg raising test (Ortho). The examining physician, if it appears that the patient is not cooperating in the straight leg raising test or is malingering, will pretend to examine the patient's feet but actually will be noting how high up the patient's feet will go with the legs extended. Usage: "There is negative concealed straight leg raising at 90° bilaterally."

Concept bipolar coagulator—an electronic coagulator for hemostasis of tiny bleeders (Neuro); effective in a wet field (under irrigation or in a bloody field).

Concept hand-held cautery.

concomitant—together, along with, accompanying, associated with. Cf. *comitant.*

Concorde suction cannula (Plas Surg).

conduction

air
air-bone
bone
His-Purkinje

conduit—see *ileal conduit.*

coned-down view (Radiol)—a study limited to a small area by the use of a cone that narrows and "focuses" the x-ray beam.

C1 (not subscript)—an inhibitor protein. There are also C1q, C2, and C4.

C1q assay ("C-one-q")—one of a series of complement components, numbered C1 to C9, related to antibody-antigen reactions. It is used to detect immune complexes in rheumatoid arthritis.

conformer (Oph)—that part of an eye prosthesis which covers the surface of an artificial eye sphere.

congenital dysplasia of hip (or dislocation) (CDH).

Congo red stain.

consensual light reflex—constriction of the pupil of one eye in response to stimulation by light of the retina of the other eye. See *direct light reflex.*

consensus (*not* concensus and *not* consensus of opinion). *Consensus* means general opinion, or conclusion after discussion with a number of people, so the word *opinion* is redundant.

consolidative process (Radiol)—abnormal process that increases the density of a tissue or region.

container, Medi-Vac suction collection.

contiguous images (in computed tomography scan) (Radiol)—a series of scans without intervals of unexamined tissue between them.

continent supravesical bowel urinary diversion (Urol)—for bladder reconstruction to treat invasive bladder cancer. Examples: Camey reservoir,

continent urinary diversion *(cont.)*
Kock pouch, Mainz pouch, Rowland pouch, and sigmoid colon reservoir.

continuous arteriovenous hemofiltration (CAVH).

continuous passive motion (CPM).

continuous positive airway pressure (CPAP).

contractionssee *Braxton Hicks contractions.*

contracture—see *Volkmann's contracture.*

contrast material-enhanced scan—MRI term (Radiol).

contrast medium—see *medication.*

contrast-to-noise ratio (C/N)—MRI term.

contrecoup injury—referring to an injury, as to the brain, occurring at a site opposite the point of contact.

control—see *dermatophyton control.*

Control-Release pop-off needle.

conus medullaris—cone-shaped lower end of spinal cord.

convergence test (Oph)—locates breaking point of fusion at near vision.

Converse nasal tip scissors (Plas Surg).

converter
analog to digital
digital to analog

convex linear array—term used in B-scan, Doppler, and color Doppler imaging (Radiol). See *B-scan.*

convolutions of Gratiolet (''grah-tee-olay'')—small convolutions that are buried beneath the lateral surface of the occipital lobe of the brain.

Cook endoscopic curved needle driver (Surg)—allows endoscopic suturing using standard curved needle sutures so that tissue approximation, anatomical reconstruction, and hemostasis can now be performed endoscopically.

cookie—see *Gelfoam cookie.*

cookie cutter—see *Freeman.*

Cook TPN catheters (total parenteral nutrition) (single and double lumen).

Cooley-Derra anastomosis clamp.

Cooperman event probability (Cardio)—a clinical scoring system used to predict cardiac morbidity.

Coopervision irrigation/aspiration handpiece. ''The residual cortex was aspirated with the Coopervision irrigation/aspiration handpiece.''

COP (colloid oncotic pressure) (Neuro)—a measurement of brain edema after cryogenic (vasogenic) brain injury.

COPBLAM (Cytoxan, Oncovin, prednisone, bleomycin, Adriamycin, Matulane)—chemotherapy protocol used to treat lymphocytic lymphomas.

COP-BLEO (Cytoxan, Oncovin, Platinol, bleomycin)—chemotherapy protocol.

COPE (Cytoxan, Oncovin, Platinol, etoposide)—chemotherapy protocol.

Cope crushing clamp (GI)—used in bowel resection.

Copeland radial pan-chamber intraocular lens (Oph).

Cope modification of a Martel intestinal clamp—used in GI surgery.

Cope nephrostomy tube (Nephrol).

copper-binding protein test (CBP).

copper wire effect (or copper-wiring) (Oph)—narrowing of arterioles in the retina; seen in the funduscopic examination of some patients with arteriosclerosis.

cor (noun)—the heart. Cf. *core, corps.*

coracoacromial—pertaining to coracoid and acromial processes.

coral
Biocoral madreporic
madreporic
Porites

cord blood (Neonat)—blood drawn from from the umbilical cord at birth; used to determine blood type, chemistries, and blood gases.

cordate—heart-shaped. Cf. *caudate, chordate.*

Cordis Gemini cardiac pacer (Cardio).

Cordis-Hakim shunt—used in the Kasai procedure for biliary atresia. See *Kasai procedure.*

Cordis Sequicor cardiac pacer (Cardio).

Cordonnier ureteroileal loop.

cordotomy, chordotomy. These words are used interchangeably by many dictionaries and journals, although *cordotomy* seems to be the preferred spelling. See *Rosamoff cordotomy.*

cord, vocal (*not* chord) (ENT).

core (noun)—the central part of something; (verb)—to take out the core of something. Cf. *cor, corps.*

Cor-Flex wire guides—used with Cook Micropuncture catheter system.

Corgard (nadolol)—cardiovascular medication, for hypertension.

Cormed ambulatory infusion pump—permits outpatient therapy in patients receiving chemotherapy, heparin, hyperalimentation, or any ambulatory infusion treatment.

cornea guttata (Oph)—degenerative condition of the cornea caused by dystrophy of the endothelial cells.

corneae, limbus—see *limbus corneae.*

corneal reflex—closure of the eyes on stimulating the cornea.

coronal orientation—MRI term.

coronary atherectomy (Cardio)—an alternative to balloon angioplasty. It works on the Roto-Rooter principle, with suction apparatus utilized to remove the excised plaque.

Corpak feeding tube.

corps ("core") (noun)—corpus; also, a group or body of individuals organized and under common direction (e.g., the medical corps). Cf. *cor, core, corpse.*

corpse—a dead body. Cf. *corps.*

corpus callosum (Neuro)—mass of white matter in the depths of the longitudinal fissure connecting the two cerebral hemispheres.

corpus Luysii—see *body of Luys.*

corpuscles—see *malpighian corpuscles.*

corset platysmaplasty (Plas Surg)—cosmetic surgery for the aging neck. The platysma is used to contour the neck like a corset, producing fewer contour irregularities.

Corti, organ of.

cortical mapping (of the brain).

cortical spoking.

cortical thumb (Neuro). The thumb lies flat on the palm, with the fingers over it; this is suggestive of a corticospinal lesion.

cor triatriatum—a cardiac anomaly in which there are three atria. Also, triatrial heart.

cor triatriatum dexter—rare congenital anomaly in which an obstructive membrane is located in the right atrium.

Corynebacterium—a gram-positive organism that causes infection in immunosuppressed patients, particularly pneumonia in AIDS patients.

Cosman ICP Tele-Sensor (Neuro)—implantable telemetric pressure sensor used in hydrocephalus shunts to measure intracranial pressure and to diagnose shunt blockage and function. Also, Cosman Tele-Monitor System.

costosternal angle.

cot—see *finger cot.*

Cotrel-Dubousset instrument system—implanted for correction of scoliosis (Ortho).

Cotrel traction (Ortho)—treatment for adult scoliosis. Uses a leather head halter, pelvic girdle, and a system of pulleys. Also, Cotrel-Dubousset.

Cotton procedure (ENT)—a cartilage graft to the cricolaryngeal area; for subglottic stenosis.

cotton-wool exudates of retina (Oph)—microinfarcts of nerve fiber layer that resemble tufts of cotton.

cottonoid patty (or paddy) (Neuro)—used to stem hemorrhage and to protect the exposed brain in surgery.

cotyledon—subdivision of the uterine surface of a discoidal placenta.

coudé catheter—bent (or elbowed).

cough CPR (Cardio)—a technique used in cardiac catheterization and emergency medicine in which the patient forcefully and repeatedly coughs. Coughing converts ventricular arrhythmias to a normal sinus rhythm.

Coulter counter—for platelet count.

Councill catheter (Nephrol).

Councilman bodies (Path)—seen in hepatocytes in viral hepatitis.

countercurrent immunoelectrophoresis test (CIE).

counterflow centrifugal elutriation—a technique which removes some lymphocytes from patients who had allogenic bone marrow transplant to decrease the incidence of graft-versus-host disease (GVHD).

counting fingers (or count fingers)—in eye examination. "Visual acuity was limited to counting fingers in the right eye, and hand movements in the left eye."

counts, kick—see *kick counts.*

coup de sabre (Fr., "stroke of a sword")—linear scleroderma usually found over the scalp or forehead.

coupled suturing (Surg)—a technique for microvascular anastomosis which is an adaptation of a type of continuous stitch used in the garment industry, generally using 9-0 and 10-0 nylon.

Courvoisier's sign—a palpably enlarged gallbladder, sometimes a sign of pancreatic carcinoma.

Cover-Roll adhesive gauze.

Cover-Strip wound closure strips—have a hypoallergenic adhesive and in some wounds these may be an alternative to sutures. They have a porous gauze strip that permits air to enter and exudate to pass through.

cover-uncover test (Oph)—assesses muscle deviation.

Coverlet—trade name for an adhesive dressing (Surg).

COWS (ENT)—a mnemonic device to help remember the Hallpike caloric stimulation response. ("Caloric testing produced COWS.") Stands for "cold to the opposite, warm to the same." See *caloric testing.*

Coxiella burnetii—rickettsia that causes Q fever. See *Q fever.*

coxsackievirus, A and B—a virus that causes meningitis and paralytic disease.

CP angle (costophrenic).

CPAP ("see-pap")—continuous positive airway pressure. Provides positive pressure in lungs even when the patient exhales fully, to prevent lungs from collapsing.

CPB (Cytoxan, Platinol, BCNU)—chemotherapy protocol.

CPC (Cytoxan, Platinol, carboplatin)—chemotherapy protocol.

CPD (cephalopelvic disproportion)—used in obstetrics.

CPD (citrate phosphate dextrose)—an anticoagulant solution for autotransfusions.

CPD syndrome—chorioretinopathy and pituitary dysfunction—characterized by severe, early-onset chorioretinopathy, trichosis, and evidence of pituitary dysfunction.

CPK (creatine phosphokinase)—a serum enzyme that can be chemically distinguished into three isoenzymes or fractions: the MB isoenzyme, elevated in myocardial infarction; the MM isoenzyme, elevated in cerebral infarction; and the BB isoenzyme, sometimes elevated in uremia and other conditions. When separated in the laboratory by electrophoresis, these isoenzymes appear as distinct bands in a visual display. Hence the expression *MB band* is roughly synonymous with *MB isoenzyme.* Do not confuse *creatine* with *creatinine.*

CPK isoenzymes:
BB bands—uremia
MB bands—myocardial infarction
MM bands—cerebral dysfunction

CPM devices (continuous passive motion) (Ortho); e.g., Autoflex II.

CPPD (calcium pyrophosphate deposition; disease).

CPS system (cardiopulmonary support) —heart-lung machine.

crack—street name for rock cocaine, a a concentrated, smokable form of the drug which is highly addicting. Cf. *crank.*

cracked pot sound—(1) a percussion sound like that heard when striking a cracked pot and indicates a pulmonary cavity; (2) a sound on percussion caused by the separation of cranial sutures in children with increased cranial pressure, e.g., as seen in hydrocephalus. See *Macewen's sign.*

cracker test (for the presence of Sjögren's disease). "She has a negative cracker test in the sense that if we were to give her a soda cracker, she would easily be able to swallow without drinking water."

cradle cap—seborrheic dermatitis manifested as thick yellowish scales, often seen on the scalp of infants.

Crafoord clamp.

Crafoord-Senning heart-lung machine.

cranial nerves, twelve—written with Roman numerals, I to XII.
I olfactory
II optic
III oculomotor
IV trochlear
V trigeminal
VI abducens
VII facial
VIII vestibulocochlear (acoustic)
IX glossopharyngeal
X vagal
XI accessory
XII hypoglossal

cranial perforator, Acra-Cut.

cranioplastic powder (Neuro)—used for repair of cranial defects.

crank—slang term for the street drug methamphetamine ("speed"), which is snorted or injected. Cf. *crack.*

Crasnitin (C-asparaginase)—antineoplastic agent.

Crawford-Adams acetabular cup arthroplasty.

Crawford low lithotomy crutches.

creatine—a nitrogenous substance that is found in muscles, brain, and blood of vertebrates. Cf. *carotene, creatinine, keratin.*

creatine phosphokinase—see *CPK.*

creatinine clearance, 24-hour—a measure of kidney function, calculated

creatinine *(cont.)* from the serum creatinine level and the amount of creatinine excreted in the urine in 24 hours. Cf. *creatine, creatinine.*

creatinine, serum—a waste product of protein metabolism, elevated in kidney disease. Cf. *creatine.*

C-reactive protein (CRP)—a protein which is high when there is an inflammatory response and returns to undetectable as the response clears.

Credé maneuver (''kre-day'') (Urol)—massaging the lower abdomen over the bladder to promote complete emptying in patients with neurological damage; e.g., ''Bladder Credé was ordered.'' Cf. *Credé method.*

Credé method (Obs)—expressing the placenta from the uterus by pushing the uterus down into the pelvis and squeezing it. Cf. *Credé maneuver.*

Creed dissector (Neuro).

creola bodies (lowercase *c*)—balls of desquamated epithelium; often found in the sputa of asthmatics.

crescendo-decrescendo murmur—increases from quiet to louder and then decreases again. May be diagnostic of aortic stenosis when heard as a systolic murmur. In aortic insufficiency it is heard as a diastolic murmur.

CREST syndrome (See also *CRST.*)
- C calcinosis cutis
- R Raynaud's phenomenon
- E esophageal dysmotility
- S sclerodactyly
- T telangiectasia

cribogram (ENT). An infant who is suspected of hearing loss is placed on a special mattress wired with sensing devices and a computer compares the baby's movements with the stimulation.

crick—painful spasm, usually in the neck.

cri du chat (cat's cry)—an indication of a chromosomal irregularity causing mental retardation; the name derives from the catlike cry emitted by these children.

Crikelair otoplasty (ENT).

crisis—see *Dietl's crisis.*

crisscross heart—a heart with crossing of the atrioventricular valves.

"crit"—slang for *hematocrit.*

criteria (pl.)—standards or means by which conclusions are arrived at. ''On EKG there were voltage criteria for left ventricular hypertrophy.'' See *Jones criteria, revised.*

Critikon balloon thermodilution catheter.

Crohn's disease—regional enteritis; a chronic granulomatous inflammatory disease.

Cröhnlein procedure (Oph).

Cronassial (Oph)—a drug used to treat retinitis pigmentosa.

Crosby-Kugler capsule—suction biopsy instrument.

cross-cover test (Oph)—measures degree of eye deviation.

crossed coil—MRI term.

crossed reflex—in which stimulus applied to one side produces a response on the contralateral side.

crosshatch pattern (Oph). See *fishbone pattern.*

cross-tunneling incision (Plas Surg)—used in performance of lipectomy. ''A cross-tunneling incision was made and a 1.8 and a 2.4 mm triple-hole cannula used.''

CRS (Counter Rotation System)—a type of brace used to correct internal and external tibial torsion in children. Consists of a hinged device with rods that attach to footplates glued onto

CRS *(cont.)*
both shoes. It allows kicking and crawling, and children can sleep in it comfortably.

CRST syndrome (See also *CREST.*)
C calcinosis cutis
R Raynaud's phenomenon
S sclerodactyly
T telangiectasia

cruciate incision—cross-shaped.

crude coal tar *(not* cold tar)—used in treatment of psoriasis (Derm).

crutches, Crawford low lithotomy.

Crutchfield skeletal traction tongs.

cryocrit (Lab)—the percentage of red and white blood cells re-added to arrive at this value.

cryomagnet—MRI term.

cryophake (Oph)—an instrument using extremely cold temperatures to remove a cataract. Also, Keeler cryophake.

cryoprobe—an instrument used to apply extreme cold to tissues, as in cryosurgery.

cryostat (Path)—a device containing a microtome for sectioning frozen tissue.

"crypto"—slang term for *cryptococcosis,* infection with *Cryptococcus neoformans,* or *cryptosporidiosis,* which is seen in AIDS patients. As with all slang, when in doubt, ask the dictator for clarification.

cryptosporidiosis antibody—immunostimulant for AIDS patients, obtained from cow's milk.

Cryptosporidium—a protozoan parasite. Sometimes referred to by slang term "crypto."

crystalloid—a substance in solution that can pass through a semipermeable membrane. "Fluids: 1600 cc of crystalloid." Normal saline solution and lactated Ringer's solution are crystalloids used as blood replacement.

crystals
Charcot-Leyden
Reinke

CSF (cerebrospinal fluid).

CSQI (continuous subcutaneous infusion)—a pain-control method utilizing a butterfly needle inserted subcutaneously and connected to an intravenous line. It is used for patients who will be receiving narcotic medication for more than 48 hours and who cannot receive intravenous medication due to poor veins or other problems. The system can be coupled with a patient-controlled analgesia pump which allows the patient to select the time when the medication is most needed for pain control and administer it. Sub-Q-Set is the trade name for one continuous subcutaneous infusion device.

CT (computed tomography).

CTCb (Cytoxan, thiotepa, carboplatin) —chemotherapy protocol used to treat metastatic breast carcinoma.

CTCL (cutaneous T-cell lymphoma). Also called mycosis fungoides.

C-terminal assay for PTH (parathormone; parathyroid hormone).

CT gantry—the bridgelike frame on a CT scanner on which the traveling crane of the scanner moves.

C_3F_8 gas (perfluoropropane)—used in pneumatic retinopexy, for correcting detached retina.

C.Ti. Brace (Ortho)—a six-point knee support especially for ACL (anterior cruciate ligament) deficient knees.

CTR (cardiothoracic ratio).

CTS (carpal tunnel syndrome).

CT scanner
cine CT scanner
General Electric CT/T 8800 scanner
Somatom DR 1 CT scanner
Somatom DR 2 CT scanner
Somatom DR 3 CT scanner

cubital tunnel syndrome—caused by compression of the ulnar nerve at the elbow. Cf. *carpal tunnel syndrome.*

cuirass (''kwe-ras''')—a covering for the chest.

CUI tissue expander (Cox-Uphoff International).

cul-de-sac—a blind pouch; a saclike cavity or tube open at only one end, e.g., the rectouterine pouch, or pouch of Douglas.

Cullen's sign—bluish discoloration around the umbilicus, indicative of a ruptured ectopic pregnancy or acute hemorrhagic pancreatitis.

culture and sensitivity (C&S) (Lab)—a lab test in which an organism is grown on a nutrient medium containing several antibiotic-laden disks. A lack of growth around a disk shows that the organism is sensitive to that antibiotic.

cup-to-disk ratio (Oph).

Curdy blade (Oph).

curet, curette
- fine-angled
- Hebra corneal
- Kushner-Tandatnick endometrial biopsy
- Laufe aspirating
- McElroy
- Skeele chalazion
- Vacurette suction

Curling's ulcer—gastric or duodenal ulcers seen in patients who have suffered severe burns over large areas of the body.

current, pulsing—MRI term.

Curschmann's spirals—formed elements that have been found in the sputa of asthmatic patients.

curve of Spee (Oral Surg)—a curved line extending along the summits of the buccal cusps from the first premolar to the third molar; named for a German embryologist, Ferdinand von Spee.

curvilinear incision (*not* curvalinear)—a curved incision.

CUSA (Cavitron ultrasonic aspirator) (Neuro)—used in tumor decompression.

cushingoid (*not* cushinoid)—having the appearance or symptoms of Cushing's disease, as in ''cushingoid facies.''

Cushing's response (Neuro). As intracranial pressure increases, the systolic blood pressure also increases noticeably, while the diastolic pressure changes little, if at all. The increased difference between the two blood pressures is significant as an indication of the onset of late-stage intracranial pressure. Not to be confused with Cushing's syndrome.

Cushing's syndrome—a symptom complex including moon facies, buffalo hump, abdominal distention, hypertension, amenorrhea (in women), impotence (in men), muscle wasting and weakness, fat pad formation, skin darkening, and skin thinning. More common in women than men. Caused by taking large amounts of steroids for long periods of time or by the excess production of cortisol. Not to be confused with Cushing's response.

cushion, Carter.

Custodis sponge, implant (Oph).

cut—a CT (computed tomography) section or image; a scan. See *tangential cut.*

cut-biopsy needle—see *PercuCut* (Radiol).

cutdown catheter—inserted in the cutdown to a vein when no veins are accessible to a needle in an emergency situation.

Cutinova Hydro—hydrocolloid transparent and flexible dressing that does not leave a residue on the wound.

Cutivate (fluticasone).

Cutler-Beard bridge flap—used in upper eyelid reconstruction, with flaps from the lower lid and the median forehead (Plas Surg).

Cutter-Smeloff cardiac valve prosthesis (Cardio).

cutting loops, used with resectoscopes.

CVA (cerebrovascular accident, called "stroke")—the result of a severe cerebrovascular occlusion in which symptoms do not resolve within 24 hours, and in which there is a long-term residual deficit. See *TIA*.

CVAD (Cytoxan, vincristine, Adriamycin, dexamethasone)—chemotherapy protocol used to treat non-Hodgkin's lymphoma.

CVB (chorionic villi biopsy)—used in prenatal diagnosis of many birth defects. It can be performed at 8 to 11 weeks, rather than the 17 to 20 weeks needed for amniocentesis.

CVC—see *central venous catheter.*

CVD (cisplatin, vinblastine, dacarbazine)—chemotherapy protocol used to treat metastatic malignant melanoma.

CVP (Cytoxan, vincristine, and prednisone)—chemotherapy protocol used to treat adult non-Hodgkin's lymphoma and breast carcinoma.

CVPP (Cytoxan, vinblastine, procarbazine, prednisone)—chemotherapy protocol.

C-wire Serter—a hand-held, battery-driven device for inserting C-wires into place in bones in hand and foot surgery (Ortho).

cyanoacrylate (Superglue)—a tissue adhesive.

Cyberlith—a pacemaker manufactured by Intermedics.

Cybex test (Ortho)—apparatus used in testing and measuring the strength of a muscle as it is involved by a joint going through range-of-motion testing, as in shoulder girdle muscles or hip and thigh muscles.

cyclocytidine—chemotherapeutic agent.

cycloergometer, Mijnhard electrical.

cycloplegia (Oph)—pathologic or induced paralysis of the ciliary muscle of the eye; paralysis of accommodation.

cycloplegic refraction (Oph).

Cyclops procedure (Ob-Gyn, Plas Surg)—technique used to cover a large soft tissue defect after excision of a breast, chest wall muscles, and clavicle or ribs. The opposite breast, which must be large, is rotated intact across the chest wall to completely cover the surgical defect.

cyesis ("si-e'-sis")—pregnancy. "Her symptoms of acute nausea and vomiting are probably secondary to cyesis."

CyHOP (Cytoxan, Halotestin, Oncovin, prednisone)—chemotherapy protocol used to treat lymphoma.

cysticercosis—infestation with a larval form of tapeworm.

cystitis, Hunner's interstitial.

cystitome (Oph)—an instrument used to open the capsule of the lens of the eye. Cf. *cystotome.*

cystoid macular edema (CME).

cystometrogram (CMG).

cystotome (Urol)—an instrument used for incising the bladder. Cf. *cystitome.*

Cytadren (aminoglutethimide).

cytarabine (Ara-C, Cytosar-U)—chemotherapy drug.

cytoblast—the cell nucleus. Cf. *cytoplast.*

cytocidal—cell-killing or destroying. "The cytocidal properties of this drug could be useful if those we are trying should prove less than effective."

cytocrit—the sum of the percentage of white blood cells and the percentage of red blood cells.

CytoGam (cytomegalovirus immune globulin)—used to treat CMV infections and CMV enteritis.

cytology, fine-needle aspiration.

cytomegalic inclusion body.

cytomegalovirus (CMV)—a herpesvirus that causes several diseases in AIDS: a retinitis which can lead to blindness, intestinal disease, and other problems.

cytomegalovirus hepatitis.

cytomegalovirus immune globulin (CytoGam).

cytomegalovirus retinitis (Oph)—an infection of the retina caused by one of a group of herpesviruses; one of a number of opportunistic infections seen in AIDS.

cytoplasmic inclusion body.

cytoplast—a cell whose nucleus has been removed, but which remains viable for a period of time. Cf. *cytoblast.*

cytosine arabinoside—see *cytarabine.*

cytostatic—bringing to a halt; stopping or suppressing the growth of cells and their reproduction; also, an agent that accomplishes this.

cytotoxic cells—"killer" T-cell lymphocytes, also called T-8 cells. T-4 cells are the lymphocytes affected by the virus, but they are needed to activate the cytotoxic cells. As AIDS research has shown, loss of one piece of the immune system makes it ineffective, as the interactions are multiple and complex.

Cytovene (ganciclovir)—used to treat CMV retinitis.

CYVADIC ("si-va-dick")—chemotherapy protocol combining Cytoxan, vincristine, Adriamycin, DTIC.

D, d

dacarbazine (DTIC-Dome)—an alkylating agent used in chemotherapy.

Dacomed snap gauge (Urol)—used in testing impotence; will break if an erection occurs during sleep, thus indicating that the impotence is not organic in nature.

Dakin's solution (Surg)—used as an antibacterial agent and in irrigating wounds.

Dalgan (dezocine).

Dalkon shield—intrauterine device.

D'Allesandro serial suture-holding forceps.

Dall–Miles cable grip system (Ortho)—cerclage application for bone grafting and fracture fixation.

Dalrymple's sign (''dal-rimplz'')—the widened eyelid opening typical of the ''stare'' in hyperthyroidism.

dalton—unit of measurement of the molecular weight of proteins (measured in kilodaltons), which constitute aeroallergens.

Dance's sign—a slight retraction of the tissue in the right iliac region in some cases of intussusception.

Dandy scissors (Neuro). *Dandy* is a proper name, not an opinion.

Dandy-Walker syndrome—congenital hydrocephalus caused by blockage of the foramina of Magendie and Luschka. Can be diagnosed on fetal ultrasound.

dapiprazole (Rev-Eyes) (Oph)—an ophthalmic solution used to reverse mydriasis.

dapsone (Avlosulfon)—previously used to treat leprosy; now used against *Pneumocystis carinii* pneumonia in AIDS patients.

DAP/TMP (dapsone plus trimethoprim) —used in therapy for *Pneumocystis carinii* pneumonia.

Darco medical-surgical shoe and toe alignment splint by Richards (Ortho).

Dardik Biograft (Vasc Surg)—modified human umbilical vein graft; used as a substitute for saphenous vein graft in revascularization procedures on the lower extremities.

Darier's disease; sign (Derm).

Darin intraocular implant lens.

dark-field microscopy—a microscopic technique using special lighting that makes it easier to identify *Treponema pallidum,* the organism that causes syphilis.

Darkschewitsch, nucleus of—also, depending on which dictionary you consult, spelled *Darkshevich, Darkschevich.*

Darrach procedure (Ortho)—ulnar resection.

DASA (distal articular set angle) (Ortho).

D'Assumpcao rhytidoplasty marker (Plas Surg).

DAT (daunomycin, Ara-C, thioguanine) —chemotherapy protocol used to treat acute myeloid leukemia.

Datascope catheter (Cardio)—used to position an intra-aortic balloon pump.

DATVP (daunomycin, Ara-C, thioguanine, vincristine, prednisone)—chemotherapy protocol.

daunorubicin HCl (Cerubidine)—chemotherapy drug.

Daunoxome (liposomal daunorubicin)—a drug used to treat Kaposi's sarcoma.

Dautery osteotome (Ortho, Oral Surg, Plas Surg).

DAVA (desacetyl vinblastine amide)—see *vindesine.*

Daviel lens spoon (Oph).

Davol drain—see *Relia-Vac.*

Davydov procedure (Ob-Gyn)—a technique used to create a new vagina in patients with congenital vaginal aplasia, or males having a sex change operation. Other techniques include Frank and McIndoe. See also *colocolponeopoiesis.*

dawn phenomenon—hyperglycemia occurring before dawn in both type I (insulin dependent) and type II (non-insulin dependent) diabetics; an early morning hyperglycemia.

DBM (demineralized bone matrix).

D_{CO}—pulmonary diffusion capacity.

DCS (dorsal column stimulator, or stimulation)—implanted for relief of pain (Neuro).

ddC (dideoxycytidine, HIVID)—a drug approved by the FDA to treat AIDS and ARC. Also used for patients who cannot tolerate Retrovir.

ddI (dideoxyinosine, Videx)—see *didanosine.*

Deaver retractor.

DeBakey-Semb clamp; forceps

debris ("duh-bree") (Path)—amorphous and necrotic material.

debulking—a process in which the inner "core" (or bulk) of a tumor is removed. This permits the outer portion to, in effect, "cave in" a bit, thereby permitting easier removal of the whole tumor. If the "outer wall" portion of the tumor does not readily separate from the attached tissue, at least the total volume of the tumor is somewhat reduced and hence does not exert as much pressure on the adjacent structures as it did before.

Decabid (indecainide) (Cardio)—antiarrhythmic drug.

DECAL (dexamethasone, etoposide, cisplatin, Ara-C, L-asparaginase)—chemotherapy protocol.

deceleration—slowing, as in "deceleration of contractions."

decerebrate rigidity (Neuro)—seen in metabolic disorders that affect upper brain stem function, evidenced by clenched teeth, and arms and legs stiffly extended. Cf. *decorticate rigidity.*

decidua—that part of the endometrium of the pregnant uterus that is shed at parturition.

decision—the settling of a controversy; a conclusion arrived at or a choice made. Cf. *discission.*

Decker pituitary rongeur.

decorticate rigidity (Neuro)—seen in lesions which damage the internal capsule of the brain and nearby structures, evidenced by flexion of the fingers, wrist, and arm, plantar flexion, and internal rotation of the leg. Cf. *decerebrate rigidity.*

decubitus ulcer—bed sore, pressure sore, trophic ulcer. Decubitus means "lying down" and these synonymous terms refer to the ulcerated areas of ischemic necrosis on the tissues that overlie bony prominences (sacrum, hips, greater trochanters, lateral malleoli, heels, and other areas where there may be pressure and friction). They are usually seen in patients who have been bedridden for long periods of time, who are emaciated or paralyzed, or in whom pain sensation is absent.

Dedo-Pilling laryngoscope (ENT).

deep tendon reflexes:
- 4+ brisk, hyperactive, clonus
- 3+ is more brisk than normal, but does not necessarily indicate a pathologic process.
- 2+ normal
- 1+ is low normal, with slight diminution in response
- 0 no response.

deep venous thrombosis (DVT).

defect, secundum atrial septal.

defibrillator
- AID implantable
- Cadence AICD
- Porta Pulse 3 portable
- Res-Q AICD

deformity
- boutonnière
- digitus flexus
- gibbous
- Haglund's

deformity *(cont.)*
- hallux abductovalgus
- hammer toe
- Hill-Sachs
- Michel
- sabre shin

degeneration
- cobblestone
- lattice
- paving stone
- striatal nigral
- Terrien's
- wallerian

deglutition mechanism (Radiol)—the coordinated sequence of muscular contractions in the mouth, pharynx, and esophagus involved in normal swallowing, as demonstrated in a barium swallow or upper GI series.

dehydroemetine (Mebadin)—used to treat amebiasis in immunocompromised patients.

déjà vu (Fr., "already seen") (Neuro, Psych)—the incorrect feeling that one has seen or experienced something before, a feeling which frequently precedes seizures. Cf. *jamais vu.*

Deklene—blue monofilament polypropylene suture used in cardiovascular surgery and in neurosurgery.

Deknatel (Shur-Strip)—a sterile wound closure tape.

Delaborde tracheal dilator (ENT).

De La Caffinière trapeziometacarpal prosthesis.

Delbet splint (Ortho)—used for heel fractures.

De Lee retractor (Ob-Gyn).

delirium—see *black patch delirium.*

"dellovibrio"—a phonetic spelling of *Bdellovibrio,* a genus of parasitic gram-negative organisms that live on certain other gram-negative bacteria.

"dellovibrio" *(cont.)* Although this is not a word you will often hear, who would think to look under the *B*'s?

delta—When a dictator gives a lab value such as "delta of 35," the reference is to the anion gap.

delta hepatitis (hepatitis D). Apparently a patient has to have been exposed to hepatitis B to get delta hepatitis.

delta OD_{450}—in amniocentesis, testing for bilirubinemia in erythroblastosis fetalis.

demineralization (Radiol)—reduction in the amount of calcium present in bone, due to disease or immobilization.

demineralized bone matrix (DBM).

De Morgan's spots, or Campbell de Morgan spots (Derm). See *cherry angiomas.*

de Morsier's syndrome—agenesis of the olfactory lobes, hypoplasia of the thalamus, dystrophy of the cerebral hemispheres, and absence of development of the gonads at puberty. Also, de Morsier-Gauthier syndrome.

Demser (metyrosine)—used in treatment of patients with pheochromocytoma for preoperative preparation, for management of those patients for whom surgery is contraindicated, and long-term treatment in patients with malignant pheochromocytoma.

de Musset's sign—rhythmic shaking of the head caused by carotid artery pulsations; a sign of aortic insufficiency.

dendritic lesion—having a branched appearance.

dengue hemorrhagic fever (DHF)—a disease on the increase in the U.S. and Latin America. The recent introduction of the *Aedes albopictus* mosquito to the U.S. will increase the probability of more severe disease, according to the CDC.

Denis Browne clubfoot splint; talipes hobble splint (Ortho). Named for Dr. Denis Browne, Hospital for Sick Children, London, England.

Dennis-Brown pouch (Urol).

Dennis tube (Surg)—plastic tube used like the Miller-Abbott tube.

Dennis-Varco pancreaticoduodenostomy.

dens view of cervical spine (Radiol). (The word *dens* is not an eponym; it is the odontoid process of axis, the second cervical vertebra.)

densitometry
- dual photon
- Norland-Cameron photon

Denver Developmental Screening Test (Peds)—rating scale for development of fine motor skills, gross motor skills, language, and personal/social skills in infants and preschool children.

Denver hydrocephalus shunt (Neuro).

Denver nasal splint—a quickly applied adhesive nasal splint (Plas Surg).

Denver pleuroperitoneal shunt (Thor Surg)—for control of chronic pleural effusions.

Deon hip prosthesis (Ortho)—made of a titanium alloy which can be implanted with or without cement.

deoxy-D-glucose—an antiviral glucose analogue which may be useful in treating herpes.

deoxynojirmycin (butyl-DNJ)—a drug used to treat patients with AIDS and ARC.

Depage-Janeway gastrostomy.

DePuy orthopedic implant.

de Quervain's disease—inflammation of the long abductor and short extensor tendons of the thumb, with accompanying tenderness and swelling. Also called *Quervain's disease.*

Dercum's disease—see *adiposis dolorosa.*

Dermablend—a cover cream used to cover vitiligo, birthmarks, etc.

dermabrasion (Derm)—an abrasion procedure for acne scars, performed after anesthetizing and freezing the skin with Freon; scars are abraded with fine sandpaper, diamond fraises, or abrasive brushes. See *diamond fraise.*

Dermalene—linear polyethylene monofilament suture material.

Dermalon—monofilament nylon suture material.

dermatome
- Brown
- Duval disposable
- Hall
- Padgett
- Reese
- Tanner-Vandeput mesh

Dermatophagoides farinae—a mite; it may be one of the principal sources of antigen in house dust in some areas. Cf. *Dermatophagoides pteronyssinus.*

Dermatophagoides pteronyssinus—a mite; it may be one of the principal sources of antigen in house dust in some areas. Cf. *Dermatophagoides farinae.*

dermatophyton control—used as a control with PPD testing.

D'Errico
- malleable brain spatula
- perforator drill
- skull trephine

DES daughter—a female exposed in utero to diethylstilbestrol (DES), formerly prescribed for bleeding and other complications of pregnancy and now known to affect fetal development of the genital tract.

Descemet's membrane—a fine membrane between the endothelial layer of the cornea and the substantia propria.

descemetocele—herniation of Descemet's membrane.

describe—to explain or characterize in words. Cf. *ascribe.*

desflurane—an anesthetic agent that appears to allow more rapid recovery than other agents, thus permitting patients to leave the hospital sooner.

desiccated (*not* dessicated)—dried.

Desilets-Hoffman introducer—used to introduce balloon, electrode, and other catheters.

Desjardin forceps (''day-zhar-dan'').

Desmarres corneal dissector (Oph).

Desmarres retractor (Oph).

desmoid lesion.

DeSouza exercises (Obs)—to encourage position change of fetus.

detachment
- retinal
- rhegmatogenous retinal

detergent worker's lung—extrinsic allergic alveolitis caused by exposure to detergent powder.

Detsky modified risk index score (Cardio)—a clinical scoring system used to predict cardiac morbidity.

De Vega tricuspid annuloplasty (Cardio)—performed on children.

developmental milestones (Peds)—the mastery of activities or skills expected at a certain age for normal child development.

Devic's disease—neuromyelitis optica, a form of acute multiple sclerosis.

device; instrument; system
- Accu-Chek II Freedom
- Accu-Line knee instrument
- Acland-Banis
- A.C.S. (Alcon Closure System)
- Acufex arthroscopic
- AICD (automatic internal cardioverter defibrillator)
- Aloka color Doppler system
- Aloka 650 ultrasound machine
- Ambu bag

device *(cont.)*
Anspach Cement Eater
applanometer
arch bar
Arthro-Flow
ArthroProbe laser
A-scan ultrasound device
Aspen laparoscopy electrode
ASTRA profile analyzers
Automator
Auto Suture Multifire Endo GIA 30 stapler
Auto Suture Premium CEEA stapler
BackBiter
Baggish hysteroscope
Bailliart's ophthalmodynamometer
Bard Biopty gun
Bateman UPF II bipolar system
beam splitter
Berman locator
Betatron I.V. insulin infusion pump
BiLAP bipolar cautery unit
Biliblanket phototherapy jacket
Bili mask
Biofix
biomicroscope (slit lamp)
Bioport collection and transport
Biopty gun
Bosker TMI system
BPM^2 (blood perfusion monitor)
Brown-Roberts-Wells stereotaxic
Buretrol volume control
BVM resuscitating device
Calandruccio triangular compression fixation
capnograph
C-arm fluoroscopy
Carolina rocker
Carter pillow
Cath-Finder
Cavitron ultrasonic aspirator (CUSA)
C Cap
celltrifuge
Cervex-Brush

device *(cont.)*
Charriere bone saw
ChemoCap
CHICK fracture table
CircOlectric bed
clam-shell brace
Clinitron bed
Clot Stop drain
Coopervision irrigation/aspiration handpiece
Cotrel-Dubousset spinal system
Crosby-Kugler pediatric capsule
cycloergometer
C-wire Serter
Dacomed snap gauge
Dalkon shield
diamond bur
diamond fraise
Diamond-lite cardiovascular
direct mechanical ventricular actuation (DMVA)
Doppler
Dyonics arthroscopic
ear oximeter
Easi-Lav gastric lavage
EBI bone healing system
EBI SPF-2 implantable bone stimulator
echogastroscope
Eclipse TENS unit
Ectra system
electro-oculogram apparatus
electronic fetal monitor
Ellik kidney stone evacuator
emergency infusion (EID)
Endoloop
Endopath ES stapler
Endotak C lead
EPL (extracorporeal piezoelectric lithotriptor)
ErecAid system
EX-FI-RE system
extracorporeal piezoelectric lithotriptor (EPL)
extractor

device *(cont.)*
FACS (Fluorescence activated cell sorter)
Faulkner folder
filiforms and followers
Fletcher applicator
Fletcher-Suit applicator
Fluorescence activated cell sorter (FACS)
fog reduction/elimination (FRED)
Fujinon colonoscope
G-suit
Gamma knife (radiosurgical instrument)
Gentle Touch colostomy appliance
Girard Fragmatome
Glassman stone extractor
Glucometer II
Goldmann applanation tonometer
gonioscope
Gottschalk Nasostat
Gould electromagnetic flowmeter
Grieshaber manipulator
Guibor canaliculus intubation
Gullstrand's slit lamp
Haag-Streit slit lamp
Haemonetics Cell Saver
Hall neurosurgical craniotome
Hall sternum saw
Hall valvutome
Handtrol electrosurgical pencil
Harrison-Nicolle polypropylene pegs
Hasson graspers
Heartmate
HeatProbe water irrigation/lavage device
Hebra fixation hook
Hemo-Cue photometer
hemodialyzer
hemostatic eraser
heparin lock
Hewlett-Packard ear oximeter
Hoffmann external fixation
Honan balloon
Honan manometer

device *(cont.)*
Hot/Ice System III
Howmedica instruments
Hubbard tank
HUI uterine injector
Hunter tendon rod
Hydrocollator
Hyfrecator
hypothermia blanket
hysteroscope
Hysteroser
Illumina PROSeries
IMED infusion device
Inspiron training device
Insuflon indwelling device
IntraDop probe
Intra-Op autotransfusion system
Intrel II spinal cord stimulation
Iowa trumpet
IVAC electronic thermometer
IVAC volumetric infusion pump
IVOX (intravascular oxygenator)
J-wire
Jamar dynamometer
Karl Storz Calutript
Karl Storz ureteropyeloscope
Killip wire
KineTec hip CPM machine
KinetiX ventilation monitor
Koch phaco manipulator/splitter
Küttner blunt dissecting instrument
Landolt ring vision test
Landry Vein Light Venoscope
LaserSonics EndoBlade
LaserSonics Nd:YAG Laser Blade scalpels
LaserSonics SurgiBlade
Leksell stereotactic frame
Leukotrap red cell storage system
Light Talker
lingoscope
Lithostar
lithotriptor or lithotripter
lithotrite
Littleford/Spector introducer

device *(cont.)*
Luedde exophthalmometer
Lumiwand
Luque rod and instrumentation
Lusk pediatric endoscopic sinus instrument
Luxtec fiberoptic system
Maddacrawler Crawler
Madsen Tympan-O-Scope
malleus nipper
Mascot indirect ophthalmoscope
Mayo stand
Medicon surgery instruments
MediPort implanted vascular
Medstone STS shock wave generator
mercury-in-Silastic gauge
MicroTeq portable belt
Microvasive biliary
Midas Rex pneumatic instrument
Mijnhard electrical cycloergometer
Mitek anchor
MixEvac bone-cement mixer
MNES
Molnar disk (or disc)
Multileaf Collimator
Myobock artificial hand
NeoKnife electrosurgical instrument
Neuro-Trace
Nevyas drape retractor
Nezhat-Dorsey Trumpet Valve hydrodissector
NovolinPen
Olympus endoscope
Optacon
Optiscope
Optotype eye testing
Ortho-evac autotransfusion
Ortholav lavage and suction
OrthoPak II bone growth stimulator
orthoplast jacket
oximeter
pachometer
PAM (potential acuity meter)
P.A.S. Port Fluoro-Free system
peakometer

device *(cont.)*
Pentax flexible sigmoidoscope
PercuGuide
permanent lead introducer
Phaco-Emulsifier aspirator
Piezolith-EPL
Polar-Mate bipolar microcoagulator
potential acuity meter (PAM)
Precision Osteolock
Premium CEEA circular stapling
Primbs-Circon indirect video ophthalmoscope
Pro-Trac cruciate reconstruction measurement
Protocult stool sampling
Pulmo-Aide nebulizer
pulse oximetry device
PulseSpray
Quinton suction biopsy instrument
ReAct NMES
Redy 2000 hemodialysis
Respiradyne
Respiragard II nebulizer
Respironics CPAP machine
Rhino Rocket
Rizzuti iris expressor
roentgen knife radiosurgical device
Rogozinski spinal fixation system
Roho mattress
Rotablator
Scaphoid-Microstaple
Silastic bead embolization
Simpson atherectomy
Simpulse lavage
Skin Scribe
slit lamp (biomicroscope)
Smith-Petersen osteotome
snap gauge band
Solcotrans drainage/reinfusion
Soluset
SONOP ultrasonic aspiration
spinal fixation system
Splintrex
Statak
Statham electromagnetic flow meter

device *(cont.)*
stimulator
subclavian peel-away sheath
Surgitron
Symbion pneumatic assist device
SynchroMed Infusion
Takata laser interferometer
Taylor pinwheel
TCPM pneumatic tourniquet
Terry keratometer
thermistor
Thermoscan Pro-1-Instant thermometer
ThinPrep processor
TLSO
Travenol infuser
Tubex injector
Tum-E-Vac
Ultra-Drive bone cement removal
UNILINK
Urocyte diagnostic cytometry
VAD (ventricular assist device)
Valleylab electrosurgical instrument
ventricular assist device (VAD)
vertebral body impactor
Vickers microsurgical instrument
Vidal-Ardrey modified Hoffmann
Visitec nucleus hydrodissector
visuscope
VitaCuff
Vital Vue suction and irrigation
vitreous cutter
Vitrophage Peyman
Volkmann's spoon
Von Lackum surcingle
Vozzle Vacu-Irrigator
VPL thalamic electrode
V-Vac apparatus
Wallach pencil
Watzke Silicone sleeve
Weck-Baggish Hysteroscopy
Welch Allyn AudioScope
Yasargil instruments
Zeiss instruments
Zelsmyr Cytobrush

dewlap—redundant skin hanging below the chin.

DeWecker iris scissors (Oph).

Dexon mesh—a synthetic (polyglycolic acid filaments) and stretchable fabric used in surgery on soft-tissue organs, e.g., liver, spleen, that do not hold sutures well. The idea is to salvage the organ by enclosing it within the mesh, suturing the mesh to the organ at ¼ to ½ inch intervals. The mesh is absorbed by the body tissues in four to six weeks, by which time healing should have taken place.

Dexon II suture—an improved Dexon suture which, according to the manufacturer, ties more securely and has better overall strength.

dextran sulfate (Uendex)—a drug used to treat AIDS.

Dextrostix—trade name of plastic strip with reagent areas that change color in the presence of glucose in a drop of capillary blood (usually obtained from the ear lobe or finger stick). Used in monitoring and control of diabetes. Made by Ames (Miles Laboratory). Cf. *Chemstrip bG.*

Deyerle pin (Ortho).

Dey-Wash skin wound cleanser (Derm)—a saline solution in an aerosol can which sprays under pressure to gently debride and cleanse wounds.

dezocine (Dalgan)—a narcotic-like drug which relieves pain as well as morphine but is not derived from natural opium, and is not a controlled substance like morphine. Similar to Talwin, Stadol, Nubain, and Buprenex, but with fewer side effects of disorientation, hallucinations, and increase of cardiac work load. Given to orthopedic patients for trauma and postoperative pain control. Given I.M. and I.V., not orally.

DFA test (direct fluorescent antibody) —specific test for *Legionella pneumophila.* See also *IFA.*

DFMO (difluoromethylornithine)—see *eflornithine.*

DFMO-MGBG (Oncol)—chemotherapy protocol consisting of difluoromethylornithine (eflornithine) and MGBG, a polyamine synthesis inhibitor used in the treatment of brain tumors.

d4T (didehydrodideoxythymidine)—see *stavudine.*

DFV (DDP [cisplatin], fluorouracil, VePesid)—chemotherapy protocol.

DG Softgut suture—a surgical chromic suture (packaged without fluid). (DG, Davis & Geck.)

DHAC (dihydro-5-azacytidine, azacitidine) (Oncol)—chemotherapy drug.

DHAP (dexamethasone, high-dose Ara-C, Platinol)—a chemotherapy protocol used to treat Hodgkin's lymphoma.

DHE (dihematoporphyrin ether) (Oncol)—a photosensitizing agent given by injection in conjunction with a laser to provide prophylactic treatment to patients with transitional cell carcinoma of the bladder following surgical resection.

DHE, DHE-45 (dihydroergotamine) (Neuro)—used in treating headaches, including migraine, and a positive response is diagnostic of migraine. "The patient uses daily ergotamine and lithium for his cluster headaches, and took two doses of DHE at home prior to coming to the hospital."

DHPG (dihydroxypropoxymethylguanine; ganciclovir)—a drug used in treatment of cytomegalovirus infections in immunosuppressed patients and those with AIDS.

DiaBeta (glyburide)—oral drug for type II diabetics (NIDDM) who do not respond to diet alone. In advertisements the *B* is written as the Greek letter ß (beta). The beta cells of the pancreas produce insulin.

diabetes, bronze—see *bronze diabetes.*

diabetes mellitus classifications—from the American Diabetes Association to replace the terms *juvenile onset* and *adult onset*, as follows:

type I–IDDM (insulin dependent diabetes mellitus) refers to the type of diabetes that requires insulin to sustain life.

type II–NIDDM (non-insulin dependent diabetes mellitus) refers to the type of diabetes that does not require insulin to sustain life. This category includes two subgroups: obese and non-obese.

Other re-defined categories include:

impaired glucose tolerance which replaces *borderline, chemical,* or *latent* as a description of glucose levels which fall between normal and diabetic.

gestational diabetes which refers to women who develop diabetes during pregnancy. Applicable only during pregnancy.

diabetes associated with certain conditions or syndromes such as diabetes secondary to pancreatic disease or endocrine disease.

diabetes mellitus, classifications in pregnancy:

class A (gestational diabetes)—transient diabetes that reverts to normal after the delivery. Usually is well controlled by diet.

class B—onset after age 20, duration less than 10 years; has been controlled by diet, but patient may

diabetes *(cont.)*
become insulin dependent during the pregnancy; may not need insulin after the delivery.
class C—onset between 10 and 19 years of age (formerly called juvenile-onset diabetes). The patient has been insulin dependent and will need increased doses during pregnancy, but will usually return to the pre-pregnancy dosage after delivery.
class D—onset at less than 10 years of age, with duration more than 20 years. Hypertension, diabetic retinopathy, and peripheral vascular disease are noted.
class E—calcification of pelvic vessels is present.
class F—diabetic nephropathy is present.
Infants of class A, B, and C diabetic mothers are likely to be large for gestational age (LGA).
Infants of class D, E, and F diabetic mothers are likely to be small for gestational age (SGA).

Diacyte DNA ploidy analysis (Oncol)—a way to identify aneuploid tumors of the prostate which may require aggressive treatment, such as tumors with intermediate Gleason scores.

Diagnex Blue test (Lab)—for gastric acid. (Diagnex Blue is a trademark.)

dial a haptic (Oph).

dialysis—continuous ambulatory peritoneal dialysis (CAPD). See *Drake-Willock automatic delivery system.*

diamagnetic—MRI term.

diamond bur (Ortho)—instrument used to abrade or smooth; for example, to resect an osteophyte.

diamond fraise (Derm)—an instrument used in dermabrasion of acne scars.

Diamond-Lite—titanium cardiovascular surgical instruments.

diamond-shaped murmur (Cardio)—a systolic heart murmur that first grows louder and then softer, the same as a crescendo-decrescendo murmur. Named for diamond-shaped tracing on phonocardiogram.

Dianon prostate profile and diagraph (Oncol)—an oncology trend report showing results over time of PSA, PAP, and LASA-P in patients with prostate cancer.

diaphanous—see through, transparent. See *diaphanoscope.*

diaphanoscope—instrument for transilluminating a body cavity.

diaphanography—transillumination of the breast, with photography of the transilluminated light on infrared-sensitive film.

diaphysis—the shaft of a long bone between the ends (the epiphyses). Cf. *diastasis, diathesis.*

diastasis—separation (or dislocation) of two bones that are normally attached without the presence of a true joint; sometimes refers to the separation of muscles, as in diastasis recti abdominis. Cf. *diaphysis, diathesis.*

diastatic fracture—involves separation of the bones at the suture line of the skull, or marked separation of the bone fragments.

diathesis—constitution of the body that predisposes one to certain diseases or conditions, as "The patient appeared to have a hemorrhagic diathesis, although there was no family history of hemophilia." Cf. *diaphysis, diastasis.*

diaziquone (AZQ)—a chemotherapy drug used to treat lymphoma, leukemia, brain tumors (astrocytomas).

dibenzodiazepines—a class of antipsychotic drugs. See *clozapine.*

dibromodulcitol (DBD, mitolactol)—a chemotherapy agent.

DIC (diffuse, or disseminated, intravascular coagulation).

DIC microscopy (differential interference contrast).

Dickerson intraocular implant lens.

didanosine (ddI, Videx)—a drug approved by the FDA to treat HIV-positive patients who cannot tolerate zidovudine (Retrovir) or who have strains of HIV that are resistant to zidovudine.

didehydrodideoxythymidine (d4T)—see *stavudine.*

didelphys—see *uterus didelphys.*

dideoxycytidine (ddC, HIVID)—a drug approved by the FDA to treat patients with AIDS and ARC.

dideoxyinosine (ddI)—see *didanosine.*

Didronel (etidronate).

diener (''dee-ner'')—an assistant in a laboratory or morgue.

Diener forceps.

diethyldithiocarbamate (Imuthiol)—a drug used to treat AIDS.

Dietl's crisis—when a kidney twists on its pedicle, cutting off blood flow.

"diff"—medical slang for WBC differential. See *differential.*

differential in white blood cell count
- polymorphonuclear neutrophils (PMNs or polys)—range 50-70% of total white blood cells
- eosinophils—range 5-6%
- basophils—range 0-1%
- monocytes—range 0-7%
- lymphocytes—range 20-40%

differential interference contrast microscopy (DIC).

Diflucan (fluconazole).

difluorodeoxycytidine (gemcitabine).

difluoromethylornithine (DFMO)—a drug used to treat AIDS.

"dig" (''dij'')—slang for digoxin, digitoxin, or digitalis. If you cannot ask the dictator and the chart does not show which drug is intended, you may transcribe *digitalis.*

DiGeorge syndrome—thymic hypoplasia. Congenital aplasia of the thymus and parathyroid glands; pure T-cell deficiency, but with B-cell function intact. Cf. *Nezelof syndrome.*

Digibind (digoxin immune Fab [ovine] fragments)—for treatment of life-threatening digoxin intoxication.

Digidote (digoxin immune Fab). See *Digibind.*

Digikit (Surg)—finger and toe pneumatic tourniquet that prevents nerve trauma that could occur with the use of a Penrose drain as a tourniquet.

digital subtraction angiography (DSA)—an interventional radiological procedure which allows visualization of the small vessels. Iodinated contrast material is injected via venous catheter, and a computer subtracts out all the tissues until only the vessels visualized by contrast material are left; any vessels blocked by occlusion or stenosis are then readily apparent.

digital to analog converter—MRI term.

Digitron—a digital subtraction imaging system.

digoxin immune Fab (Digibind, Digidote).

dihematoporphyrin ether (DHE) (Oncol). Selectively retained by malignant cells, DHE is given intravenously. An argon laser is then used to produce a photochemical reaction in the malignant cells which destroys them.

dihydroergotamine—see *DHE.*

Dilamezinsert penile prosthesis (Urol).

Dilapan (Ob-Gyn)—synthetic laminaria for cervical dilatation. See *Laminaria* (genus).

dilator
- Amplatz
- Bakes
- Bozeman
- Brown-McHardy
- Delaborde tracheal
- Dotter
- Eder-Puestow metal olive
- Garrett
- Hayman
- Hurst mercury
- Kohlman urethral
- Maloney esophageal
- Rigiflex balloon
- Soehendra

DILE (drug-induced lupus erythematosus).

dilevalol (Unicard) (Cardio)—a beta blocker drug used to treat mild to moderate hypertension.

dilutional hematocrit (Lab)—when too much water or crystalloid dilutes the blood, lowering the hematocrit. *Not* delusional.

DIMOAD syndrome—diabetes insipidus, diabetes mellitus, optic atrophy, and deafness.

Dinamap blood pressure monitor and Oxytrak pulse oximeter—to measure oxygen saturation (Surg).

Dingman breast dissector; mouth gag.

dinitrochlorobenzene. See *DNCB.*

Dipentum (olsalazine).

dipslides—see *Uricult dipslides.*

dipstick—see *OvuStick dipstick.*

dipyridamole—coronary vasodilator.

dipyridamole echocardiography test—for detection of coronary artery disease. It may demonstrate exercise-induced myocardial ischemia, which might be "EKG-silent," by providing evidence of the ischemic event. Also an agent to reduce blood viscosity.

direct fluorescent antibody test (DFA).

direct light reflex—light reflex in which the response occurs in the eye that was stimulated. See *consensual light reflex.*

direct vision internal urethrotomy (DVIU).

disc, var. spelling of *disk.* The *disk* spelling is preferred in most dictionaries, but *disc* has long been used in names of anatomic structures, and some physicians insist on its use in their transcription.

discharges, periodic lateralized epileptiform (PLEDs) in EEG.

discission—the incision, or cutting into, as of a capsule of a cataract, or of a soft cataract, or of the cervix uteri. Cf. *decision.*

discoloration, heliotrope infraorbital.

disconjugate gaze—when the eyes do not work in unison. Alternate spelling, *dysconjugate.* Apparently either spelling is acceptable.

discreet—circumspect, prudent, using or showing good judgment in conduct and in speech, as "I hope you will be most discreet in using this information." Cf. *discrete.*

discrete—separate, composed of distinct parts or discontinuous elements, as "There were large, discrete nodules noted in the neck." (A mnemonic device to help you remember this spelling: "discrete" means separate, and notice that the "t" separates the two e's.) Cf. *discreet.*

disease (See also *syndrome.*)
- *Acanthamoeba* keratitis
- achondroplastic dwarfism

disease *(cont.)*
acute fatty liver of pregnancy (AFLP)
acute intermittent porphyria (AIP)
acute lymphoblastic leukemia (ALL)
acute monoblastic leukemia (AMOL)
acute myelomonoblastic leukemia (AMMOL)
acute myeloblastic leukemia (AML)
acute poststreptococcal glomerulonephritis (APSGN)
acute tubular necrosis (ATN)
adenosis
adiposis dolorosa
agranulocytosis
AIDS (acquired immunodeficiency syndrome)
AIDS-related complex (ARC)
AIDS-related syndrome (ARS)
air-space
Alström's
Alzheimer's
angiolymphoid hyperplasia with eosinophilia (ALHE)
apocrine metaplasia
ARDS (adult respiratory distress syndrome)
ariboflavinosis
arteriosclerotic retinopathy
arteriovenous malformation (AVM)
arteritis
asymmetric septal hypertrophy (ASH)
atriovenous malformation (AVM)
babesiosis
bagassosis
Barrett's esophagus
Bartter's
Bassen–Kornzweig abetalipoproteinemia
Batten
Beckwith-Wiedemann
Behçet's
Benedikt's ipsilateral ocular paralysis
Berger's

disease *(cont.)*
Bible printer's lung
bilharziasis
bipolar affective illness
bipolar disorder
Blackfan-Diamond
blue diaper
blue rubber-bleb nevus
blue toe
blunt duct adenosis
Boerhaave's
branch retinal vein occlusion (BRVO)
breast fibrocystic
brittle bone
Brodie's abscess
bronze diabetes
Brown's tendon sheath
Brown-Séquard
Budd's
Budd-Chiari
Budd's jaundice
bulimia nervosa
bulimorexia
Burkitt's lymphoma
Burkitt-type acute lymphoblastic leukemia
caisson
calcium pyrophosphate deposition (CPPD)
cameral fistula
carcinoma in situ (CIS)
cataract
central serous retinopathy
cervical intraepithelial neoplasia (CIN)
chalazion
Charcot-Bouchard aneurysm
Cheatle-Henry hernia
cheese worker's lung
Chiari's
Chlamydia trachomatis infection
chloroquine retinopathy
chondromalacia patellae
chondroplastic dwarfism

disease *(cont.)*
chordee
chordoma
chorioretinopathy and pituitary dysfunction (CPD)
choristoma
Christmas
chronic active hepatitis
chronic fatigue syndrome (CFS)
chronic granulocytic leukemia (CGL)
chronic lymphocytic leukemia (CLL)
chronic myelocytic leukemia (CML)
chronic persistent
circinate retinopathy
Cobb's
congenital dysplasia (or dislocation) of the hip (CDH)
cornea guttata
coronary artery (CAD)
cor triatriatum
cor triatriatum dexter
Crohn's
Curling's ulcer
Cushing's
cytomegalovirus (CMV)
cytomegalovirus hepatitis
cytomegalovirus retinitis
Dandy-Walker
Darier's
decubitus ulcer
deep vein (or venous) thrombosis (DVT)
degenerative joint disease (DJD)
delta hepatitis (hepatitis D)
de Morsier's
de Morsier-Gauthier
dengue hemorrhagic fever (DHF)
de Quervain's
Dercum's
detergent worker's lung
Devic's
diabetic retinopathy
diffuse idiopathic skeletal hyperostosis (DISH)

disease *(cont.)*
DiGeorge
disseminated lupus erythematosus
drug-induced hepatitis
drug-induced lupus erythematosus (DILE)
Duchenne's paralysis
Eales
Ehlers-Danlos
ENANB hepatitis (enterically transmitted non-A, non-B hepatitis)
endolymphatic hypertension
endophthalmitis
ependymitis granularis
ependymoma
Epstein-Barr
Erb's palsy
Erb-Duchenne paralysis
erythema migrans
erythroplasia of Queyrat
Ewing's sarcoma
Fabry's
Fallot's pentalogy
Fallot's trilogy
farmer's lung
fat embolism
fibrocystic breast
fibromuscular dysplasia (FMD)
fish meal lung
Fitz–Hugh and Curtis
florid adenosis
Fort Bragg fever
fragile X
Freiberg's
fungemia
furrier's lung
gastroesophageal reflux (GERD)
Gianotti-Crosti
giant cell arteritis (GCA)
giant papillary conjunctivitis (GPC)
Gilles de la Tourette's
glaucoma
glioblastoma multiforme
Goldenhar
graft–versus–host (GVHD)

disease *(cont.)*
Gudden's atrophy
Guillain-Barré
Haemophilus influenzae type B (HIB)
hairy-cell leukemia (HCL)
Halbrecht's
Hamman-Rich
Haverhill fever
hemangiopericytoma
hemophilia A
hemophilia B
Henoch-Schönlein purpura
hepatic venous web
hepatitis
hepatitis C
hepatitis D (delta hepatitis)
hepatitis F
herpes whitlow
HIB (*Haemophilus influenzae* type B)
Hill-Sachs
Hirschsprung's
HIV-associated thrombocytopenia
housemaid's knee
Hunner's interstitial cystitis
Hunner's ulcer
hyperlipoproteinemia (HLP)
hypertensive retinopathy
idiopathic hypertrophic subaortic stenosis (IHSS)
idiopathic thrombocytopenic purpura (ITP)
immunoglobulin-complexed enzyme (ICE)
immunoproliferative small-intestinal (IPSID)
infantile motor neuron
intraretinal microangiopathy (IRMA)
intraretinal microvascular abnormalities (IRMA)
Ivemark's
jacksonian epilepsy
Kaposi's sarcoma
Kasabach-Merritt

disease *(cont.)*
Kawasaki
Kaznelson's
Kearns-Sayre
Kearns-Sayre-Shy
Kienböck's
Kimmelstiel–Wilson (K–W)
König (Koenig)
Kostmann's infantile agranulocytosis
kraurosis vulvae
Krukenberg's tumor
Kugelberg–Welander
Landry-Guillain-Barré-Strohl
Laurence-Moon-Biedl
Leber's
legionnaires'
Lejeune's
lenticular nuclear sclerosis
Lesch–Nyhan
Letterer–Siwe
Lhermitte–Duclos
lipoid nephrosis
Löffler's (Loeffler's)
Louis-Bar's
Lown-Ganong-Levine
Ludwig's angina
Lyme
lymphedema praecox
lymphocytic interstitial pneumonitis (LIP)
lymphogranuloma venereum (LGV)
MAC infection (*Mycobacterium avium* complex)
Madura foot
MAI infection (*Mycobacterium avium-intracellulare*)
malaria
maple bark stripper's
maple–syrup urine (MSUD)
Marchiafava–Bignami
Marie's ataxia
Martorell hypertensive ulcer
mature cataract
maturity onset diabetes of the young (MODY)

disease *(cont.)*
meat wrapper's asthma
meibomian cyst
meralgia paresthetica
Merzbacher
Miege's
miliaria
milk leg
Milroy's
mitochondrial cytopathy
mitral valve prolapse (MVP)
mixed connective tissue (MCTD)
MJA degenerative
Mondini's dysplasia
monoblastic leukemia (MOL)
mucocutaneous lymph node
multiple colloid adenomatous goiter (MCAG)
multiple endocrine adenopathy (MEA)
multiple endocrine neoplasia (MEN)
multiple evanescent white dot (MEWD)
mushroom worker's
myalgic encephalomyelitis (ME)
Mycobacterium avium complex (MAC)
Mycobacterium avium-intracellulare (MAI)
mycosis fungoides
myxoma
NANB hepatitis (non-A, non-B)
necrotizing enterocolitis (NEC)
neurilemmoma
Nezelof
Niemann–Pick
nil
no appreciable (NAD)
no evidence of (NED)
non-A hepatitis
non-A, non-B hepatitis (NANB)
non-B hepatitis
nonspecific urethritis (NSU)
Norrie's
nosocomial

disease *(cont.)*
null cell lymphoblastic leukemia
null-type non-Hodgkin's lymphoma
obsessive-compulsive disorder (OCD)
oculocraniosomatic neuromuscular
ophthalmoplegic plus
optic neuritis
organic brain syndrome (OBS)
Ormond
osteoarthritis
osteoarthritis dissecans
osteochondritis dissecans
painter's encephalopathy
pantaloon embolus
papilledema
papular acrodermatitis of childhood (PAC)
paroxysmal nocturnal hemoglobinuria (PNH)
Patella's
pectus excavatum
peliosis hepatis
Pelizaeus–Merzbacher
peptic ulcer (PUD)
perilymphatic fistula (PLF)
persistent hyperplastic primary vitreous (PHPV)
Peutz-Jeghers
Peyer's patches
phthisis bulbi
pink tetralogy of Fallot
pinkeye
pleural effusion
Pneumocystis carinii pneumonia (PCP)
podagra
polycystic ovary (PCO)
Pontiac fever
posterior polymorphous dystrophy (PPMD)
Pott's puffy tumor
presbyopia
Prinzmetal's angina

disease *(cont.)*
progressive multifocal leuko-encephalopathy (PML)
progressive systemic sclerosis (PSS)
psammoma
Q fever
Quervain's
ratbite fever
Rector-Gordon-Healey-Mendoza-Spitzer type IV renal tubular acidosis
renal tubular
respiratory distress syndrome (RDS)
retinal commotio
retinal detachment
retinopathy of prematurity (ROP)
retinoschisis
retrobulbar neuritis
retrolisthesis
reversible obstructive airway disease (ROAD)
Reye's
rhabdomyolysis
Richter's hernia
Riedel's struma
Roger's
Rokitansky's
rolandic epilepsy
Roth–Bernhardt
Rothmund-Thomson
rubeosis iridis
saddle embolus
Saethre-Chotzen
Sandifer
Scheuermann's
sexually transmitted (STD)
Sinding-Larsen-Johannson
slim
Sly
squamous cell carcinoma (SCC)
Schlichting posterior polymorphous dystrophy
Schönlein-Henoch purpura
scleroderma

disease *(cont.)*
sclerosing adenosis
senile dementia of the Alzheimer type (SDAT)
Sertoli-cell-only
severe combined immunodeficiency (SCID)
Sézary
Sheehy
short-limb dwarfism
single-stripe colitis (SSC)
solar keratosis
Spitzer
spontaneous bacterial endocarditis (SBE)
Stewart-Treves
Still's
straddling embolus
strep throat
subacute bacterial endocarditis (SBE)
subacute bacterial peritonitis (SBP)
subarachnoid hemorrhage (SAH)
subcortical atherosclerotic encephalopathy (SAE)
suberosis
Sudeck's atrophy
syndactyly
syndrome of inappropriate antidiuretic hormone secretion (SIADH)
systemic lupus erythematosus (SLE)
tailor's bunion
Takayasu's arteritis
Taussig-Bing
tendinitis
Terrien's degeneration
tetralogy of Fallot
thromboembolic (TED)
thrombosis
thrombotic thrombocytopenic purpura
Tolosa-Hunt
Tornwaldt's bursitis
Tourette's

disease *(cont.)*
- transient ischemic attack (TIA)
- transposition of the great arteries (TGA)
- trichinosis
- trichosis
- trophic ulcer
- tularemia
- typhlitis
- Van Bogaert's
- venous thromboembolic
- venous web
- vipoma
- viral hepatitis
- vitelliform macular degeneration
- Voerner's
- Vogt-Koyanagi-Harada
- von Hippel-Lindau
- von Recklinghausen's
- von Rokitansky's
- VTED (venous thromboembolic d.)
- Waldenström's macroglobulinemia
- Warthin's tumor
- Wegener's granulomatosis
- Weir Mitchell's
- Werdnig-Hoffmann
- Wernicke's
- Wharton's tumor
- wheat weevil
- Whipple's
- Wiskott-Aldrich
- Wolff-Parkinson-White
- wood pulp worker's lung
- yuppie flu
- Zollinger-Ellison

DISH (diffuse idiopathic skeletal hyperostosis).

disk, disc (Gr., *diskos,* L., *discus*)—a circular or rounded flat plate. Note: *Disk* appears to be the preferred spelling, although *disc* is also used, especially in names of anatomic structures.

disk, choked (Oph)—edema and hyperemia of the optic disk, usually associated with increased intracranial pressure. Also called papilledema.

disk diameter (dd or DD) (Oph)—1.5 mm (the diameter of the optic nerve head); used in measuring the size of a fundal lesion or in describing its location. Also, disc diameter.

diskectomy with Cloward fusion. *(Not* discectomy.)

disk plication.

disorder
- attention deficit (ADD)
- bipolar
- immunoglobulin-complexed enzyme (ICE)
- manic-depressive
- obsessive-compulsive (OCD)
- systemic lupus erythematosus (SLE)

disproportion—see *cephalopelvic.*

dissecans—see *osteochondritis.*

dissection, dissector
- blunt
- Cavitron
- Creed
- Desmarres corneal
- Dingman breast
- Falcao suction
- finger
- Kitner
- Küttner blunt
- Neivert
- Nezhat-Dorsey Trumpet Valve hydrodissector
- Pearce nucleus hydrodissector
- Rhoton
- sharp and blunt
- spud
- Trumpet Valve

disseminated lupus erythematosus (*not* erythematosis). See *systemic lupus erythematosus* (SLE).

dissociated vertical divergence (DVD).

distal articular set angle (DASA) (Ortho).

distension—see *distention.*

distention—the state of being expanded, stretched. Also, distension.

distribution, Boltzmann—MRI term.

Diulo (methyl metolazone).

Dix-Hallpike test for paroxysmal positional nystagmus (Oph).

DJD (degenerative joint disease) (Ortho).

DLCO (**d**iffusing capacity of the **l**ung for **CO**) (carbon monoxide).

DMARDs (disease-modifying antirheumatic drugs)—thought to slow down the basic destructive rheumatoid arthritis process, e.g., oral or injectable gold, methotrexate, azathioprine (Imuran), cyclophosphamide (Cytoxan), hydroxychloroquine (Plaquenil).

DMVA (direct mechanical ventricular actuation) (Cardio)—a type of ventricular assist device which has several advantages over other methods. It can begin biventricular support in as little as three minutes because insertion is technically easy, there is no need for systemic anticoagulation because it has no cannulas in any blood vessels, it decreases the need for drug support for a failing heart, it can provide prolonged circulatory support without causing cardiac trauma, and it dramatically increases cardiac output. Currently DMVA is used as a temporary measure to sustain patients whose hearts fail while they wait for a suitable donor heart for heart transplantation. Before the DMVA device is surgically inserted, a transesophageal echocardiogram is done to determine cardiac dimensions in order to size the assist cup of the DMVA, which fits snugly around the whole heart. Cup sizes range from 90 to 150 mm. A left anterior thoracotomy is performed. After the heart is exposed, the cup slides onto the heart from the bottom up to fit over both ventricles. A vacuum system within the cup causes it to attach to the surface of the heart without the need for sutures. In an emergency, the DMVA device can be applied in as little as three minutes. Once in place, an alternating vacuum/pressure pump causes the heart to contract and relax. Drive lines and a chest tube protrude through the incision, which is then closed.

DNA, complementary (cDNA).

DNA polymerase-alpha (Oncol)—a tumor marker. When found in frozen tissue sections of patients who have had an exploratory thoracotomy for early nonsmall-cell lung cancer, the presence of this marker can be used to indicate those patients who will most likely suffer an early relapse of the disease and a poorer prognosis.

DNCB (dinitrochlorobenzene)—used in the treatment of conjunctival papillomas resistant to surgery and cryosurgery. After sensitization of the patient's lymphocytes to DNCB, the tumor can be debulked, followed by painting the base of the tumor with DNCB. Also used in treating AIDS.

DNJ (N-butyl-deoxynojirmycin)—drug used to treat AIDS.

DNS (dysplastic nevus syndrome)—can lead to malignant melanoma.

DOA (dead on arrival). The patient had already expired upon arrival at the medical facility.

Dobbhoff feeding tube.

Docke's murmur—diastolic murmur associated with stenosis of left anterior descending artery of the coronary distribution.

docking needle.

Döderlein's bacillus—a strain of lactobacillus normally seen in the vagina. It is considered a benign bacterium and maintains the normal acid pH of the vagina.

Dohlman incus hook (ENT).

Dohlman plug—used to treat perforated corneal ulcers.

dolichocephalic—long head.

doll's eye sign (Neuro)—dissociation between movements of the eyes and those of the head. A positive sign indicates damage to cranial nerves III, IV, and VI.

domperidone (Motilium).

DonJoy Goldpoint knee brace (Ortho)—for resisting tibial translation in a patient with deficient anterior or posterior ligaments. Note: Both *DonJoy* and *Donjoy* may be used.

DonJoy knee splint (Ortho). "A dry sterile dressing was then applied, followed by a DonJoy splint holding the knee out in extension."

donor island harvesting—a method of obtaining micro- and minigrafts from a hairbearing strip.

donor-specific transfusion (DST).

Doppler
- blood flow detector
- fetal heart monitor
- IntraDop
- IntraDop intraoperative
- intraoperative
- ultrasonic blood flow detector
- ultrasonic fetal heart monitor

Dopplette—a small Doppler monitor.

Doptone monitoring (Obs)—of fetal heart tones.

Doral (quazepam).

Dorello's canal (Neuro)—an opening in the temporal bone which is the point of entry of the sixth cranial nerve into the cavernous sinus.

Dorendorf's sign—of aortic arch aneurysm, evidenced by fullness of supraclavicular groove.

Dormia stone basket.

Dornier gallstone lithotriptor.

dorsal (adj.)—referring to the back or to any posterior part or surface, e.g., the dorsal surface of the hand is the back of the hand. See *dorsum.*

dorsal column stimulator (DCS)—a device implanted near the spinal column to control chronic pain through percutaneous electrical stimulation; used in some patients with amyotrophic lateral sclerosis to increase contraction of the diaphragm.

dorsal lithotomy position (*not* dorsolithotomy).

dorsal penile nerve block (DPNB)—a technique to reduce behavioral stress and modify the adrenocortical stress response in neonates undergoing circumcision.

dorsum (noun)—back; posterior aspect. See *dorsal.*

Dos Santos needle for aortography (Vasc Surg).

dothiepin (Prothiaden)—an antidepressant drug.

Dotter dilator (Urol).

Dotter-Judkins PTA (percutaneous transluminal angioplasty)—involves dilatation of the lumen of a stenotic femoral artery in patients who are not good risks for femoral-popliteal bypass surgery. It involves the use of a special catheter which is directed to the site of the atheromatous lesion under fluoroscopy, and then progressively larger catheters are introduced over a guide wire. See *PTA.*

double-armed suture—a suture with a needle at each end. See *suture.*

double-blind study—a study in which neither the patient nor the physician knows if the drug being administered is a test medication or a placebo.

double bubble flushing reservoir—used in patients with hydrocephalus (Neuro).

double bubble sign (Radiol)—seen in infants with choledochal cysts and obstructive jaundice. "Plain films show the double bubble sign, with a large air bubble that represents the stomach; the second bubble represents air dilating the duodenum that is proximal to the point of blockage."

double contrast technique (Radiol)—a modification of the barium enema procedure. After the standard barium enema examination has been completed, the patient expels most of the barium, and the colon is then inflated with air. The coating of barium remaining on the surface may outline masses or defects not seen during the standard examination.

Double-J indwelling catheter stent—trademark, from Surgitex (Urol).

double-threaded Herbert screw.

Douvas roto-extractor (Oph).

dowager's hump—kyphosis due to osteoporosis of the spine.

Dow hollow fiber dialyzer.

downgoing toes—in a normal response to the Babinski test, the great toe curls downward when the sole of the foot is stroked; thus, a negative Babinski is a flexor plantar response: "The toes are downgoing." Cf. *upgoing.*

doxacurium chloride (Nuromax)—a long-acting neuromuscular blocker used in conjunction with a general anesthetic. Provides skeletal muscle relaxation. Most useful in patients with heart disease who are undergoing surgery because, unlike Pavulon, it does not cause tachycardia.

doxazosin mesylate (Cardura) (Cardio). An alpha$_1$-adrenergic blocker, doxazosin acts by blocking alpha$_1$-adrenergic receptors and reducing the production of the natural neurotransmitter norepinephrine. This causes blood vessels to dilate and blood pressure to decrease. It is used as an antihypertensive drug and is similar to prazosin (Minipress).

Draeger high vacuum erysiphake (Oph).

Draeger tonometer (Oph)—a hand-held applanation tonometer; used to measure intraocular pressure.

drain, drainage system
- Blair silicone
- butterfly
- Chaffin-Pratt
- Clot Stop
- Davol
- endoscopic retrograde biliary (ERBD)
- Nélaton rubber tube
- Penrose
- Quad-Lumen
- Relia-Vac
- Thora-Drain III three-bottle chest drainage unit
- Thora-Klex chest drainage system

Drake clip (Neuro)—used in clipping intracranial aneurysms.

Drake-Willock automatic delivery system—used in peritoneal dialysis in association with Tenckhoff catheter.

drape
- fenestrated
- Ioban antimicrobial incise
- Opraflex incise
- Steri-Drape

Draw-a-Bicycle test (Psych)—a mental status examination. Also, DAB test.

Draw-a-Flower test (Psych)—mental status examination. Also, DAF test.

Draw-a-House test (Psych)—mental status examination. Also, DAH test.

Draw-a-Person test (Psych)—mental status examination. Also, DAP test.

drawer sign (Ortho)—in testing for ligamentous instability or for rupture of the cruciate ligaments of the knee.

drawn ankle clonus.

dressing (See also *adhesive, bandage.*)
- Acu-Derm I.V./TPN
- Acu-Dyne wound
- Allevyn
- Bioclusive transparent
- BlisterFilm transparent
- ClearSite transparent wound
- Coban
- CollaCote
- CollaPlug
- CollaTape
- Comfeel Ulcus
- Coverlet adhesive surgical
- Cutinova Hydro
- DuoDerm
- DuoDerm CFG
- Elastikon
- Elastomull
- Flexinet
- Fuller shield
- Glasscock ear
- Inerpan
- IntraSite gel
- Kaltostat wound packing
- Kling adhesive
- Koch-Mason
- LYOfoam
- LYOfoam C
- LYOfoam tracheostomy
- Medipore Dress-it
- Mesalt
- Mitraflex multilayer wound

dressing *(cont.)*
- Nu Gauze
- Nu-Gel
- O'Donoghue
- OpSite
- Sof-Wick
- Sorbsan topical wound
- Synthaderm
- Tegaderm transparent
- Tube-Lok tracheotomy
- Ultec hydrocolloid
- Uniflex polyurethane adhesive surgical
- Vari/moist
- Veingard
- Velpeau
- Viasorb
- Vigilon
- wet-to-dry
- Wound-Span Bridge II
- Xeroform

Drews forceps (Oph).

Drews intraocular implant lens (Oph).

DREZ lesion (dorsal root entry zone) (Neuro).

DREZ-otomy (Neuro)—a surgical procedure to treat spasticity and pain in the lower limbs.

drill
- Cement Eater
- D'Errico perforator
- Fisch
- Gray
- Hall air
- Mathews
- Osteone air
- Shea
- Stille cranial

Dripps-American Surgical Association score (Cardio)—a clinical scoring system used to predict cardiac morbidity.

dromperidone (Motilium)—an antiemetic drug.

dronarinol (Marinol)—an antiemetic drug given with chemotherapy; also used to treat loss of appetite in AIDS patients. The active ingredient is derived from the marijuana plant.

drop attacks—episodes of dropping objects but remaining conscious; a form of petit mal epilepsy. Also may be experienced by narcoleptics who have sudden brief periods of unconsciousness.

drug-induced lupus erythematosus (DILE).

drusen—small hyaline globular pathological growths formed on Bruch's membrane (Oph).

dry heaves—gagging or retching without emesis.

DSA (digital subtraction angiography).

DSM (degradable starch microspheres) (Oncol)—microspheres of glucose polymers injected into an artery at the same time as a chemotherapy drug to temporarily block the blood flow at the capillary level (chemoembolization). The chemotherapy drug is then concentrated in the region of the cancer and high tissue uptake is achieved. DSM has a short half-life and does not occlude the local circulation long enough to produce ischemia, and in conjunction with a chemotherapy drug can be administered repeatedly.

DST (donor-specific transfusion)—used before kidney transplantation, to identify any possible incompatibility between donor and recipient and thus possibly prevent rejection of a transplant.

"D-stix"—slang for Dextrostix.

D-Tach needle—see *pop-off needle.*

DTIC-Dome (dacarbazine) (Oncol)—a single drug used in the treatment of malignant melanoma.

DTPA (diethylenetriamine-penta-acetic acid or acetate) (Radiol)—used in combination with gadolinium as a contrast medium in MRI scans.

dual-lock total hip replacement system.

dual photon densitometry—test recommended for diagnosis of osteoporosis through comparative height measurements. Loss of height means the patient is losing trabecular bone and should undergo further testing for osteoporosis.

Duane's classification of convergence insufficiency (Oph).

Duane's retraction syndrome (Oph)—a congenital, usually unilateral, disorder of eye movement, affecting females more often than males. The affected eye usually has complete absence of abduction, and partial absence of adduction (sometimes the reverse). The involved eye retracts into the orbit on adduction, and demonstrates pseudoptosis. There is also paresis or failure of convergence. Also known as Stilling-Türk-Duane syndrome.

Dubowitz scale for infant maturity (Peds), as in "The infant was 38 weeks' gestational age by Dubowitz." It takes about 24 hours to perform the testing, in which neurological function is correlated with the fetus' gestational age.

duck waddle—a test of the integrity of the knee joints and menisci, in which the patient is required to "walk" in a squatting position.

Ducrey's bacillus. See *Haemophilus ducreyi.*

ductions (Oph)—monocular rotations (with the other eye covered):
abduction—outward rotation

ductions *(cont.)*
adduction—inward rotation
infraduction—downward movement
supraduction—upward movement

ductions and versions (Oph).

Duecollement maneuver—in hemicolectomy.

Duffy blood antibody type—factor in agglutination. See also *Kell, Kidd, Lewis, Lutheran.*

Duhamel pull-through procedure—for correction of Hirschsprung's disease. It involves excision of the aganglionic segment of the proximal colon and anastomosis between the normal remaining bowel and the posterior wall of the healthy segment of the rectum. Cf. *Lester Martin modification of Duhamel procedure.*

Duke bleeding time (Lab)—the number of minutes it takes for a small incision in the skin (by puncture of the earlobe), made with a lancet, to stop bleeding.

Dukes' classification of carcinoma—named for Cuthbert E. Dukes, a British pathologist. Classes:
A invading mucosa and submucosa
B invading muscularis
C spread to regional lymph nodes; distant metastasis

Dulaney intraocular implant lens.

dullness, shifting (GI). In abdominal examination, a change in the percussion note as the patient rolls from his back to his side is called shifting dullness and confirms the presence of ascitic fluid.

dumbbell-shaped shadow (Radiol).

Dumon-Harrell bronchoscope.

Dumon-Harrell trachea tube.

dumping syndrome (GI)—symptoms of palpitations, sweating, and weakness, sometimes seen after gastrectomy, and caused by rapid emptying of gastric contents into the small intestine (hence "dumping").

Dunlop synoptophore test (Oph)—for eye vergence.

Dunlop thrombus stripper.

duodenal bulb (Radiol)—an onion-shaped dilatation of the duodenum immediately below its origin at the pylorus.

duodenal C-loop (Radiol)—C-shaped loop formed by the duodenum as it courses around the head of the pancreas.

duodenal sweep (Radiol)—the normal course of the duodenum, from the pylorus and around the head of the pancreas to the ligament of Treitz, as visualized with contrast medium in an upper GI series.

duodenal switch (GI)—a procedure for pancreaticobiliary diversion that eliminates the need for the antrectomy and vagotomy that must be done with a Roux-en-Y gastrojejunostomy.

duodenostomy—see *Witzel duodenostomy.*

duodenum deformed by scarring (Radiol).

DuoDerm dressing—a wound dressing used in treatment of leg ulcers, pressure sores, and superficial wounds. Also, DuoDerm CGF dressing (control gel formula).

Duo-Lock—see *Mueller Duo-Lock hip prosthesis.*

duplex pulsed-Doppler sonography (Cardio).

duplex ultrasound (Radiol)—used in the diagnosis of deep venous thrombosis instead of venography. Shows areas of blood flow in color contrast on a video screen to demonstrate

duplex ultrasound *(cont.)* movement of blood. Does not require use of contrast media, so is less painful, less expensive, and quicker than venogram. Individuals who are allergic to certain contrast media will be spared allergic reactions.

DuP 937 (Oncol)—a drug used in treating patients with solid tumors when other chemotherapy is ineffective.

Duragesic—see *fentanyl.*

Durapatite (hydroxyapatite).

Duraphase prosthesis (Urol)—inflatable penile prosthesis.

Duraprep surgical solution.

Dura-T contact lens—trade name of an extra-hard plastic contact lens.

Duret hemorrhage—blood effusion in the brain stem due to herniation.

Duroziez' sign.

dusky, duskiness—a bluish skin color from cyanosis.

Duval disposable dermatome (Plas Surg).

DuVal distal (caudal) pancreaticojejunostomy (GI)—a drainage technique that was used more in the past than at present. The term may be encountered in a patient's past history.

DuVries hammer toe repair.

DVD (dissociated vertical divergence). The eyes do not move together, and the deviating eye tends to move up and out.

DVI (deep venous insufficiency)—see *Hunter tendon rod.*

DVI (digital vascular imaging).

DVIU (direct vision internal urethrotomy) (Urol).

DVP (daunomycin, vincristine, prednisone)—chemotherapy protocol.

DVPL-ASP—chemotherapy protocol: daunorubicin, vincristine, prednisone, and L-asparaginase.

DVT (deep venous thrombosis) (Ortho, Vasc Surg).

dwarf—see *Russell dwarf.*

dwarfism
achondroplastic
chondroplastic
short-limb

Dwyer cable and screws (Ortho).

Dwyer correction of scoliosis (Ortho)—a procedure using an internal device of clips, screws, and a cable to straighten the spinal column. A clip is applied to each vertebra involved; a screw with a screwhead that has a hole in it is screwed through a hole in the clip and into the bone. A braided titanium cable is run through the holes protruding from the screwheads and tightened (after grafts of cancellous iliac bone or pieces of rib bone have been placed between the vertebrae). Tension is then applied to the cable.

Dwyer osteotomy (Pod)—calcaneal osteotomy as seen in ankle surgery.

dye—see *Berwick's dye* (Gyn).

dye laser—a type of laser used to remove birthmarks such as port wine stains by pinpointing and vaporizing the abnormal blood vessels which cause these marks. No anesthesia is necessary, as the procedure is essentially painless. The yellow-orange dye inside the laser is sensitive to the color red, therefore zeroing-in on the blood vessels with light energy that turns into heat, thus vaporizing the vessels, or on skin tumors consisting of blood vessels. It cannot be used for correction of varicose veins.

DynaCirc—see *isradipine.*

Dynagrip blade handle.

dynamic computerized tomography—rapid sequential CT scanning after an

dynamic CT *(cont.)*
intravenous bolus injection of contrast medium—for detection of microadenomas that are isodense with surrounding tissues on conventional (delayed) CT scans.

dynamic graciloplasty (GI)—a technique for correcting fecal incontinence in which the gracilis muscle is wrapped around the anus to create a new sphincter. Several weeks later, a standard cardiac pacemaker is implanted in the lower abdomen and electrodes placed on the gracilis muscle. Continued stimulation of the muscle by the pacemaker actually changes the type of muscle fibers to ones which resist fatigue and can maintain a sustained contraction around the anus. When the patient needs to defecate, the pacemaker is temporarily turned off with an external magnet.

dynamometer—see *Jamar.*

Dyonics arthroscopic instruments.

DyoVac suction punch—for arthroscopy.

dysconjugate gaze—see *disconjugate.*

dysfunctional (*not* dis-)—abnormality of function of an organ.

dyskaryosis—aberrant nuclear arrangement or structure; may be seen in malignancy or cell death. Cf. *dyskeratosis.*

dyskeratosis—aberrant keratin production and/or deposition. Cf. *dyskaryosis.*

dysphagia—difficulty in swallowing due to mechanical problems with the GI tract, esophageal infection or ulcers, or strokes. Cf. *dysphasia.*

dysphasia—impairment or loss of the power to use or understand speech; caused by disease of, or injury to, the brain. Cf. *dysphagia.*

dysplasia
congenital d. of hip (CDH)
fibromuscular (FMD)
Mondini's

Dysport—see *Clostridium botulinum toxin.*

dysthymia (Psych)—mood disorder. ''Secondary to her disabling organic illness, she has developed a chronic dysthymia.''

dystrophy
fingerprint
posterior polymorphous (PPMD)
reflex sympathetic
Schlichting posterior polymorphous

E, e

EAC (expandable access catheter) (Cardio)—used to facilitate embolectomy and angioplasty procedures. In its collapsed state, the EAC is inserted into either the iliac, femoral, or popliteal artery. In its expanded state, the lumen of the EAC is large enough so that an angioscope with either a Fogarty embolectomy catheter or an angioplasty balloon can be placed inside it.

EAEC (enteroadherent *E. coli*) (GI).

Eagle-Barrett syndrome (''prune-belly syndrome''), in which one or more layers of the abdominal wall musculature may be absent at birth, often accompanied by other congenital anomalies.

Eagle equation (Cardio)—a clinical scoring system used to predict cardiac morbidity.

Eagle straight-ahead arthroscope.

Eagle Vision-Freeman punctum plug (Oph). See *Freeman punctum plug.*

Eales disease (Oph)—seen principally in young men, characterized by neovascularization and recurrent hemorrhage of retinal vessels.

EAP (etoposide, Adriamycin, Platinol)—chemotherapy protocol to treat gastric adenocarcinoma.

ear—may easily be confused with ''air'' when the dictator says ''air-bone gap'' in audiology *(never* ''ear bone gap'' or ''airborne gap'').

ear oximeter *(not* air)—a photoelectric device which is attached to the ear and measures the oxygen saturation of the blood that passes through the ear. See *Hewlett-Packard ear oximeter.*

earring, Brent pressure—used to treat earlobe keloids.

Easi-Lav (GI)—a system for gastric lavage. Used in patients with upper GI bleeding, it delivers a greater volume of lavage in less time than standard methods.

EAST test (Vasc Surg)—an acronym for **e**xternal rotation, **a**bduction, **st**ress test. With the hands/arms held straight up (as in a holdup), the hands are opened and closed. In a positive EAST test, the patient reproduces the symptoms for which medical care was sought.

eating cell (phagocyte).

Eaton agent (*Mycoplasma pneumoniae*)—used thus in dictation: "primary atypical pneumonia, possibly due to the Eaton agent."

EBI bone healing system—noninvasive system for treating nonunion and failed arthrodesis with electromagnetic fields. (EBI stands for Electro Biology, Inc.).

EBI SPF-2 implantable bone stimulator (Ortho).

EBL (estimated blood loss) (Surg). This is estimated by measuring blood in the suction bottle and weighing the sponges that have soaked up blood.

EBNA (Epstein-Barr nuclear antigen) **test.**

Ebstein's cardiac anomaly *(not* Epstein, as in *Epstein-Barr virus).*

eburnated bone; eburnation.

EBV (Epstein-Barr virus)—the herpes-like virus known to cause mononucleosis, with evidence that it plays a part in susceptibility to Burkitt's lymphoma, and possibly to AIDS.

E-CABG—endarterectomy and coronary artery bypass grafting.

echo characteristics (ultrasonography) (Radiol)—the frequency, intensity, and distribution of echoes produced by a structure or region.

echocardiography—a noninvasive cardiac diagnostic procedure; it uses the principle of sonar (or depth sounding, as in locating submarines in the ocean) in which pulsing high-frequency sounds are bounced off the patient's chest and cardiac structures. From the pattern of these waves are determined the dimensions, position, and movements of the chamber walls and valve leaflets, and any possible deformities. Also, M-mode, sector scan, transesophageal echocardiogram. See *two-dimensional echocardiography.*

echocolonoscope (GI)—combines the Olympus CF-UM3 colonoscope with the EU-M3 endoscopic ultrasound system.

echogastroscope (GI)—used for endoscopic ultrasonography.

Echols retractor (Neuro).

EchoMark catheter (Cardio)—angiographic catheter that contains a wire and transducer sensitive to ultrasound signals. As the catheter is advanced, ultrasound (rather than x-rays) is used to correctly position the catheter in the vessel.

echo planar imaging—MRI term.

echo sign (Psych)—repetition of the last word of a sentence or phrase, indicating brain pathology.

echo time (TE)—an MRI term given in milliseconds (msec).

EC-IC bypass (extracranial-intracranial) (Neuro)—surgery for complete carotid occlusions or intracranial carotid stenosis not treatable by endarterectomy.

Eckhout vertical gastroplasty (named for Clifford V. Eckhout, M.D.).

Eclipse TENS unit—see *TENS.*

ECMO ("ek-mo") (extracorporeal membrane oxygenation) (Peds)—a technique used in infants with serious lung problems at birth with poor prognosis for survival. The baby's blood is circulated through a machine that removes carbon dioxide and adds oxygen, thereby functioning for the lungs while they mature, or heal.

ECMV (etoposide, Cytoxan, methotrexate, vincristine)—chemotherapy protocol used to treat small-cell lung carcinoma.

***E. coli* L-asparaginase** (Oncol)—a chemotherapy drug used to treat acute lymphoblastic leukemia. *E. coli* is a gram-negative bacterium which provides the enzyme L-asparaginase aminohydrolase contained in this version of L-asparaginase. Some people who are allergic to the *E. coli*-derived version of the drug can be given *Erwinia* L-asparaginase, derived from the gram-negative bacterium *Erwinia*.

ECRB (extensor carpi radialis brevis) (Ortho).

ECRL (extensor carpi radialis longus) (Ortho).

ECS (extracellular-like, calcium-free solution). See *cardioplegic solution*.

ecstatic (Psych)—exhibiting great elation or enthusiasm. Cf. *ectatic*.

ECT (electroconvulsive therapy).

ectatic—stretched or distended. Cf. *ecstatic*.

Ectra system (Ortho)—for endoscopic release of the transverse carpal ligament in carpal tunnel syndrome.

EDAM (10-ethyl-deaza-aminopterin, 10-EdAM) (Oncol)—a single agent chemotherapy drug.

EDAP (etoposide, dexamethasone, Ara-C, Platinol)—chemotherapy protocol used to treat multiple myeloma.

EDC (extensor digitorum communis) (Ortho).

eddy currents; eddies—MRI term.

edema
brawny
pitting

Eder-Puestow metal olive dilator (Surg).

Edgeahead phaco slit knife (Oph)—used during cataract surgery.

Edinger-Westphal nucleus—the parasympathetic nucleus from which arises the oculomotor nerve (cranial nerve III), for constriction of the pupil and accommodation of the lens for near vision.

Edmondson Grading System in small hepatocellular carcinoma; it is written EdGr II, etc.

EEA stapler (end-to-end anastomosis) (Neuro, Surg).

EEC syndrome—ectrodactyly-ectodermal dysplasia-clefting syndrome, including hypertelorism, cleft lip or palate, or both, and possibly seizures.

effacement—abnormal flattening of the contour of a structure.

effect—(verb)—to execute, accomplish, bring to pass, as "This therapy should effect a cure"; (noun)—an immediate result produced by an agent or cause, as "The surgical procedure produced a good cosmetic effect." Also, proarrhythmic; Somogyi; Tyndall effect. Cf. *affect*.

efferent—moving away from the center. Cf. *afferent*.

E5 monoclonal antibody—a drug obtained from mice and found to be effective against gram-negative sepsis (a virulent and deadly multisystem disease caused by the endotoxins released in the blood stream by gram-negative bacteria). E5 binds to the endotoxins, inactivating them.

effusion—escape of a fluid into a part. Examples: pericardial and pleural. Cf. *infusion*.

eflornithine (DFMO, Ornidyl)—used to treat *Pneumocystis carinii* pneumonia in AIDS patients. It has an antiprotozoal action and is also used to treat sleeping sickness.

EFM (electronic fetal monitoring) (Obs) uses telephone transmission of data and remote sensory devices for patient monitoring.

Egan's mammography (Radiol)—a set of procedures for mammographic examination developed by Robert L. Egan, M.D., the author of a standard textbook and many articles on mammography.

EG/BUS (external genitalia/Bartholin's glands, urethra, and Skene's glands).

EGD (esophagogastroduodenoscopy).

Ehlers-Danlos syndrome—increased laxity and elasticity in the supporting structures of the joints; can also follow neurosyphilis or severe rheumatoid arthritis.

EIA (enzyme-linked immunoassay)—used in the detection of AIDS-associated retroviruses.

eicosapentaenoic acid (EPA)—a marine fatty acid, an analogue of arachidonic acid that is found in fish, some other marine oils, and also possibly in seaweeds. Some researchers think that a diet rich in EPA may be protection against thrombosis in patients with high serum cholesterol and triglyceride levels.

EID (Emergency Infusion Device)—percutaneous central venous large-bore catheter.

Eifrig intraocular implant lens.

Einhorn regimen of chemotherapy.

Eisenmenger complex—congenital heart anomaly.

EIWA (Escala Inteligencia Wechsler Para Adultos) (Psych). The Wechsler Adult Intelligence Scale for administration to adults who speak only Spanish.

ejection fraction, Teicholz.

EKG leads (electrocardiograph)
cardiac leads—I, II, III, V_1 to V_6
augmented leads: aVF, aVL, aVR

Ektascan laser printer (Radiol)—used in digital imaging.

elastic fibers stain (Weigert)—a special tissue stain to reveal the presence of elastin (a fibrous microscopic cell protein) found in skin and vessels.

elastica-van Gieson's stain.

Elastikon elastic tape—for pressure dressings.

Elasto-Gel shoulder therapy wrap (Phys Ther)—used for giving heat treatments for shoulder injuries.

Elastomull—an elastic gauze bandage—a double-woven stretch dressing.

Eldisine (vindesine) (Oncol)—chemotherapy drug.

electroconvulsive therapy (ECT).

electrode. When a neurosurgeon says: "The electrode was connected with zero two zero negative polarity," it should be written 0-2/0 negative.
Types of electrodes:
Aspen laparoscopy
Bioplus dispersive
esophageal pill
Greenwald flexible endoscopic
Levin thermocouple cordotomy
Megadyne/Fann E-Z laparoscopic
Nashold TC
scalp
ventroposterolateral thalamic
VPL (ventroposterolateral) thalamic

electrogalvanic stimulation (Ortho)—used in treatment of fractures. See *pulsing current.*

electromechanical dissociation (EMD) **of the heart.**

electronic fetal monitoring (EFM).

electro-oculogram apparatus—used in determining saccadic velocity (Oph).

electrophoresis—a process in which charged particles (such as ions), suspended in liquid, are moved under the influence of an applied electrical field. Note the different root words in electrophoresis *(phoresis,* carrying, transmission) and plasmapheresis *(apheresis,* separation).

electrophysiologic study (EPS).

electroretinogram, -graphy (ERG).

electrostimulation—see *pulsing current.*

electrotransfer test—see *Western blot electrotransfer test.*

elemental diet—for burn patients, a diet which is a high-nitrogen liquid which requires almost no digestion and produces little residue.

elevator
- Aufricht
- Boies nasal fracture
- Buec uterine
- Freer
- Hough hoe
- Somer uterine
- Soonawalla uterine
- Tessier

ELF (etoposide, leucovorin, fluorouracil)—chemotherapy protocol used to treat gastric carcinoma.

elicit—to draw out, as "We could elicit little information as to the patient's past medical history." Cf. *illicit.*

Elipten (aminoglutethimide).

ELISA (enzyme-linked immunosorbent assay)—the first "AIDS test" used by the blood banks to diminish the chance of HIV infection through a blood transfusion, but ELISA can also be used to test for things other than the HIV antibody.

Elite dual-chamber rate responsive pacemaker (Cardio)—marketed by Medtronic, weighing only 1½ oz., and using CapSure SP leads.

Ellestad protocol—treadmill stress test (Cardio).

Ellik kidney stone basket; evacuator (Urol).

Ellingson intraocular implant lens (Oph).

Ellsworth, in *Reese-Ellsworth classification of retinoblastoma.*

Eloesser flap (Cardio).

ELP broach (Surg).

ELP femoral prosthesis (Ortho).

ELP stem for hip arthroplasty (Ortho).

Elsberg cannula (Neuro).

EL10—a drug used to treat AIDS.

elusion—an adroit or clever escape; escape notice of, as "Elusion of a fourth parathyroid gland indicated its possible congenital absence." Cf. *allusion, illusion.*

embolization, Silastic bead.

embolus
- pantaloon
- polyurethane foam
- saddle
- straddling

embryoscopy (Ob-Gyn)—the use of a fiberoptic endoscope to visualize a fetus in the first trimester. This technique allows greater access to very tiny fetuses than ultrasonographically guided prenatal diagnostic testing.

Emcyt ("m-site") (estramustine phosphate sodium)—used in treatment of prostatic carcinoma that is unresponsive to estrogen therapy.

EMD (electromechanical dissociation) (Cardio)—"He was defibrillated into asystole and treated with atropine, but he went into an EMD and we were unable, despite continued and adequate CPR, to resuscitate him."

Emergency Infusion Device (EID). See *EID.*

Emmet-Studdiford method of perineorrhaphy.

Eminase (anistreplase).

eminence (Ortho)—a bony projection. Cf. *imminent.*

EMI scanner (''emmy'')—the original CT scanner. EMI (Electrical Musical Instruments, a British company.)

empty nest syndrome—restlessness and depression in parents whose children have grown up and left home.

empty sella syndrome (Neuro)—diagnosed in patient with an enlarged sella turcica, where there is no tumor present and the sella fills with air on pneumoencephalogram.

EMS (eosinophilia-myalgia syndrome).

Emulsifier. See *Phaco-Emulsifier-aspirator* used in cataract extractions.

E-MVAC (escalated methotrexate, vinblastine, Adriamycin, cisplatin or Cytoxan)—chemotherapy protocol used to treat tumors of the urothelial tract.

EMV grading, Glasgow Coma Scale; E = eyes; M = motor; V = voice. Written as $E_2M_4V_2$. The Glasgow Coma Scale goes to 8. See *Glasgow Coma Scale.*

ENA (extractable nuclear antigen).

ENANB hepatitis—enterically transmitted non-A, non-B hepatitis.

ENBA (Epstein-Barr virus nuclear antigen).

encainide (Enkaid) (Cardio)—temporarily withdrawn from the market by the manufacturer in 1992. Used in treating premature ventricular contractions.

encapsulated liposomes. See *liposomes.*

encephalomyelitis, myalgic.

encephalopathy, painter's (Neuro)—a chronic organic brain syndrome secondary to exposure to fumes from some types of paints.

endarterectomy and coronary artery bypass grafting (E-CABG).

Ender nail or rod fixation (Ortho)—for fixation of long bone fractures.

endogenous morphine (endorphins).

Endoloop (Surg)—disposable chromic ligature suture instrument.

endolymphatic hypertension.

Endo-Model rotating knee joint prosthesis (Ortho)—permits flexion of the joint up to 165°.

Endopath ES (GI)—reusable endoscopic stapler.

endophthalmitis (Oph)—inflammation of the internal structures of the eye or the adjacent tissues.

Endo-P-Probe (Surg, Urol)—used in combination with standard ultrasound machines for endorectal ultrasonography.

endoprosthesis, Wall stent biliary.

endorphin (**end**ogenous m**orphine**)—natural morphine-like compound produced by the brain.

endoscope, endoscopy
echocolonoscope
echogastroscope
embryoscopy
Karl Storz Calcutript
Karl Storz flexible
lingoscope
Messerklinger
Olympus CF-UM3 colonoscope
velolaryngeal

endoscopic laser cholecystectomy—see *laparoscopic laser cholecystectomy.*

endoscopic retrograde cholangiopancreatogram (ERCP).

endoscopic transpapillary catheterization of the gallbladder (ETCG) (GI)—a procedure to dissolve gallstones. The gallbladder is catheterized using an ERCP catheter. The catheter with a hydrophilic guide wire is passed through the nose and

endoscopic transpapillary cath *(cont.)* advanced via a retrograde approach through the common bile duct. The ERCP catheter is then exchanged for a radiopaque Teflon biliary dilating catheter that allows the guide wire to be inserted into the cystic duct and gallbladder. The next day the patient undergoes both extracorporeal shock-wave lithotripsy and infusion of solvent through the catheter to dissolve gallstones.

endoscopic ultrasonography (EUS) (GI)—examination of the esophagus and stomach with ultrasound using an echogastroscope. It can measure the thickness of the gastric folds and determine the depth to which carcinoma has invaded the stomach wall in order to stage esophageal and gastric carcinomas. It produces the different layers of the gastrointestinal wall.

endoscopic variceal sclerotherapy (EVS).

Endosol (Oph, ENT)—balanced salt solution for eye or ENT irrigation in surgery.

Endotak C lead (Cardio)—a combination transvenous catheter and lead used with automatic implantable cardioverter defibrillators.

endotracheal tube, Lanz low-pressure cuff.

Enduron acetabular liner (Ortho)—a ball liner made with UHMWPe (ultra-high molecular weight polyethylene) for extra strength to prevent cracking.

enema, air contrast barium (ACBE).

en face ("ahn fahs")—Fr. "in front" or "head on." "X-rays revealed left chest wall and diaphragmatic pleural plaques, the former seen both in profile and en face."

engaged, engagement (Obs)—said of the fetal head as it enters and becomes lodged in the superior pelvic strait.

enisoprost—a drug given in conjunction with cyclosporine (Sandimmune) to decrease its toxicity in patients who have an organ transplant.

Enkaid (encainide).

Enlon-Plus—a drug combination of atropine and edrophonium which blocks the effects of muscle relaxants used during general anesthesia.

enoxacin (Comprecin, Penetrax)—a fluoroquinolone type of antibiotic used to treat gonorrhea and urinary tract infections. It has a broad spectrum of antibacterial activity similar to Cipro.

ENP (extractable nucleoprotein).

Ensure Plus—a liquid diet formula.

Entamoeba histolytica—parasite which can be very virulent in AIDS.

Entera-Flo (GI)—enteral feeding pump for use with Entera closed tube feeding products that look like boxed drink containers.

enteral (GI)—pertaining to the small intestine or to administration of a drug or solution via the small intestine. Example: enteral feedings via tube. Cf. *parenteral.*

enterically transmitted non-A, non-B hepatitis (ENANB).

Enterobacter gergoviae.

Enterobacter liquefaciens, now *Serratia liquefaciens*—has been isolated from the intestinal tract, respiratory tract, blood, and urine.

Enterobacter sakazakii—formerly *E. cloacae.*

enterocleisis—closure of a wound in the intestine. Also, occlusion of the lumen of the intestine. Cf. *enteroclysis.*

enteroclysis—the injection of a nutritional or medicinal liquid into the bowel. Cf. *enterocleisis.*

enterokinase—an enzyme of the small intestine.

enteroscopy, small-bowel (SBE).

Entero-Test—a method for retrieving duodenal contents without intubation; the patient swallows a nylon line coiled inside a gelatin capsule.

entity, new chemical (NCE).

enucleation (Oph)—removal of the eyeball, without taking the eye muscles or the remaining orbital contents. Also, shelling out a tumor from its bed without rupturing it.

enuresis (Urol)—bed-wetting. Enuresis differs from incontinence in that enuresis more commonly refers to involuntary discharge of urine during sleep. Cf. *anuresis.*

Envacor—Abbott's trade name for a lab test of two HIV proteins.

enzyme, cathepsin D.

enzyme immunoassay technique—screens drugs in the urine that have been present for up to 7 days.

enzyme-linked immunoassay (EIA).

enzyme-linked immunosorbent assay (ELISA).

EOG (electro-oculogram)—used in sleep studies, as in "EOG does show some rapid eye movement."

eosinophilia-myalgia syndrome (EMS)—the correct name for the group of symptoms resulting from the use of the amino acid L-tryptophan. The clinical picture of severe myalgia, fever, and arthralgias can be confused with myositis or trichinosis unless a history of L-tryptophan use is established.

EP (evoked potential)—a noninvasive way to examine the functional integrity of the central nervous system. It demonstrates the response of the brain to electrical stimulation. EPs are used as indicators, both diagnostic and prognostic, in patients with head injuries. See *brain tests, noninvasive.*

EPA (eicosapentaenoic acid).

Ependorf angiocatheter.

ependyma—cells lining the fluid-filled central cavity of the brain and spinal cord.

ependymitis granularis—granular inflammation of the lining membrane of the ventricles of the brain.

ependymoma—tumor originating from ependymal cells lining the ventricular system of the central nervous system.

EPI (epirubicin).

"epi"—slang term for epinephrine (Adrenalin); also, epithelial cell seen in urinalysis. See *Eppy.*

epi-ADR, epi-Adriamycin (epirubicin).

epicritic—two-point sensation (Neuro).

epidermal growth factor (Oph, Plas Surg)—given to increase the rate of corneal healing after corneal transplant surgery. Used to accelerate wound healing in partial-thickness wounds and second-degree burns.

epihidrosis—excessive perspiration.

epinephrine—used as an adjunct with local anesthetic to prolong the effectiveness of the anesthetic agent used and to constrict superficial blood vessels. Also, racemic epinephrine. Cf. *"epi," Eppy.*

epiphysis—the end of a long bone, usually wider than the long portion of the bone. Cf. *apophysis, hypophysis, hypothesis.*

epirubicin (epi-Adriamycin, epi-ADR, EPI)—a chemotherapy drug.

episiotomy, in *Matsner median episiotomy and repair.*

Epistat double balloon (ENT)—used in treatment of uncontrolled epistaxis.

epistaxis—nasal bleeding.

epithelium, retinal pigment (RPE).

Epitrain (Ortho)—an elastic elbow support with contoured silicone inserts.

EPL (extracorporeal piezoelectric lithotriptor) (Urol)—a device with a single-focus dish which directs all of the shock waves to the renal stone or gallstone, eliminating any unfocused shock waves that could cause the patient pain or discomfort (thus eliminating the need for anesthesia). The stone is then reduced to fragments 2 mm or less in size which are then readily passed by the patient. Trade name: Piezolith-EPL.

EPO—a synthetic form of erythropoietin. It is given to stimulate RBC production in AIDS patients taking zidovudine (Retrovir). See also *epoetin alfa.*

EPOCH (etoposide, prednisone, Oncovin, Cytoxan, Halotestin)—chemotherapy protocol. Used to treat refractory lymphoma.

epoetin alfa (*not* alpha) (erythropoietin; Epogen; Procrit)—a genetically engineered erythropoietin used in treatment of severe anemias (such as those that are a side effect of AZT therapy, and dialysis), and anemia found in patients who are in chronic kidney failure.

Epogen (epoetin alfa).

Eppy—the Barnes-Hind brand of epinephrine borate; used to treat glaucoma. Cf. *"epi."*

Eprex (erythropoietin)—a recombinant human erythropoietin used to treat anemia in AIDS patients.

EPS (electrophysiologic study)—used to assess ventricular arrhythmias.

Epstein-Barr virus. See *EBV.*

equilibratory ataxia—the disturbance of equilibratory coordination, with abnormal gait and station. On testing gait and station, the physician is ruling in/out lesions of the vermis, labyrinthine-vestibular apparatus, and frontopontocerebellar pathways.

equivalent—as in anginal equivalent, migraine equivalent. An atypical pain syndrome, in which the location or character of the pain differs from that usually experienced. "It is not clear whether this left shoulder discomfort radiating down his arm is arthritic or may be an anginal equivalent." Cf. *milliequivalent.*

ER (estrogen receptor)—a cytoplasmic protein. Estrogen receptor tests of breast cancer tissue reflect the degree of hormone dependency of that particular breast cancer. If there is a high degree of hormone dependency, an oophorectomy may be performed to alter the course of the disease.

ER (evoked response) (Neuro).

ERBD (endoscopic retrograde biliary drainage).

Erb's palsy—injury to the fifth and sixth cervical roots, causing flaccid paralysis of the entire arm, without involving the small muscles of the hand. Also called *Erb-Duchenne paralysis* and *Duchenne's paralysis.*

Erb-Duchenne paralysis—see *Erb's palsy.*

ERCP (endoscopic retrograde cholangiopancreatography)—study of the gallbladder, pancreas, and biliary system through an endoscope and a special cannula.

ErecAid system (Urol)—nonsurgical treatment for erectile impotence.

ERG (electroretinography) (Oph).

Ergamisol (levamisole).

ergonovine maleate test for detection of coronary artery disease (Cardio).

Erhardt lid forceps (Oph).

Ernst, in *Lepley-Ernst tube.*

Ergos 02 pacemaker (Cardio)—a dual-chamber rate responsive pacemaker.

Erika dialyzer.

erogenous zones (Psych)—areas of the body that produce feelings of sexual desire when stimulated. Cf. *aerogenous.*

E-rosette receptor.

ERT (estrogen replacement therapy).

***Erwinia* L-asparaginase** (Oncol)—a chemotherapy drug used to treat acute lymphoblastic leukemia. *Erwinia* is a gram-negative bacterium which provides the enzyme L-asparaginase aminohydrolase contained in this version of L-asparaginase. *Erwinia* is used as a source of this enzyme rather than the original source, the gram-negative bacterium *E. coli*, because some patients exhibit sensitivity to the *E. coli*-derived version of L-asparaginase.

ERYC (pronounced "Eric" or "airy-C")—an erythromycin capsule containing enteric-coated little pellets, or beads; an antibiotic.

erysiphake, in *Draeger high vacuum erysiphake.*

Ery-Tab—trade name for an enteric-coated erythromycin tablet.

erythema migrans (EM)—a rash that appears after a bite of the tick (*Ixodes dammini*) that transmits the organism (*Borrelia burgdorferi*) that causes Lyme disease. The rash is circular in form, target-like, may disappear and reappear, often in another site (hence *migrans*). It may be the first symptom of Lyme disease. See *target lesion.*

Erythroflex—a hydromer-coated central venous catheter that resists thrombus formation.

erythroplasia of Queyrat.

erythropoietin, recombinant human (Eprex, Marogen)—used to treat anemia in patients with AIDS or end-stage renal failure.

Escala Inteligencia Wechsler Para Adultos (EIWA).

escape pacemaker (Cardio). Unless an escape pacemaker takes over pacing the ventricles, ventricular standstill occurs, and you will see only P waves on the EKG tracing.

Esmarch bandage ("Ez-mark")—used as a tourniquet.

eso deviation ("ee-so")—inward deviation of the eye; also, esotropia, esophoria (Oph).

esophageal dysmotility (Radiol)—seen on upper GI series; abnormality in the strength or coordination of peristaltic movements in the esophagus.

esophageal pill electrode (Cardio)—a disposable EKG lead encased in a gelatin capsule which is swallowed by the patient. Two attached wires exit through the patient's mouth and are attached to an EKG machine. When the gelatin capsule dissolves, electrical activity from the heart can be detected. The esophageal electrode is thus better able to record the electrical activity of the atrial contraction which is obscured with standard EKG leads.

esophagectomy, Lewis-Tanner.

esophagogastroduodenoscopy (EGD)—examination of the esophagus, stomach, and duodenum using an endoscope.

esophagoscope, Schindler.

esophagus, Barrett's.

esotropia—turning inward of the eye; crossed-eye.

estazolam (ProSom)—a sedative drug of the benzodiazepine group (similar to Dalmane and Restoril). Used for treatment of insomnia.

Esterman visual function score—used as the standard, adopted by the American Medical Association, for rating visual field disability (glaucoma). Obtained from the patient's responses to a disability questionnaire. Scores range from I-4-e to V-4-e. (Benjamin Esterman, M.D.)

Estland flap.

estramustine phosphate sodium (Emcyt)—hormonal chemotherapy drug. See *Emcyt.*

estrogen receptor (ER)—used in test of tumor tissue for its response to estrogen therapy; if the membrane accepts estrogen, the estrogen will be used in treatment of the tumor.

estrogen replacement therapy (ERT).

ESWL (extracorporeal shock-wave lithotripsy) (Urol). See *lithotriptor.*

etafilcon A (Acuvue)—disposable contact lens (Oph).

ETCG (endoscopic transpapillary catheterization of the gallbladder).

E_TCO_2 (end-tidal carbon dioxide) (Pulm)—used in addition to arterial blood gas values to assess the patient's ventilatory status.

ethambutol (Myambutol)—a drug used to treat tuberculosis, and now used to treat MAC infection in AIDS patients.

ethanol—alcohol, EtOH.

ethers—see *dihematoporphyrin ethers.*

Ethibond—polyester suture with prethreaded Teflon pledgets.

Ethicon—Teflon paste.

Ethiflex—a synthetic suture material. (Ethibond, Ethiflex, and Ethilon sutures are all manufactured by Ethicon, but they have different coating materials.)

Ethilon—a monofilament nylon suture with extremely low tissue reactions. It comes in black, green, and clear and is a nonabsorbable suture.

ethiofos (amifostine, Ethyol, gammaphos, WR-2721) (Oncol)—used to treat advanced ovarian carcinoma. Acts as a protective agent when cisplatin is used for chemotherapy.

Ethmozine (moricizine).

Ethodian (iophendylate) (Radiol)—a radiopaque contrast medium and diagnostic aid.

ethylene vinyl alcohol (EVAL).

Ethyol (ethiofos).

etidronate (Didronel). This drug, when taken with calcium supplements, has been found to increase bone mass in women with osteoporosis; it can also reduce the incidence of spontaneous fractures experienced by these patients.

E to A changes—on chest examination the patient's "e" sounds like "a" through a stethoscope.

etodolac (Lodine, Ultradol) (Ortho)—an analgesic and nonsteroidal anti-inflammatory drug (NSAID) for use in pain relief and for patients with osteoarthritis. Its side effects are similar to those of other NSAIDs, including abdominal pain and nausea.

etoglucid (Oncol)—a chemotherapy drug for transitional cell bladder carcinoma, administered intravesically.

EtOH (lowercase "t")—ethanol, ethyl alcohol.

etoposide (VP-16, VePesid)—a chemotherapy drug used in treatment of Kaposi's sarcoma and other cancers.

ETT (exercise tolerance test). See *MPHR* and *Bruce protocol.*

EUA (examination under anesthesia).

Eucerin—proprietary name of wool fat-based cream (Derm).

Eulexin (flutamide).

Euro-Collins multiorgan perfusion kit—used for organ procurement and preservation.

EUS (endoscopic ultrasonography).

euthymic—normal thymus gland function.

euthyroid—normal thyroid gland function.

EVA (etoposide, vinblastine, Adriamycin)—chemotherapy protocol used to treat Hodgkin's disease.

Evac-Q-Kwik—administered orally as a bowel prep to clean the colon prior to x-ray.

evacuator, Ellik.

EVAL (ethylene vinyl alcohol) (Neuro). Used for liquid embolization of spinal angiomas (as in Cobb's syndrome). EVAL, not a glue, is used in the same way as cyanoacrylate.

Evans tenodesis (Ortho)—reconstruction of the peroneus brevis tendon to treat chronic lateral ankle instability by reattaching the tendon to the muscle in a slightly overlapped fashion.

Evermed catheters.

evisceration —(1) removal of the contents of the eyeball, but leaving the shell of sclera (Oph); (2) disemboweling; exenteration; splitting open of a surgical wound and subsequent spillage of its contents (Surg).

evoked potential (EP) (Neuro). See *EP.*

evoked response (ER) (Neuro). See *brain tests, noninvasive;* also *EP.*

EVS (endoscopic variceal sclerotherapy) (GI, Surg)—to control variceal hemorrhage, particularly due to portal hypertension.

Ewald total elbow replacement (Ortho).

Ewald tube—used in gastric lavage (Med).

Ewart's sign—pericardial effusion.

Ewing's sarcoma—osteosarcoma.

ExacTech blood glucose meter—for self-testing by diabetics.

examination—see *test.*

excavatum, pectus. (*Not* excurvatum).

excess—the degree or state of surplus, or beyond the usual, as "There was excess peritoneal fluid present." See *base excess.* Cf. *access, axis.*

excision—removal, as of an organ, by cutting. Cf. *incision.*

Exelderm (sulconazole nitrate).

exercise
- Calleja
- Codman
- DeSouza
- Kegel
- Regen's flexion
- Stryker leg

exercise tolerance test (ETT).

EX-FI-RE external fixation system (Ortho)—for reduction and fixation of long bones and for limb lengthening.

exo deviation (Oph)—outward deviation of the eye; also, exotropia, exophoria.

Exosurf Pediatric (colfosceril palmitate) (Neonat)—a synthetic surfactant used to supplement low levels of natural surfactant in the lungs of premature infants suffering from respiratory distress syndrome (RDS), also known as hyaline membrane disease. Surfactant maintains surface tension to prevent the lungs from collapsing with each breath. It is administered via an endotracheal tube. It is also being tested in patients with cystic fibrosis, apnea of prematurity, adult respiratory distress syndrome, and asthma. See *RDS, Survanta.*

expander
AccuSpan tissue
Becker tissue
CUI tissue
Hespan plasma volume
Heyer-Schulte tissue
Intravent tissue
plasma (Hespan, or hetastarch)
PMT AccuSpan tissue
Radovan tissue
Silastic H.P. tissue

expire—(1) to exhale; (2) to take one's last breath, i.e., to die.

expressor, Rizzuti iris.

Express PTCA catheter (percutaneous transluminal coronary angioplasty) (Cardio).

exquisite—said of extremely severe pain or tenderness, as "exquisite tenderness of the breast."

exstrophy—congenital eversion of an organ, as of the bladder.

extension *(not* extention).

extinction phenomenon (Neuro)—when the patient is touched in the same area on both sides of the body and perceives it on only one side; may be indicative of a lesion of the sensory cortex.

extracellular-like, calcium-free solution (ECS).

extracorporeal circulation—using the heart-lung machine to provide circulation outside the body during heart surgery.

extracorporeal membrane oxygenation therapy (ECMO).

extracorporeal piezoelectric lithotriptor (EPL)—see *EPL.*

extracorporeal shock-wave lithotripsy (ESWL). See *lithotriptor.*

extractor (Ortho)—an instrument to remove a metal implant from bone. See *Glassman stone extractor.*

extravasation of contrast (Radiol)—leakage of contrast medium from the structure into which it is injected through a perforation or other abnormal orifice.

extremis, in—at the point of death.

exudate, cotton-wool.

ex vivo (L., outside of the living body). "He mentioned that in the near future there will be a commercial concern which is able to grow blood ex vivo and to have the cells then harvested for therapeutic transfusions."

eye chart; test
Berens 3-character
Birkhauser
Ferris
HRL screening plates
Ishihara color vision
Jaeger
Landolt ring chart
Mentor BVAT
octopus
Snellen
Sonksen-Silver visual acuity
Teller acuity cards (TAC)

eyes
doll's
raccoon
sunset

F, f

Fab—acronym for **f**ragment, **a**ntigen-**b**inding, as in Fab fragment, Fab region, Fab segment. See *digoxin immune Fab (ovine) fragments.*

FAB (French/American/British)—morphologic classification of acute nonlymphoid leukemia:
- M1—myeloblastic, with no differentiation
- M2—myeloblastic, with differentiation
- M3—promyelocytic
- M4—myelomonocytic
- M5—monocytic
- M6—erythroleukemia

FAB staging of carcinoma, as "FAB $T_2N_1M_0$." See *TNM classification.*

fabere sign—acronym for the maneuvers of Patrick's test for hip-joint disease: **f**lexion, **ab**duction, **e**xternal **r**otation, **e**xtension.

Fabry's disease (Oph)—verticillate keratopathy (whorl-shaped); a lipid-storage disease.

FAC (5-fluorouracil, Adriamycin, Cytoxan)—chemotherapy protocol used to treat breast carcinoma.

facial (Derm, ENT)—pertaining to the face. Cf. *falcial, fascial.*

FAC-M (fluorouracil, Adriamycin, Cytoxan, methotrexate)—chemotherapy protocol.

factor (See *cogulation factors.*)
- autocrine motility (AMF)
- blood coagulation
- cardiac risk
- coagulation
- epidermal growth
- fibroblast growth
- nerve growth (NGF)
- Rh (Rhesus)
- rheumatoid (RF)
- Stuart
- thymic humoral
- tumor necrosis (TNF)
- von Willebrand's

Factor III multimer assay, as "The patient's Factor III multimer assay is still pending."

Faden retropexy (Oph)—posterior fixation suture procedure used in strabismus surgery.

fadir sign—acronym for maneuvers used to test the hip joint: **f**lexion, **ad**duction, **i**nternal **r**otation.

Fagan test (Psych, Peds)—used to detect retardation in infants. A six-month-old is shown a picture for a

Fagan *(cont.)* certain period of time. Later, the infant is shown the same picture and a new picture. The amount of time the infant looks at the new picture correlates with overall intelligence.

failed back surgery syndrome (FBSS) (Ortho)—seen in patients who have persistent back pain following back surgery. Further testing often reveals a migrated disk fragment, another disk herniation at a different level, previously undetected lateral recess syndrome (stenosis), a tethered nerve root, an anomalous root or tumor above the level of the previous surgery.

Fajersztajn's crossed sciatic sign (Ortho).

Falcao suction dissector (ENT).

falcial—see *falcine region.* Cf. *facial, fascial.*

falcine region—either the region of the falx cerebelli or the falx cerebri. Also *falcial.*

Fallot's pentalogy—tetralogy of Fallot plus atrial septal defect. See *Fallot's trilogy, tetralogy of Fallot.*

Fallot's trilogy—congenital cyanotic heart disease that includes pulmonary stenosis, atrial septal defect, but does *not* have any ventricular septal defect. See *Fallot's pentalogy, tetralogy of Fallot.*

Falope ring (Ob-Gyn).

false labor. See *Braxton Hicks contractions.*

false negative—a test result that is normal or negative despite the presence in the patient of a disease or condition that would be expected to produce an abnormal or positive test result.

false positive—an abnormal or positive test result in a patient who is healthy or free from the condition tested for.

falx cerebri (Neuro)—a sickle-shaped fold of tough connective tissue partially separating the two cerebral hemispheres.

FAM (Oncol)—a chemotherapy protocol used to treat recurrent gastric, biliary tract carcinoma, and large-cell undifferentiated carcinomas. Consists of the drugs 5-fluorouracil, Adriamycin, and mitomycin C.

FAM-CF (fluorouracil, Adriamycin, mitomycin, citrovorum factor)—chemotherapy protocol.

FAME (fluorouracil, Adriamycin, MeCCNU)—chemotherapy protocol.

FAMP (fludarabine monophosphate).

FAMTX (fluorouracil, Adriamycin, methotrexate [MTX])—chemotherapy protocol used to treat gastric carcinoma.

FANA (fluorescent antinuclear antibody).

Fansidar (sulfadoxine-pyrimethamine). Used for prophylaxis and treatment of chloroquine-resistant falciparum malaria. Now used as an AIDS drug.

Fanta eye speculum (Oph).

FAP (Oncol)—a standard chemotherapy protocol used to treat gastric carcinoma. Consists of the drugs 5-fluorouracil, Adriamycin, and Platinol.

FAPs (fibrillating action potentials).

Faraday shield—MRI term.

faradic (electrical) **stimulation.** Named for Michael Faraday, English physicist, 1791-1867.

farmer's lung disease—extrinsic allergic alveolitis caused by exposure to moldy hay.

Farr test—a specific test for anti-DNA antibodies in screening for systemic lupus erythematosus (SLE). High titers of anti-DNA antibodies would be diagnostic of SLE.

farsightedness—see *presbyopia.*

fascial (Surg)—pertaining to the subcutaneous layer of fascia found throughout the body and encountered during surgery. Cf. *facial, falcial.*

fast low-angle shot (FLASH)—MRI term (Radiol).

fast-Fourier transform (FFT)—MRI term (Radiol).

fast-twitch fibers—fast runners have relatively more of these than the rest of the population in their skeletal muscles.

fat depot ("de-po")—area in the body of deposit of stored fat. "The face was very bony, showing loss of fat depots."

fat embolism syndrome (FES).

fat pad sign (Ortho)—"X-rays of the right elbow show no acute bony injury or any posterior fat pad sign per the radiologist's interpretation."

fat towels (or wound towels) (Surg). Used in surgery to protect tissues, to keep them from losing moisture.

Faulkner folder (Oph)—an instrument which holds an intraocular lens in a folded position for insertion during cataract surgery.

Favoloro sternal retractor (Surg).

FAZ (foveal avascular zone) (Oph).

FBI (food-borne illness).

FBSS (failed back surgery syndrome).

FCAP (fluorouracil, Cytoxan, Adriamycin, Platinol)—chemotherapy protocol used to treat breast carcinoma.

FCU (flexor carpi ulnaris) (Ortho).

FDI (frequency domain imaging)—in ultrasound (Radiol).

FEC (fluorouracil, epirubicin, Cytoxan)—chemotherapy protocol used to treat breast carcinoma.

Fechner intraocular implant lens (Oph).

F_ECO_2 (fraction of expired carbon dioxide)—recorded numerically on a capnograph.

FED (fluorouracil, etoposide, DDP [cisplatin])—chemotherapy protocol.

Federici's sign—a sign of gas in the abdomen, or peritonitis, when cardiac sounds are heard on abdominal auscultation.

feeding solution—see *medication.*

feeding tube—see *tube.*

$FEF_{25\text{-}75\%}$ (forced midexpiratory flow)—a measure of the rate at which the patient can expel air from the lungs. Flow is measured in liters per second during the median half of forced expiration—that is, from the time that 25% of total volume has been expelled to the time that 75% has been expelled. This study is more sensitive to mild airway obstruction than other tests of pulmonary function. "Spirometry obtained at this time reveals a normal examination, with the exception of the $FEF_{25\text{-}75\%}$ which is reduced to 50% of predicted. These findings are sometimes considered indicative of some degree of small airway disease."

Fein antrum trocar needle (ENT).

Felig insulin pump—worn externally.

fellow—the holder of a fellowship for teaching or research, an academic appointment carrying a stipend and providing facilities for postdoctoral study or research. Teaching fellow, research fellow.

felodipine (Plendil) (Cardio)—a once-a-day calcium channel blocker for mild to moderate hypertension.

felon—an abscess of the fingertip. See *herpes whitlow.*

femtoliter (fL)—unit of measurement in mean corpuscular volume (MCV)—one-quadrillionth of a liter.

fenestra ovalis; fenestra vestibuli. See *vestibular window.*

fenestrated Drake clip (Neuro)—for clipping of intracranial aneurysm.

fenestrated drape—sterile surgical drape with round opening to expose just the operative site.

fenestrated tracheostomy tube—tracheostomy tube with an opening on its upper surface that permits the patient to talk while still keeping the airway open.

fenestrating—the making of openings. Cf. *festinating.*

fenestration—a window-like inclusion in a cell caused by large cellular spaces called vacuoles.

fenoterol (Berotec) (Pulm)—drug used to prevent bronchial asthma attacks.

fentanyl (Duragesic) (Oncol)—a narcotic available in a transdermal patch designed to provide 72 hours of continuous pain control in patients with cancer. Prior to development of the transdermal patch, fentanyl (Sublimaze) was commonly used in combination with inhaled anesthetics to maintain general anesthesia.

fentanyl citrate (Peds)—a narcotic drug previously given by injection with regional or general anesthesia. Available in a candy-like oral tablet (to be sucked); for pediatric patients to relieve severe pain. Oral transmucosal fentanyl citrate is abbreviated OTFC.

fern test—used in obstetrics to determine the level of estrogen secretion; so-called because of the fernlike appearance of the cervical and uterine mucus when it dries on the glass slide.

Ferris chart—measures visual acuity (Oph).

ferromagnetic—MRI term.

fertilization, in vitro (IVF).

FES (fat embolism syndrome) (Pulm). A complication of long-bone fracture or trauma to fatty tissues, FES occurs when an embolus of fat lodges in the lungs. FES is a type of ARDS (adult respiratory distress syndrome).

$FeSO_4$—chemical symbol for iron sulfate.

festinating gait—the short, accelerating steps seen in patients with Parkinson's disease. Cf. *fenestrating.*

fetal-pelvic index (Ob-Gyn)—a method of determining the presence of fetal-pelvic disproportion which is more accurate than estimated fetal weights by ultrasonography, the use of the Mengert index, or x-ray pelvimetry. A positive fetal-pelvic index indicates fetal-pelvic disproportion and the need for a cesarean section. A false negative result can occur in the presence of a malpositioned fetus.

fetal small parts—the extremities of a fetus as felt through the mother's abdominal wall.

Feuerstein myringotomy drain tube (ENT).

FEV (forced expiratory volume). The subscript, as in FEV_1, indicates the number of seconds in which the forced expiratory volume is measured.

fever
dengue hemorrhagic (DHF)
Fort Bragg

fever *(cont.)*
Haverhill
Pontiac
Q
ratbite
spiking

FFP (fresh frozen plasma).

FFT (fast-Fourier transform)—MRI term. See *Fourier analysis.*

FGF (fibroblast growth factor).

FIAC (fiacitabine).

fiacitabine (FIAC)—drug used to treat AIDS and ARC patients, HIV-positive patients, and CMV infections.

fialuridine (FIAU)—drug used to treat patients with AIDS and ARC, HIV-positive patients, and herpesvirus infections.

FIAU (fialuridine).

fiberoptic bronchoscopy (FOB).

fiber
C-fiber
James
Purkinje's
Remak
Rosenthal
Sharpey's

fiberoptic, fiber optic, fibreoptic—these three different versions appear in different books and journals, with *fiberoptic* the most common. *Fibreoptic* is a British spelling. See *Luxtec fiberoptic system.*

fibrillating action potentials (FAPs).

fibrin glue—a surgical adhesive (Surg, Neuro). "I reconstituted the anterior wall of the sella with a piece of nasal septal cartilage, and then over this I applied fibrin glue in which I placed a piece of subcutaneous fat."

fibroblast growth factor (FGF).

fibrocystic breast disease—see *breast fibrocystic disease, stages of.*

fibromuscular dysplasia (FMD).

fibrose—a verb meaning to form fibrous tissue. Cf. *fibrous.*

fibrous—an adjective describing something composed of fibers.

Fick method (Cardio). The oxygen content of exhaled air is measured to determine oxygen consumption in a patient undergoing cardiac catheterization. This is then compared to the oxygen levels from an arterial blood sample and a venous blood sample. The differences in oxygenation are used to calculate the cardiac output.

Fick sacculotomy (ENT)—a procedure for treatment of progressive endolymphatic hydrops (Ménière's disease). Picks are introduced through the footplate of the stapes to puncture the saccule, thus producing a permanent fistula in the saccular wall to drain endolymph into the perilymphatic space. See *Cody tack operation.*

FID (free induction decay)—MRI term.

field gradient; field lock—MRI terms.

FIGO (Fédération Internationale de Gynécologie et Obstétrique)—used in staging adenocarcinoma of the endometrium, e.g., FIGO II. It was originally *FEGO* (**F**ederation of **G**ynecology and **O**bstetrics) but now the French abbreviation is used.

figure 4 position (Ortho)—so-called because in this position the patient lies with the right side of the body up and brings the right ankle up to rest on the left knee, forming the figure 4.

fil d'Arion silicone tube (Oph).

filiforms and followers (Urol)—used to dilate a urethral stricture.

filgrastim (Neupogen) (Oncol)—a white blood cell stimulator that counteracts the myelosuppression caused by chemotherapy. See *G-CSF.*

filling defect (Radiol)—a zone within a tubular structure that is not filled by injected contrast medium (usually a tumor or abnormal mass).

filling factor—MRI term.

filmy adhesion (Surg).

filter
Gianturco-Roehm bird's nest vena cava
Greenfield IVC
Kim-Ray Greenfield caval
Mobin-Uddin umbrella
Vena Tech LGM vena cava

filter replacement fluid (FRF).

filtered-back projection (Radiol).

filtering bleb (Oph)—a tiny, surgically coated vesicle, or blister, placed over a passageway into the eye to provide drainage in treatment of open-angle glaucoma.

filum terminale—thread-like extension of the spinal cord from conus medullaris to the tip of the dural sac.

finasteride (MK-906) (Oncol)—a chemotherapy drug given to prostatic cancer patients who have already had a radical prostatectomy.

fine-angled curet (*not* Fine) (Neuro).

fine-needle aspiration biopsy (FNAB). Also, *skinny needle, Chiba needle.*

finger cot—surgical glove material to fit just one finger.

finger fracture (Surg)—blunt dissection performed with the surgeon's fingers.

finger friction (ENT)—"She cannot hear finger friction in either ear." Rubbing thumb and index finger together makes an audible—well, *rubbing* sound. It may not be heard by someone with hearing loss.

fingerprint dystrophy—a corneal dystrophy characterized by fine, wavy, concentric lines that may be associated with a map- or dot-like pattern.

fingerstick devices for blood glucose testing: Autoclix, Autolet, Monojector.

finger-to-nose test (F to N) (Neuro). The patient is asked to touch his nose with the index finger of one hand and then the other, with the eyes closed, alternating hands and increasing speed. In a variation of this test, the patient is asked to touch his nose and then the examiner's finger at a distance of 12 to 18 inches, with increasing speed. This test is used to evaluate the patient's coordination, and may be one of the neurologic tests administered in the physical examination.

Finkelstein's sign; test (Ortho)—for synovitis of the abductor pollicis longus tendon.

Finney Flexi-Rod penile prosthesis (Urol).

Finochietto rib retractor.

FIRDA (frontal irregular rhythmic delta activity)—in EEG. "Since the amplitude of the FIRDA was greatest over the left hemisphere, it may in this instance also suggest a possible left frontal structural lesion."

first pass effect—metabolic action of the liver on drugs. A drug that is taken orally first passes through the liver before reaching the general circulation to exert any systemic effect. For some drugs the first-pass effect is so extensive that almost all of the drug dose is immediately metabolized. Some drugs are not metabolized and are excreted unchanged through the kidneys. A decreased rate of drug metabolism occurs in patients with liver diseases and hepatitis, impaired liver function due to aging, or immature liver function in premature infants.

first pass view (in multiple gated acquisition scan, or MUGA) (Radiol)—an image or set of images obtained immediately after injection of radionuclide into the circulation, when its concentration in the blood pool is at its highest.

first-toe Jones repair (Ortho).

Fisch drill (ENT)—named for Professor Ugo Fisch of University of Zurich.

fishbone pattern of sclerotic white retinal arterioles and venules—often seen in lattice degeneration of the retina (Oph). Also called crosshatch pattern.

fish meal lung disease—extrinsic allergic alveolitis caused by exposure to fish meal.

fissula—a little groove. Cf. *fissura, fistula.*

fissura—fissure, a general reference to a groove or cleft, e.g., fissura cerebri lateralis (fissure of Sylvius). Cf. *fissula, fistula.*

fistula (cf. *fissula, fissura)*—aberrant passage from one organ to another, or from an organ through to the outside surface of the body. Types:
AV (arteriovenous)
brachioaxillary bridge graft
brachiosubclavian bridge graft
Brescio-Cimino AV
cameral
perilymphatic (PLF)

Fitz-Hugh and Curtis syndrome—gonococcal perihepatitis in women with a history of gonorrheal salpingitis.

5-ASA (5-aminosalicylic acid)—see *mesalamine.*

5-azacytidine—see *azacitidine.*

5-FU (5-fluorouracil)—antineoplastic chemotherapeutic agent.

5-HIAA (hydroxyindoleacetic acid)—substance found in the urine of patients with carcinoid tumors of intestine.

5-HT$_1$ and **5-HT$_2$ receptors** (Psych)—two types of serotonin receptors present in the central nervous system which are stimulated by certain drugs such as buspirone (BuSpar) to relieve anxiety. Serotonin is also known as 5-hydroxytryptamine (5-HT).

5-HT$_3$ receptors (Oncol)—a serotonin receptor found in the chemoreceptor trigger zone of the brain and in the GI tract. The stimulation of these receptors is thought to trigger the vomiting reflex. The antiemetic drug ondansetron (Zofran) is the first drug in the class of 5-HT$_3$ receptor blockers and is used to prevent vomiting in chemotherapy patients.

5'nucleotidase (5'NT) ("five prime nucleotidase").

566C80—drug used to treat *Pneumocystis carinii* pneumonia and toxoplasmosis in AIDS patients.

five-view chest x-ray (*not* 5-U)—AP, PA, lateral, and both oblique views. "A five-view chest x-ray series was obtained."

fixation, fixator
Ace-Fischer
Ace Unifix
Calandruccio triangular compression
cementless
Ender nail or rod
EX-FI-RE external
Georgiade visor halo
Hoffmann external
hydroxyapatite
LPPS hydroxyapatite
Luque rod
Monticelli-Spinelli leg

fixation *(cont.)*
Orthofix
Pennig dynamic wrist fixator
Precision Osteolock
Rogozinski spinal
Seidel intramedullary
TiMesh implantable hardware
Versa-Fx femoral
Vidal-Ardrey modified Hoffmann
Wolvek sternal approximation
Zickel nail
ZMS intramedullary

fixation device (Ortho)—any appliance placed surgically in or on a bone to stabilize a fracture during healing. See *fixation.*

fixation hook, Hebra.

fixation ring, in *McNeill-Goldmann blepharostat fixation ring.*

fixative (Path)
glycol methacrylate
Hollande's solution
Zenker's

FK-506 (GI)—an antibiotic which suppresses the action of lymphocytes and prevents rejection of a newly transplanted liver. It is significantly more effective than cyclosporine and causes fewer side effects.

FK-565—a drug used to treat HIV-positive patients.

fL (femtoliter).

FLAC (fluorouracil, leucovorin calcium, Adriamycin, Cytoxan)—chemotherapy protocol used to treat breast carcinoma.

Flack's node—see *sinoatrial node.*

flail chest *(not* frail)—movement of the chest wall inconsistent with respirations; caused by fractures of the ribs.

flap
Abbe-Estlander
axial

flap *(cont.)*
Bakanjian
butterfly
Byers
Chinese
cross-finger
Cutler-Beard bridge
distant pedicle
Eloesser
Estland
free
Gunderson conjunctival
Iselin flag
island
latissimus dorsi myocutaneous
Limberg
liver
meilolabial
Moberg advancement
neurovascular
non-island
radial
Sewell-Boyden
thenar
Thom
TRAM
transposition
transverse rectus abdominis myocutaneous (TRAM)
tummy tuck
V-Y island

FLAP (fluorouracil, leucovorin calcium, Adriamycin, Platinol)—chemotherapy protocol used to treat gastric adenocarcinoma.

flare—sudden exacerbation; a sudden outburst; a spreading out. Also a term used in ophthalmology, as in *aqueous flare, cell and flare, Tyndall effect. Not* flair, which means an aptitude or bent, as in "She has a flair for writing."

flaring, nasal or alar. See *alar flaring.*

Flarex (fluorometholone acetate) (Oph)—a steroid in ophthalmic solution.

FLASH (fast low-angle shot)—an MRI term (Radiol). "FLASH images were obtained with gradient echo technique."

flat or flattened affect—diminished emotional response; apathy.

Flatt finger/thumb prosthesis (Ortho).

Fleischer ring (Oph)—a deposit of iron, ring-shaped, in the cornea; seen with keratoconus. See *Kayser-Fleischer ring.*

Fletcher-Suit applicator (Oncol)—an appliance used for the insertion of radiation sources for treatment of carcinoma of the endometrium. Also, Fletcher applicator.

Flexeril (Ortho)—a skeletal muscle relaxant. Often misspelled "Flexoril" because of association with flexor muscles.

Flexicath silicone subclavian cannula (Nephrol).

Flexiflo gastrostomy tube enteral delivery system (GI).

Flexiflo Stomate low-profile gastrostomy tube (GI)—does not require endoscopy for removal.

Flexinet dressing.

Flexi-Rod II penile prosthesis (Urol).

Flexisplint—flexed arm board used as a restraint after brachial embolectomy or placement of an AV fistula in the forearm.

Flexon stainless steel multistrand suture.

flexor—a muscle that flexes a joint. Cf. *flexure.*

FlexStrand cable—see *Hawkins breast localization needle* (Radiol).

flexure—the bent part of an organ or structure. Cf. *flexor.*

Flexxicon and Flexxicon Blue catheters (Urol)—dialysis catheters with flexible tips.

"flick-ten-yule"—see *phlyctenule.*

Flieringa scleral ring (Oph). Application of the Flieringa ring maintains the shape of the globe when vitreous is lost.

flip angle—MRI term.

floaters (Oph)—translucent specks of various sizes and shapes that float across the visual field; due to small bits of protein on cells floating in the vitreous.

flocculation—bentonite flocculation test for trichinosis.

floppy (Peds)—general term used to describe lack of muscle tone in extremities of newborns, due to hypoxia.

floppy guide wire (Cardio)—a high torque guide wire used in catheterization. See also *high torque floppy guide wire.*

Florida pouch (Urol)—a continent urinary reservoir using a detubularized right colonic segment as the urinary reservoir, thus allowing a large-capacity, low-pressure pouch.

flow cytometry (Urol)—a method to detect recurring bladder cancer by examining the DNA of urothelial cell sediment in urine specimens. It is thought to be more accurate than urine cytology.

flowmeter
Gould electromagnetic
Statham electromagnetic

flow rate, maximum midexpiratory.

flow volume loop—a term used in spirometry reports.

Floxin (ofloxacin).

floxuridine—see *FUdR.*

Floxyfral (fluvoxamine).

FLT (fluorothymidine).

fluconazole (Diflucan)—an antifungal drug similar in its action to ketoconazole (Nizoral) and amphotericin B but with fewer side effects. Used for severe fungal infections, particularly candidiasis, in immunocompromised patients with AIDS, cancer, or organ transplants.

flucytosine (5-FC, Ancobon)—used to treat fungus infections in AIDS and other immunocompromised patients.

Fludara (fludarabine).

fludarabine (FAMP, fludarabine monophosphate, Fludara) (Oncol)—a chemotherapy drug used to treat non-Hodgkin's lymphoma and chronic lymphocytic leukemia.

Flu-Glow (Oph). Interesting name; it sounds as though it would be something that would make you glow in the dark if you have the flu. Not so. Actually it is the name of a fluorescein-impregnated paper strip used to diagnose corneal abrasion or the presence of a foreign body in the eye. The strip is moistened with a sterile solution and placed on the conjunctiva of the lower lid. Any break in the corneal epithelium will permit the fluorescein to be absorbed, and the defect will appear as a bright green fluorescence under appropriate lighting. No defect, no glow.

fluid output, insensible. See *insensible fluid output.*

Flumadine (rimantadine)—an antiviral agent used to prevent infections by influenza type A viruses.

flumazenil (Mazicon)—an antagonist; drug that reverses the action of benzodiazepine sedatives. Used for reversal of surgical anesthesia (particularly after endoscopy) or overdose involving benzodiazepine drugs (such as Valium).

flumecinol (Zixoryn) (Neonat)—used to treat hyperbilirubinemia in infants not responding to phototherapy.

fluorescein angiography (Oph)—evaluates the anatomic and physiologic states of blood vessels in the choroid and retina after intravenous injections of fluorescein dye.

fluorescein uptake (Oph).

Fluorescence activated cell sorter (FACS) (Lab)—an automated lab tool which separates individual cells in a sample by fluorescence and size.

fluorescent treponemal antibody absorption (FTA-ABS)—test for syphilis.

Fluor-i-Strip (Oph). See *Flu-Glow,* a similar product by another manufacturer.

fluorodeoxyglucose (FDG) (Radiol)—a radioactive tracer used to perform a PET scan to evaluate heart function at rest. It is able to differentiate between ischemic and normal myocardium.

fluorodeoxyuridine (FUdR).

fluoroquinolone—a class of antibiotics with a broad spectrum of antibacterial activity. Includes ciprofloxacin (Cipro), norfloxacin (Noroxin), ofloxacin (Floxin), and enoxacin (Penetrax).

fluoroscopy, C-arm.

fluorosilicone oil (Oph)—a type of substitute for vitreous humor, this drug is used to float and help facilitate the removal of a dislocated intraocular lens.

fluorothymidine (FLT)—used to treat patients with AIDS and ARC.

Fluoro Tip cannula (GI)—used during ERCP. Has a radiopaque distal tip for location on fluoroscopy.

Fluosol—an "artificial blood"; actually an oxygen transport medium and

Fluosol *(cont.)* plasma expander. Used in those patients who would refuse blood transfusions.

Fluosol-DA 20%—an oxygen-transport fluid used during percutaneous transluminal coronary angioplasty to increase cardiac oxygenation.

fluoxetine (Prozac)—an antidepressant chemically unrelated to any others but as effective as tricyclic antidepressants.

flupertine maleate—a non-narcotic analgesic for mild to moderate pain.

flush—method of taking blood pressure in infants.

flush aortogram (Cardio).

flutamide (Eulexin)—used to treat advanced prostatic cancer, this drug blocks the uptake of androgen by tumor cells.

fluticasone propionate (Cutivate)—a topical corticosteroid used in dermatological treatment. Similar to betamethasone (Diprosone, Valisone) and dexamethasone (Decaderm).

fluvoxamine (Floxyfral) (Psych)—a drug that is a 5HT blocker and inhibits the reuptake of serotonin by nerve cells in the brain. This results in increased levels of active serotonin which produces a therapeutic action in treating depression and obsessive-compulsive disorders.

flu, yuppie—see *yuppie flu.*

FMD (fibromuscular dysplasia).

fmoles/mg (femtomoles/mg) (Oncol)—a measurement used with estrogen and progesterone receptors to determine if a patient with breast cancer should be categorized as positive or negative. (Greater than 10 fmoles/mg is considered positive.)

FNAB (fine-needle aspiration biopsy).

FNA cytology (fine-needle aspiration).

FNM (fluorouracil, Novantrone, methotrexate)—chemotherapy protocol used to treat breast carcinoma.

FO (foot orthosis) (Pod).

foam cell (foamy histiocyte)—a cell which has a ground-glass-appearing cytoplasm due to accumulation of fat, glycogen, or other material.

foam embolus, polyurethane.

foam stability test; index (Neonat)—a determination of maturity of the fetal lungs, as demonstrated by the ability of pulmonary surfactant in the amniotic fluid to form a stable foam in ethanol after being vigorously shaken. Also called shake test.

FOB (fiberoptic bronchoscopy).

Foerster capsulotomy knife—used in plastic and reconstructive procedures on the breast to remove spherical contractures from the breast pocket during re-do breast implant procedures.

Foerster sponge forceps (Surg).

Fogarty balloon biliary catheter—for removal of gallstones from the biliary tract.

Fogarty catheter—threaded up through a vessel to remove emboli.

Fogarty Hydrogrip clamp.

folinic acid rescue—see *leucovorin rescue.*

Foltz catheter (Neuro).

Folstein's Mini-Mental Status Examination (Neuro)—a method of grading the cognitive state of patients. This is one of the tests administered to patients with symptoms suggestive of Alzheimer's disease.

Fomon retractor (Plas Surg).

Fontan modification of the Norwood procedure for hypoplastic left-sided heart syndrome (Cardio). See *Norwood; Gill/Jonas; Sade.*

Fontan procedure (Cardio)—anastomosis of the right atrial appendage to the pulmonary artery, to separate the left and right heart circulations in patients with levotransposition of the great vessels, single ventricle, atrial septal defect, coarctation of the aorta, and small left atrium.

foot
immersion
Madura
rockerbottom

foot drop—passive plantar flexion of the foot due to paralysis of dorsiflexor muscles.

foot pound—a unit of measurement related to work, or stress placed upon the extremities (Ortho).

foramen of Luschka (Neuro)—opening at the side of the fourth ventricle communicating with the subarachnoid space.

foramen ovale *(not* O'Valley, although it sounds like that)—an opening in the sphenoid bone, through which pass a branch of the trigeminal nerve and some blood vessels (foramen ovale basis cranii), and also an opening in the septum secundum of the heart of the fetus between the atria (foramen ovale cordis).

forced expiratory volume (FEV).

forced vital capacity (FVC).

forceps—an instrument with a pair of blades and handles, used in surgery to grasp tissue, and also surgical sponges, etc. Why do I give this well-known term? Simply to emphasize that, even though the word ends in "s," it is a singular (as well as plural) form—"an instrument." I have known it to be used incorrectly thus: "This was resected with a double-action bone forcep." But grasping with a single blade would be like clapping with one hand or eating with one chopstick. So, "forceps" it is. Examples:
ACMI Martin endoscopy
Acufex straight and curved basket
Aesculap
Allis
Asch septal
ASSI bipolar coagulating
Ballantine
Barnes-Crile
Berke ptosis
bipolar
bipolar coagulating
Blaydes corneal
Bonaccolto
bone-cutting
Bores
Bracken
Bracken iris
Carroll bone-holding
Caspar alligator
Castaneda suture tag
Castroviejo
Colibri
D'Allesandro serial suture-holding
DeBakey-Semb
Desjardin
Diener
Dodick Nucleus Cracker
Drews
Erhardt lid
Foerster sponge
Freeman lens fixation
Fujinon biopsy
Gradle cilia
Grieshaber iris
Halsted
Hardy microbipolar
Hartmann
Hertel rigid dilator stone
Hertel stone
Hildebrandt uterine hemostatic
Hirst placenta
Jaffee capsulorhexis

forceps *(cont.)*
Jansen-Middleton septotomy
Kelman-McPherson angled
Kevorkian-Younge
Kielland (or Kjelland)
Kraff nucleus splitter
Kraff-Utrata tear capsulotomy
Linn-Graefe iris
Llobera fixation
Malis angled-up bipolar
Malis irrigation
Max Fine tying
McPherson lens
microbipolar
Neubauer vitreous microextractor
Noyes nasal dressing
Ogura tissue and cartilage
Olympus FBK 13 endoscopic biopsy
Peyman-Green vitreous
Pierse corneal
Pollock
Poppen
Puntenney
Quire mechanical finger
Rhoton ring tumor
Rhoton titanium microsurgical ring
Rowe disimpaction
Rudd-Clinic hemorrhoidal
Russian
Sachs tissue
Schaaf foreign body
Shepard-Reinstein IOL
Sinskey
sponge
Struempel-Voss ethmoid sinus
Struycken nasal cutting
SureBite biopsy
Takahashi
Tischler cervical biopsy punch
Twisk
Utrata capsulorhexis
Walsham

forceps *(cont.)*
Wies chalazion
Yeoman uterine biopsy

Fordyce granules (Dental)—an ectopic collection of sebaceous glands or choristomas in the oral cavity that require no treatment and cause no untoward effects.

Forel, space of.

forme fruste—atypical form of disease.

FormFlex (no space) **intraocular lens.**

formication (Psych)—a sensation of insects crawling over the skin; most commonly seen in cocaine or amphetamine intoxication. Cf. *fornication.*

fornication—sexual intercourse between unmarried people. Cf. *formication.*

Foroblique lens—*not* four oblique.

Fortaz (ceftazidime).

49er brace (Ortho)—knee brace; probably first used by that football team.

Fort Bragg fever.

fortification spectrum (Neuro)—a jagged formation of bright lines sometimes seen as an aura of migraine headache and in other conditions.

foscarnet (Foscavir; trisodium phosphonoformate)—a Swedish drug, pronounced ''fos-car-net.'' An alternative to ganciclovir in treating cytomegalovirus in AIDS patients, it is also active against herpes and HIV.

Foscavir (foscarnet).

fosinopril (Monopril) (Cardio)—antihypertensive and ACE inhibitor. ACE inhibitors act to prevent angiotensin I from being converted into angiotensin II which is a powerful vasoconstrictor. Less angiotensin II acting on the blood vessels allows the vessels to dilate, thus lowering the blood pressure. See also *ramipril.*

Foss clamp.

fossa (pl., fossae)—a depression, hollow, or channel. "The pain radiates into both tonsillar fossae."

fotemustine (S 10036) (Oncol)—an investigational chemotherapy drug to treat advanced gastric carcinoma.

Fouchet's reagent ("foo-shay").

4-aminopyridine (Neuro)—used to relieve symptoms of multiple sclerosis.

4-aminosalicylic acid (Pamisyl, Rezipas)—used to treat ulcerative colitis in patients who are allergic to sulfasalazine.

fourchette (Fr., fork)—a fork-shaped object or area; usually refers to the frenulum labiorum pudendi (Gyn). "At surgery a small amount of scar was seen at the posterior fourchette."

4-epi-Adriamycin (epirubicin).

four-flap Z-plasty (Hand Surg)—for thumb web deepening, in surgery for repair of syndactyly.

4-HC (4-hydroperoxycyclophosphamide, Pergamid) (Oncol)—used to treat bone marrow in vitro before reinfusing it into patients treated for acute myelogenous leukemia.

Fourier analysis of electrocardiograms (during exercise-induced myocardial ischemia).

Fourier transform, fast-Fourier transform—MRI terms.

Fourneau 309 (suramin).

four-view chest x-ray (Radiol)—PA and lateral, and both oblique views.

fovea centralis retinae—a tiny pit in the center of the macula, composed of slim, elongated cones; it is the area of clearest vision.

foveal avascular zone (FAZ).

FPG (fasting plasma glucose).

FPL (flexor pollicis longus) (Ortho).

F (plasma)—plasma F is plasma cortisol, or a dictator may speak of "free F in the urine."

Fractura Flex—elastic plaster of Paris bandage. In applying the bandage to form a cast, the bandage material is first moistened in water and then applied in bandage-fashion to the extremity, rubbing each layer of the bandage into the layer beneath it. The cast is said to set within four minutes.

fracture
- blow-in
- blow-out
- Chance
- circumferential
- closed
- Colles'
- comminuted
- diastatic
- finger
- fulcrum
- Galeazzi f. of radius
- greenstick
- hangman's
- LeFort I, II, III
- Malgaigne's
- march
- open
- pillion
- ping-pong
- ring
- Salter
- seat belt
- SER-IV
- zygomatic-malar complex (ZMC)

fracture-dislocation, Monteggia.

fragile X syndrome (refers to X chromosome)—a form of retardation that males may inherit from the maternal side of the family.

Fragmatome tip with an ultrasound spatula (Oph).

fraise, diamond (Derm)—an instrument used in dermabrasion of acne scars.

Francisella tularensis—organism that causes tularemia.

Frankel, in *Reitman-Frankel test for SGOT and SGPT.*

Frank procedure (Ob-Gyn)—a technique to create a new vagina in patients with congenital vaginal aplasia, or in males having a sex change operation. Other techniques include McIndoe and Davydov. Also, see *colocolponeopoiesis.*

Frank-Starling law of the heart (Cardio)—the heart pumps out of the right atrium all the blood returned to it without letting any back up in the veins. Named for Otto Frank (German) and Ernest Henry Starling (British), physiologists who, in the early 20th century, formulated the concept upon which the law of muscle contraction is based. Also called Frank-Starling principle.

frappage (Resp Ther)—clapping with a cupped hand on the patient's chest and back to loosen pulmonary secretions so they can be coughed up or suctioned out. Also called percussion.

FRC (functional residual [or reserve] capacity).

FreAmine—amino acid injection; a nutrient solution for burn patients.

freckled—spotted, speckled. "There was a major intrasellar component that was a typical soft, freckled gray adenoma."

FRED (fog reduction/elimination device) (GI)—used on endoscopic instruments.

free air (Radiol)—air or gas in a body cavity where it does not belong, usually after escape from the gastrointestinal tract.

free beta test (Ob)—Down syndrome screening test that detects a specific protein marker at 14-17 weeks of gestation.

Freedom knife (Oph)—a diamond knife blade used during intraocular surgery.

free induction decay (FID); **free induction signal**—MRI terms.

Freeman cookie cutter areola markers—used in reduction mammoplasty. Cf. *mammaplasty, mammoplasty.*

Freeman lens fixation forceps (Oph).

Freeman Punctum Plug (Oph)—a small, bullet-shaped plug made of silicone that is inserted in the opening of the tear duct at the inner aspect of the lower eyelid. It prevents tears from being drained from the eye and is used to treat dry eyes.

Freeman-Swanson knee prosthesis (Ortho).

Freer elevator (Oph, ENT).

free thyroxine index (FTI).

free toe transfer (Hand Surg)—method of constructing a thumb by transplanting a toe to the hand.

Freiberg's disease (Ortho)—avascular necrosis of metatarsal head, treated with DuVries arthroplasty.

French-eye needle. The eye of the needle has a split, or spring, at the end with a little slot for the suture material to slip into, rather than the customary way, through the eye.

French scale—used for denoting size of catheters, sounds, and other tubular instruments, each unit being roughly equivalent to 0.33 mm in diameter.

frequency, angular; Larmor—MRI terms.

frequency domain imaging (FDI)—in ultrasound (Radiol).

Fresenius volumetric dialysate balancing system (Nephrol).

fresh frozen plasma (FFP).

Freund's complete adjuvant (FCA)—a water-in-oil emulsion of antigen which, when injected, induces antibody formation. Cf. *Freund's incomplete adjuvant.*

Freund's incomplete adjuvant—water-in-oil emulsion of antigen, without mycobacteria. Cf. *Freund's complete adjuvant.*

FRF (filter replacement fluid)—given intravenously during CAVH (continuous arteriovenous hemofiltration) to maintain fluid balance.

friable—crumbly; easily broken up or damaged.

friction, finger.

friction knot—see *surgeon's knot.*

Friedländer's bacillus—see *Klebsiella pneumoniae.*

Friedlander marker (Oph)—used during corneal surgery. Types: arcuate; optical zone; transverse incision.

Frigitronics probe (Oph)—used in freeze-thaw cryotherapy.

Frisium (clobazam) (Psych)—an anti-anxiety drug.

frogleg view (Radiol)—a radiographic study of one or both hip joints for which the patient lies on his back with thighs maximally abducted and externally rotated and knees flexed so as to bring the soles of the feet together.

Froment's sign (Neuro)—a simple test of ulnar nerve function. The patient puts the tips of his thumb and index finger together, and if the resulting circle is askew, this is a positive Froment's sign and points to ulnar nerve damage and loss of thumb adductor function.

fronds, sea—description of neovascularization seen on eye examination (Oph).

frondy—see *fronds.*

frontal irregular rhythmic delta activity (FIRDA)—in electroencephalogram.

frontal release sign (Neuro).

frost, synovial—see *synovial frost.*

froth, meibomian—see *meibomian froth.*

frozen section—technique by which tissue removed during an operation is quickly frozen and the pathology identified (while the patient is still on the operating table) so that the surgeons will know what they are dealing with; this will then determine their options in proceeding with the operation. Cf. *paraffin section, permanent section.*

Frykman classification of hand fractures.

FSH (facioscapulohumeral dystrophy).

FSH (follicle-stimulating hormone).

FTA-ABS—fluorescent treponemal antibody absorption test for syphilis.

FTI (free thyroxine index). "The FTI was normal at 2.6, and all other thyroid function tests were within normal limits."

F to N (sounds like *F2N*)—finger-to-nose test (Neuro).

ftorafur—a chemotherapeutic agent.

FTT (failure to thrive)—in infants or the severely debilitated, or a patient making no progress despite treatment.

FUdR (fluorodeoxyuridine, floxuridine)—halogenated thymidine analogue; a radiosensitizer. Cf. *BUdR, IUdR.*

fugue state ("fyug") (Psych)—a period of days, weeks, or years, in which a person loses memory and takes flight from a painful or untenable situation and may start a new life, new job, new marriage, etc., without memory of the past.

Fujinon biopsy forceps—used in endoscopic biopsies.

Fujinon colonoscope.

fulcrum fracture—seat belt fracture. See *Chance fracture.*

full-bladder technique (Radiol)—ultrasonographic examination of the pelvic region performed while the subject's bladder is distended with urine. This is done to improve the recognition of the bladder outline, which cannot be distinguished adequately when the bladder is empty.

full colon—dictated punctuation indicating the need for a colon mark, as opposed to a semicolon.

full-column barium enema (Radiol)—barium enema examination in which the contrast medium is injected into the colon under full pressure, by elevation of the barium reservoir to the maximum safe height.

full stop—dictated punctuation indicating the need for a period.

Fuller shield—a rectal dressing.

full-thickness skin graft (FTSG).

fundal height (Obs). "The fundal height is approximately 31 cm." The obstetrician measures the distance from the symphysis pubis to the top (dome or fundus) of the uterus. After the twentieth week of pregnancy, the fundal height in centimeters equals the number of weeks of pregnancy. If the fundal height increases more than this, it may indicate a multiple pregnancy or a fetus that is large for dates.

fundoplication
- Belsey Mark IV
- Collis-Nissen
- Nissen

fundus oculi—the posterior inner part of the eye as seen with the ophthalmoscope.

funduscopic—*not* fundoscopic.

fungemia—systemic fungal infection.

funicular suture—a term used for interfascicular or grouped fascicular repair (Neuro).

Furniss ureterointestinal anastomosis.

furrier's lung disease—extrinsic allergic alveolitis caused by exposure to animal fur and hair dust.

fusion (Oph)—coordination of images seen by both eyes into one image.

Futura wrist splint (Ortho).

FUVAC (fluorouracil [5-FU], vinblastine, Adriamycin, Cytoxan)—chemotherapy protocol.

FVC (forced vital capacity).

Fydorov intraocular implant lens.

G, g

Gabbay-Frater suture guide.

gadolinium diethylenetriamine–penta-acetate—see *Gd-DTPA.*

Gaffney joint (Ortho)—orthosis for ambulation in children with cerebral palsy and myelomeningocele. Made of stainless steel vacuformed into polypropylene in seven sizes for use in a hinged ankle joint.

gag, mouth
 Dingman
 McIvor
 Sluder-Jansen

gag reflex—contraction of the pharyngeal musculature in response to stimulation of the pharyngeal mucosa.

gait
 cogwheel
 festinating
 glue-footed
 listing
 scissors

gait and station (Neuro, Ortho)—term used in the physical examination. Gait refers to the way a patient walks, and the pattern of it. Station is a test for coordination problems. When the patient stands with feet close together and the body sways, this is one sign of incoordination.

Galand disc lens (Oph)—a rigid one-piece intraocular lens made from PMMA (polymethyl methacrylate).

Galeazzi fracture of radius (Ortho).

Galeazzi's sign (Ortho)—indicates dislocation of hip. Lying supine, with the knees bent, if one knee is lower than the other, there is dislocation of the hip, or a shortened femur.

Galen—see *vein of Galen.*

Galin intraocular implant lens.

Gallavardin phenomenon (Cardio).

galling—chafing of apposed skin surfaces, as in the groin; intertrigo.

gallium nitrate (Ganite) (Oncol)—used to prevent hypercalcemia in patients with carcinoma.

gallium scan (Radiol, Ortho)—the intravenously introduced ^{67}Ga localizes in areas of granulocyte concentration, such as in osteomyelitis, thus revealing hidden infections.

gallop—see *summation gallop.*

Galveston metacarpal brace (Ortho)—to treat fractured second through fifth metacarpals.

Galveston Orientation and Amnesia Test (GOAT)—mental status examination.

Gambee suture ("gam-bay").

Gambro Lundia Minor—brand of artificial kidney (hemodialyzer), parallel plate type.

game leg—impaired by injury or disease.

gamekeeper's thumb—instability of first metacarpophalangeal joint due to ligament tear.

gamete intrafallopian transfer (GIFT).

Gamimune N (immunoglobulin)—for intravenous administration to treat immunodeficiency symptoms in patients who are unable to produce enough IgG antibodies. Used to treat patients with AIDS and ARC.

gamma glutamyl transferase (GGT).

gamma hydroxybutyrate (GHB)—a drug to treat sleep disorders such as narcolepsy.

Gamma knife (Oncol)—not a knife, but a radiosurgical instrument used in new and advanced radiation therapy. The gamma rays are fired with such accuracy that only the diseased cells are destroyed, leaving the adjacent healthy tissues intact. Thus, more radiation can be administered to the tumor if that is indicated. Cf. *roentgen knife.*

gammaphos—see *ethiofos.*

Gamna-Gandy body of the spleen (Radiol)—organized focus of hemorrhage, caused by portal hypertension. Contains fibrous tissue, hemosiderin, and calcium. Also called siderotic nodules or bodies.

ganciclovir (Cytovene, DHPG)—used to treat cytomegalovirus (CMV) infection and CMV retinitis in AIDS patients.

ganglioglioma—a rare variety of tumor composed of ganglion cells and glial cells; prevalent in first three decades of life.

ganglioside GM1 (Neuro). A natural component of cells in the central nervous system, ganglioside GM1 has been found to allow damaged nerves to regrow. Along with the now-standard treatment of methylprednisolone following spinal cord injury, the use of ganglioside GM1 produces an increase in neurologic function one year status post injury.

Ganite (gallium nitrate).

Ganong, in *Lown-Ganong-Levine syndrome.*

gantry, CT—see *CT gantry.*

gap
  air-bone
  anion

Gardner chair (Neuro)—used as an operating table, with the patient in the sitting position.

Gardner-Wells skull tongs (Neuro).

Gardnerella vaginalis—newer name for the bacterium formerly called *Haemophilus vaginalis*; normal vaginal flora, but thought perhaps to be the cause of vaginitis infections.

Garrett dilator—used in kidney transplant surgery.

gas chromatography—an analytic technique with many applications in medicine, particularly in screening serum and urine for poisons and drugs of abuse.

gas density line (Radiol)—a linear band of maximal radiolucency, representing or appearing to represent a narrow zone of air or gas.

gas-forming organism in bowel wall (Radiol).

Gass scleral punch (Oph).

Gastaut's syndrome (HEE syndrome—hemiconvulsion, hemiplegia, and epilepsy).

gastrinoma—hormonally active tumor of pancreas or stomach.

Gastroccult—a lab test for occult blood in gastric juices; said to be more reliable than some of the earlier tests.

gastrocnemius reflex. Cf. *Achilles reflex* and *ankle jerk.*

gastroenterostomy
Billroth
Hofmeister

gastroesophageal reflux (Radiol)—on upper GI series, abnormal backflow of material from the stomach into the lower esophagus.

Gastrografin (meglumine diatrizoate), a radiopaque medium used in examination of the upper GI tract.

gastrojejunostomy, antecolic.

gastroplasty
Eckhout vertical
Mason vertical-banded
vertical-banded (VBG)

gastrostomy
Depage-Janeway
Partipilo method
percutaneous endoscope (PEG)
Stamm

Gastrozepine (pirenzepine) (GI)—drug used to treat peptic ulcer disease.

Gatch bed.

gatch—from height of setting of Gatch bed, as "45° gatch."

gated blood (pool) cardiac wall motion study—a radionuclide study.

gated view (in multiple gated acquisition scan, or MUGA) (Radiol)—an image obtained by a technique synchronized with motions of the heart to eliminate blurring.

gauge (noun)—standard measure, as of wire or needle diameter; (verb)—to find the exact measurement of. See *Dacomed snap gauge; mercury-in-Silastic strain gauge; Preston pinch gauge.* Cf. *gouge.*

gauss ("gowse")—MRI term. See *tesla.*

gaussian ("gow'-zee-en") **mode profile laser beam**—MRI term.

Gauss' sign—the marked degree of mobility of the uterus, seen during the early weeks of pregnancy (Obs).

gauze
Aquaphor
iodoform
Nu Gauze dressing
Xeroform
wick

Gaynor-Hart position (Radiol)—positioning the patient for an axial radiographic projection of the carpal tunnel. See *carpal tunnel syndrome.*

gay-related immunodeficiency disease (GRID)—an obsolete term for AIDS.

gaze—see *disconjugate gaze.*

G banding—technique of chromosome staining.

GCA (giant cell arteritis).

G-CSF (granulocyte colony-stimulating factor) (Oncol)—a naturally occurring growth factor produced by epithelial cells and monocytes that acts on the bone marrow to increase the production of neutrophils. Used in chemotherapy and in treating bone marrow depression in AIDS patients. See *filgrastim.* Cf. *GM-CSF.*

Gd-DTPA (gadolinium diethylenetriamine-pentaacetate)—a contrast agent used in MRI scans.

Geenan cytology brush (GI).

Geenan Endotorque guide wire (GI)—used for cannulation of tortuous or strictured biliary ducts.

gegenhalten ("gay'-gen-hal-ten") (Neuro)—seen in cerebral cortical disorders, when the patient involuntarily resists passive movement. "Gegenhalten increase in tone is present and noticeable during the examination."

gelatin compression boot—used in the treatment of venous ulcer and stasis dermatitis. Works on the principle of even pressure on the veins, protecting them from further trauma. See *Unna boot.*

Gelfoam—a purified gelatin product the body tissues will absorb. Used for hemostasis in surgery, and also used, in some forms, for treatment of gastric ulcer, etc.

Gelfoam cookie (Neuro). "A Gelfoam cookie was placed over the craniotomy." See *Gelfoam.*

Gelocast (Ortho)—a cast material.

gemcitabine (Oncol)—a chemotherapy drug used to treat advanced gastric adenocarcinoma or malignant melanoma. Also called difluorodeoxycytidine.

gemistocytes (Neuro, Oncol)—swollen astrocytes, either reactive or part of tumor.

GeneAmp PCR test—used to detect early HIV infection, and also now for childhood leukemia (chronic myeloid and acute lymphocytic). It is one thousand times more sensitive than previous leukemia tests and weeks faster. PCR (polymerase chain reaction)—a DNA technology.

Genentech biosynthetic human growth hormone (trade name, Protropin). Genentech, the manufacturer, produces human growth hormone by the DNA recombinant method.

General Electric CT/T 8800 scanner—analyzes stereotaxic data to obtain X, Y, and Z coordinates for each target lesion (Neuro).

Genesis total knee system (Ortho).

geniculum—sharp, knee-like bend in a structure or organ.

Genoptic (gentamicin sulfate)—a sterile ophthalmic solution.

gentamicin liposome (TLC-G-65)—a drug used to treat MAI infection in AIDS patients.

Gentle Touch (GI)—postoperative colostomy appliance.

geographic tongue—a condition of the tongue in which irregular zones of redness appear and create an appearance somewhat like a map.

Geomedic total knee prosthesis (Ortho).

Geometric knee prosthesis (Ortho).

Georgiade visor (Neuro, Ortho)—halo fixation apparatus.

GER (gastroesophageal reflux).

GERD (gastroesophageal reflux disease) (GI).

Gerdy's tubercle—in the knee.

Geref (sermorelin acetate).

germ tube test (brief form for germination tube)—a quick lab test to distinguish *Candida albicans* from other yeasts. "The patient had a yeast growing also, thought not to be *Candida albicans* by two-hour germ tube."

Germanin (suramin).

germination tube—see *germ tube.*

Gerstmann's syndrome—agraphia.

Geuder corneal needle (Oph).

Geuder keratoplasty needle (Oph).

gestational assessment, Ballard.

Gey's solution—a fixative solution used with flexible bronchoscopy.

GFAP (glial fibrillary acidic protein)—a test used for identifying some types of brain tumors (Neuro).

GFR (glomerular filtration rate) (Urol).

GGT (gamma glutamyl transferase).

GGTP (gamma glutamyl transpeptidase)—a liver function test.

Ghajar guide (Neuro)—for intraventricular catheter placement. Used in trauma, in reduction of intracranial pressure; for placement of shunts in hydrocephalus; for placement of pharmacologic agents directly into cerebral ventricles. Designed by Jamshid Ghajar, M.D.

GHB (gamma hydroxybutyrate)—drug used to treat narcolepsy and other sleep disorders.

Gherini-Kauffman endo-otoprobe—a a type of laser probe used in ear surgery.

Ghon complex—a peripheral calcified granuloma and lymph node in the lung, diagnostic of old tuberculous infection.

ghost vessels—in the cornea (Oph).

GHz (gigahertz).

Giannestras step-down procedure (Pod)—a modification of the Giannestras step-down osteotomy used to lengthen post-traumatic shortness of the metatarsals.

Gianotti-Crosti syndrome—papular acrodermatitis of childhood (PAC).

giant cell arteritis (GCA)—a systemic disease of unknown etiology; characterized by vasculitis in branches of the carotid artery, with narrowed vascular lumen and thickened intima. The artery may be occluded by thrombosis. This may be an immune-mediated abnormality. See *von Willebrand factor.*

Gianturco expandable (self-expanding) **metallic biliary stent; prosthesis** (GI)—a metal stent used to treat biliary and esophageal strictures; its wires are crisscrossed in a Z pattern. Also called a Z stent.

Gianturco-Roehm bird's nest vena cava filter (Cardio).

Gianturco wool-tufted wire coil (Vasc Surg)—used in embolization treatment of arteriovenous fistulae or pseudoaneurysms.

Giardia lamblia—a protozoan parasite. Can be transmitted in drinking water and through sexual contact. Is virulent in AIDS patients.

GIA stapler (Surg)—transects and staples. (GIA, gastrointestinal anastomosis.)

gibbous deformity (adj.) (Ortho)—humped, hump-backed, protruding. Cf. *gibbus.*

gibbus (n.)—a hump. Cf. *gibbous.*

Gibson inner ear shunt (ENT)—used to reduce inner ear pressure in patients suffering from Ménière's disease.

Giemsa-Wright stain.

GIFT (gamete intrafallopian transfer).

gigahertz ("jig'-uh-herts") (GHz)—a unit of frequency that equals 1 billion hertz (cycles per second)—10^9 Hz.

Gigli saw ("gee-lee," "jig-gly," or "gig-lee") (Ortho).

Gilles de la Tourette's syndrome. See *Tourette syndrome.*

Gillette joint (Pod)—orthosis for ambulation in children with cerebral palsy and myelomeningocele. Made of rubber vacuformed into polypropylene to provide a plantar-flexion stop and free dorsiflexion.

Gilliam's suspension of the uterus.

Gillies elevation (Plas Surg)—procedure for fractured zygoma.

Gillies horizontal dermal suture (Plas Surg).

Gill/Jonas modification—of the Norwood procedure for hypoplastic left-sided heart syndrome. See *Fontan; Sade.*

Gills intraocular implant lens.

Gilmore intraocular implant lens.

Gilvernet retractor ("Jheel-vehr-nay") (Urol).

gimpy—pejorative term for a lower extremity in which pain, spasm, or deformity causes a limp.

Girard Fragmatome—a fragmentation probe used in cataract extraction, eye surgery (Oph).

Girdlestone-Taylor procedure (Ortho).

Gittes urethral suspension procedure (Urol) (Dr. Ruben F. Gittes).

glabellar tap (Neuro). With the extended index finger, the examiner taps the patient's forehead in the midline at the level of the supraorbital ridges. The patient blinks. This maneuver is then repeated. Normally the patient, knowing what is happening, does not again blink. However, a patient with certain central nervous system pathology blinks every time the glabella is tapped. A positive glabellar tap after infancy is a sign of brain damage.

Glandosane (ENT)—flavored synthetic saliva to relieve dry mouth symptoms.

glands
- BUS
- EG/BUS
- Littre
- meibomian

Glasgow Coma Scale (GCS)—used to assess the prognosis of patients with head injuries by describing the patient's level of consciousness. It is divided into three parts:

Eyes open:
- spontaneously
- to speech
- to pain
- do not open

Glasgow *(cont.)*

Best verbal response:
- oriented
- confused
- inappropriate words
- incomprehensible sounds
- no verbal response

Best motor response:
- obeys commands
- localizes pain
- flexion to pain
- extension to pain
- no motor response

Each of the parameters is scored on a scale of 1 through 5. The total of the values added together indicates the patient's level of consciousness. Normal would be 14 or 15; 7 or less would be considered coma. A score of 3 would be considered brain death (but is not conclusive). See *EMV grading.*

Glasgow Outcome Scale
- Good recovery
- Moderate disability
- Severe disability
- Permanent vegetative state
- Death

Glassman clamp.

Glassman stone extractor (Surg)—for removal of impacted common duct stones.

glaucoma (Oph)—a disease characterized by increased intraocular pressure and impaired vision, ranging from slight abnormalities to absolute blindness.

glaukomflecken (Oph)—yeast-shaped opacities that form following acute glaucoma attack.

Gleason score (Oncol)—for carcinoma of the prostate: a grading for prognosis, on a scale of 1 through 5, from

Gleason score *(cont.)*
well differentiated to poorly differentiated. The test is done twice, in different areas, and the results added together. A score of 10, for example, would give a grave prognosis.

Gliadel (Neuro, Oncol)—an implant used to treat malignant glioma. It consists of 1.4 cm thin wafers, as many as eight of which are left in situ after surgical removal of this type of brain tumor. The wafers contain the chemotherapy drug BCNU, which is the most effective single chemotherapeutic agent currently available to treat this malignancy. However, it causes toxicity and cannot be given systemically in levels high enough to completely kill all tumor cells. Current treatment for malignant glioma involves surgical resection, radiation therapy, and chemotherapy with BCNU. With the Gliadel implant, the BCNU can be delivered in high concentrations directly to the site of the tumor, after the tumor has been surgically removed or debulked. The drug is released over a three-week period as the wafers disintegrate. The wafers are absorbed by the body and do not need to be surgically removed.

glial fibrillary acidic protein (GFAP) —a test used for identifying some types of brain tumors (Neuro).

Glidewire (GI)—trade name of a coated, kink-resistant guide wire used in procedures of the biliary tract. Also, Microvasive Glidewire. (Note: guide wire is two words, Glidewire is one.)

glioblastoma multiforme—malignant tumor usually occurring in the cerebrum of adults.

Glisson's capsule—connective tissue covering of the liver.

glitter cell.

GLNS (gay lymph node syndrome)— one of the older initialisms (and now pejorative) for AIDS.

globus hystericus—the sensation of a lump in the throat, sometimes accompanied by choking, due to emotional upset.

globus pallidus—one of the basal ganglia.

glomerular filtration rate (GFR) (Urol).

glomerulonephritis, acute poststreptococcal (APSGN).

glove
Biobrane
Repel

GLQ223 (compound Q)—a highly purified protein (trichosanthin) from a Chinese cucumber plant. It has been shown in cell cultures to selectively kill cells that are already infected with HIV, and inhibits further production of the virus without adversely affecting normal cells. Scientists working on this project have also found that HIV-infected macrophages are a reservoir of infected cells in AIDS patients, and that GLQ223 appears to block reproduction of infected T-cells and kills HIV-infected macrophages. Since both types of cells are necessary to the normal functioning of the immune system, these studies are promising. GLQ223 is a trade name.

Glucometer II—a home glucose monitoring system.

glue—see *adhesive.*

glue-footed gait—an ataxic gait in which the patient seems unable to lift either foot from the floor.

glutaraldehyde-tanned bovine collagen tubes—for vascular xenografts or heterografts.

glutaraldehyde-tanned porcine heart valve—xenograft or heterograft.

gluteal bonnet—gluteus maximus and minimus.

Glutose—convenient, single-dose tube of oral glucose for quick treatment of hypoglycemia.

glycol methacrylate—an embedding medium for pathology specimens.

glycosylated hemoglobin—an assay of diabetic control; glucose stays attached to the red cell for the life of the cell and can be measured.

Glypressin (terlipressin).

GM-CSF (granulocyte/macrophage colony-stimulating factor)—a naturally occurring growth factor which stimulates myeloid progenitor cells in the bone marrow to divide and differentiate into granulocytes and macrophages. Also stimulates mature granulocytes and macrophages to higher levels of migration towards pathogens, phagocytosis, and cytotoxic activity, thus enhancing the effectiveness of the immune system. Used in chemotherapy and in conjunction with AZT in treatment of AIDS. See *sargramostim.* Cf. *G-CSF.*

GM1 monosialotetrahexosylganglioside—see *ganglioside GM1.*

GMS stain (Gomori, or Grocott, methenamine silver)—a stain used to establish the diagnosis of *Pneumocystis carinii* pneumonia.

GnRH (gonadotropin-releasing hormone). See *LHRH* (luteinizing hormone-releasing hormone).

GOAT (Galveston Orientation and Amnesia Test).

Goeckerman regimen (Derm)—treatment for psoriasis including application of tar and tar-based medications, shampoos with tar, and two types of light treatment (shortwave ultraviolet light in increasing doses daily, and quartz light in increasing doses).

Golaski graft (Neuro)—a knitted Dacron graft used during carotid endarterectomy and carotid-subclavian artery bypass.

Golay coil—MRI term.

Goldman cardiac risk index score (Cardio)—a clinical scoring system used to predict cardiac morbidity.

Goldenhar syndrome—oculoauriculovertebral dysplasia (Plas Surg). This is a congenital anomaly involving the eye, ear, vertebrae, and mandible, temporal and zygomatic bones, and the muscles used in facial expression and mastication.

Goldmann applanation tonometer (Oph)—used to measure intraocular pressure.

Goldmann lens (Oph)—a three-mirror contact lens used in photocoagulation procedures for detached retina, or in lattice degeneration.

Golgi complex—a collection of vesicles in the cell cytoplasm where products of cell metabolism are placed into vacuoles for excretion.

Goligher retractor—modification of the Berkeley-Bonney self-retaining 3-blade abdominal retractor for use in abdominal surgery.

Goligher retractor frame.

GoLytely—gastrointestinal lavage prep for improved visualization in bowel examination.

Gomco suction tube.

Gomori (or Grocott) **methenamine silver** (GMS)—a stain used to establish the diagnosis of *Pneumocystis carinii* pneumonia.

gonadorelin acetate (Lutrepulse) (Gyn). Used to induce ovulation in women with amenorrhea resulting from dysfunction of the hypothalamus. It is

gonadorelin acetate *(cont.)* administered I.V. with a special pump. Has successfully induced ovulation in 70% of the recipients.

gonadotropin-releasing hormone (abbreviated GnRH). See *goserelin acetate* (Zoladex).

gonial angle—of the mandible.

gonioscope—an optical instrument for direct visualization of the anterior chamber through the use of a goniolens; e.g., Sussman gonioscope.

goniotomy knife, Barkan.

Gonzales blood group—a blood group character (antigen Go[a]) for which the antibody was reported in a mother (Mrs. Gonzales) of a newborn infant with erythroblastosis fetalis. This is an antibody apparently found only in individuals who are of black parentage, and it is distinct from all previously classified blood group systems.

Goodell's sign (Ob-Gyn)—softening of the cervix because of an increased blood supply, an early clue to pregnancy.

Goodenough test (Psych)—a draw-a-man test to estimate intelligence. The name of the test does not refer to the performance; it is named for Florence Goodenough.

Goosen vascular punch.

Gore-Tex—nonabsorbable surgical suture and a graft material (also used for many other purposes). Examples:
bifurcated vascular graft
cardiovascular patch
catheter
knee prosthesis
limb; shunt
soft tissue patch
surgical membrane
vascular graft

goserelin acetate (Zoladex) (Urol, Ob-Gyn)—a synthetic version of the naturally occurring gonadotropin-releasing female hormone. It is used to treat advanced prostate cancer which thrives in the presence of the male hormone androgen, and to treat endometriosis and to induce ovulation in women.

Gosset, spiral band of.

Gott shunt—used in liver transplantation.

Gottschalk Nasostat—a rubber cannula used to stop epistaxis (nosebleed).

gouge—(noun) a hollow chisel used for cutting or removing bone or cartilage; (verb) to scoop out, as with a gouge. Cf. *gauge.*

Gould electromagnetic flowmeter—records arterial blood flow rates.

Gould intraocular implant lens.

Goulian mammoplasty.

Gowers' maneuver (Neuro)—patients with weakness may find it necessary to "climb" up their legs with their hands, to rise from a sitting position.

Gowers sign (Neuro)—classical sign of Duchenne muscular dystrophy; also called *tripoding.*

GPC (giant papillary conjunctivitis) (Oph).

GPMAL (obstetrical history): gravida, para, multiple births, abortions, live births.

gp120—an AIDS vaccine.

graciloplasty—see *dynamic graciloplasty.*

gradient coil; gradient magnetic field —MRI terms.

Gradle cilia forceps (Oph).

grading, EMV (eyes, motor, voice).

graft, graft material
advancement flap
aldehyde

graft *(cont.)*
aldehyde-tanned bovine (cow)
aldehyde-tanned ovine (sheep)
autograft
autologous fat
BAGF (brachioaxillary bridge graft fistula)
bifurcated vascular
Biograft—bovine heterograft
BioPolyMeric
Bonfiglio bone
bovine heterograft
brachioaxillary bridge
brachiosubclavian bridge
CABG (coronary artery bypass)
Calcitite
Dacron
Dardik biograft
Durapatite
free
full-thickness
glutaraldehyde-tanned bovine
glutaraldehyde-tanned porcine
Golaski
Gore-Tex
Hapset bone graft plaster
Hemashield
heterograft
inlay
Interpore
Ionescu-Shiley pericardial xenograft
knitted Dacron arterial
Marlex synthetic
Meadox Microvel double velour
Milliknit
Nicoll bone
onlay
ovine (sheep)
pedicle
pigskin
porcine xenograft
Proplast
PTFE (polytetrafluoroethylene)
Pyrost
Sauvage

graft *(cont.)*
skin
Solvang
split-thickness
Tiersch
Unilab Surgibone
Wolfe
xenograft

GraftAssist vein/graft holder (Cardio) —reduces the chance of narrowing at the anastomosis site.

graft, skin (Surg, Plas Surg)
split thickness—.010 to .035 inch thick.
full thickness—greater than .035 inch thick.
free graft—does not have its own blood supply; gets blood from capillary ingrowth from underlying tissue.
pedicle graft—gets its blood supply from subcutaneous vessels that came with the pedicle portion of the graft.

graft-versus-host disease (GVHD)—caused by reaction to an allograft, from marrow transplant, etc. Following is the GVHD grading system (written as clinical grade 1, etc.):
1 Mild skin rash (generally maculopapular). No gastrointestinal or liver function abnormalities.
2 Moderately severe skin rash. Mild gastrointestinal symptoms. Slight increase in bilirubin and perhaps also in liver enzymes.
3 Moderately severe skin rash, gastrointestinal symptoms, and liver function abnormalities.
4 Severe peeling and flaking of the skin, severe gastrointestinal symptoms, and liver function abnormalities.

graft-versus-host reaction. See *graft-versus-host disease.*

Graham Steell heart murmur (no hyphen).

gram-negative organisms—*Haemophilus, Neisseria, Pseudomonas.* See *Gram's stain; gram-positive.*

gram-positive organisms—*Clostridium, Corynebacterium, Staphylococcus, Streptococcus.* See *Gram's stain; gram-negative organisms.*

Gram's stain (named for Hans Christian Joachim Gram)—a stain using the bacterial property of stain retention or loss, to help in classification and subsequent treatment. The smears are fixed to a slide by heat and stained with a solution of crystal violet, which stains all bacteria. An iodine solution then fixes the dye to the gram-positive organisms. The specimen is decolorized by washing with a mixture of acetone and alcohol, and then counterstained with a dye of another color (usually safranin). Gram-positive organisms retain the original purple stain; gram-negative organisms, however, turn pink (if safranin was used). Note: Capitalize Gram's stain, but lowercase gram-negative and gram-positive. See *gram-negative; gram-positive.*

granularis, ependymitis.

granule
  Birbeck
  Fordyce
  Much's
  Nissl's
  zymogen

granulocyte colony-stimulating factor—see *G-CSF.*

granulocyte/macrophage colony-stimulating factor—see *GM-CSF.*

granuloma, pyogenic—see *pyogenic granuloma* (granuloma pyogenicum).

granulomatosis—see *Wegener's.*

grapes—see *Carswell's.*

graph—see *capnograph.*

graphesthesia (Neuro)—relates to the perception and identification of letters or numbers written on the skin with a blunt object.

graphospasm—writer's cramp.

grasper—see *Hasson grasper.*

grasp reflex. An infant will automatically grasp a finger placed against the palmar surface of its hand.

GRASS (gradient recalled acquisition in a steady state)—technique for cardiac MRI test (Radiol).

Gratiolet, convolutions of.

gravida—the number of pregnancies a woman has had: *gravida 4,* having been pregnant 4 times; *gravida 5, para 3, ab 2,* five pregnancies, three live births, two abortions or miscarriages.

Gravindex (Ob-Gyn)—relatively sensitive pregnancy test used in physician offices.

gray (Gy)—the International System unit of absorbed dose, equal to the energy imparted by ionizing radiation to a mass of matter corresponding to 1 joule per kilogram. Used in radiotherapy. See *joule.*

Gray drill (Ortho).

gray line—in the eye.

Grayson's ligament in hand (Ortho)—it keeps the skin sleeve from twisting around the bones of the digit. You may hear this referred to in operative procedures for Dupuytren's contracture. See also *Cleland's ligament;* they are not synonymous.

great vessels (Radiol)—on chest x-ray, the major vascular trunks entering and leaving the heart: the superior and inferior venae cavae, the pulmonary arteries and veins, and the aorta.

Greene fiberoptic cystoscope.

Greene intraocular implant lens (Oph).

Greenfield IVC filter (Cardio)—a permanent inferior vena cava filter, placed via the right jugular vein into the inferior vena cava to filter out emboli that might otherwise reach the lung.

Greenwald flexible endoscopic electrodes (Surg).

Gregoire, in *Lich-Gregoire repair.*

Gregory instruments (Vasc Surg)—developed by Dr. Roger Gregory:
baby profunda clamp
carotid bulldog clamp
external clamp
forceps
stay sutures

grenz ray—long wave irradiation; used in treatment of localized neurodermatitis and in lichen simplex chronicus; a low-energy x-ray. (Not a proper noun; do not capitalize.)

Greulich and Pyle, bone age—for skeletal maturation staging (Radiol).

GRID (gay-related immunodeficiency diseases)—a pejorative term replaced by *AIDS* and *HIV.*

grid—see *Amsler grid* (Oph).

Grieshaber iris forceps (Oph).

Grieshaber light source (Oph).

Grieshaber manipulator (Oph)—multifunction instrument used in vitreous surgery. It has a light source, a suction forceps, and a coagulator.

Griesinger's sign—swelling and pain in the neck on rotation, easily mistaken for meningitis, but in this case due to thrombophlebitis of the mastoid emissary vein.

grip tester—see *Jamar.*

Grocott (or Gomori) **methenamine silver** (GMS). See *Gomori.*

Grollman catheter (Radiol).

Groshong catheter—used in central venous lines for administration of intravenous chemotherapeutic agents.

gross description (Path)—description of tissue as it appears to the unaided eye prior to fixation and paraffin embedding.

Grosse and Kempf locking nail system (Howmedica, Inc.)—femoral and tibial nails. There are two types: static locking (complete locking) and dynamic locking (partial locking). Stabilizes and controls fragment rotation and maintains desired bone length.

ground-glass cells (Path)—as seen in chronic hepatitis B.

Gruentzig—see *Grüntzig.*

grunting (Peds)—involuntary noise made by newborns with respiratory distress to try to keep lungs adequately inflated.

Grüntzig balloon catheter (Gruentzig) (Vasc Surg)—used in percutaneous transluminal dilatation and angioplasty. (An umlaut is required over the "u" in Grüntzig; if an umlaut is not available on the keyboard, the spelling is Gruentzig.)

GSB elbow prosthesis—by Gschwind, Scheier, and Bahler (Ortho).

G6PD (glucose-6-phosphate dehydrogenase)—X-linked enzyme. Used as a cell marker to study possible origin of different neoplastic disorders.

G691—chemotherapy protocol.

G-suit—an external counterpressure device used to control hemorrhage; provides tamponade of pelvic fracture-induced hemorrhage.

guaiac—test of occult blood in the stool.

Gudden's atrophy—retrograde degeneration of the thalamus after cortical lesions. Named for German neurologist, Bernhard Aloys von Gudden.

Gudden's atrophy *(cont.)*
Also, Gudden's commissure, Gudden's tract, nucleus of Gudden.

Gudden's tract—mammillotegmental tract in the brain.

Guepar hinge-knee prosthesis.

guerney. See *gurney.*

Guerry, in *Lieb–Guerry cataract implant lens.*

Guibor Silastic tube (Oph)—used in surgery of the lacrimal system.

guide, guide wire
Cor-Flex
Gabbay-Frater suture
Geenan Endotorque
Ghajar
Glidewire
Lunderquist
Lunderquist-Ring torque
Magnum
Microvasive Glidewire
Terumo
Todd-Wells

Guillain-Barré syndrome (pronounced "ge-yán bar-ráy")—acute idiopathic polyneuritis, an acute, rapidly progressive nerve inflammation, with weakness of the muscles of the legs, then weakness in the arms and face, and may also affect the muscles of respiration. It appears to be self-limiting in 90 to 95% of patients, with complete recovery, but it can result in flaccid quadriplegia or respiratory failure. Also called infectious polyneuritis, Landry-Guillain–Barré–Strohl syndrome, Landry-Guillain syndrome, and Landry's paralysis.

Gullstrand's slit lamp—see *biomicroscope.*

gun
Bard Biopty
Biopty
Cobe

Gunderson conjunctival flap (Oph).

Gunn, in *Marcus Gunn syndrome, Marcus Gunn pupil.*

Gunn crossing sign (Cardio).

GunSlinger shoulder orthosis (Ortho)—for correct positioning and immobilization of the shoulder and arm following surgery.

gurney (guerney)—high wheeled cot for moving patients.

Gusberg hysterectomy clamp—with Kapp-Beck serrations.

Gustilo-Kyle cementless total hip arthroplasty with femoral stems made of Ti6A14V alloy (Ortho).

gut-hormone profile. The pattern of hormone release may help to distinguish celiac disease from other abdominal problems.

gut, surgical (catgut).

guttata, cornea. See *cornea guttata* (Oph).

Guttmann subtalar arthrodesis (Ortho).

guy sutures (not Guy)—a steadying or guiding suture, to prevent movement.

Guyon's canal ("guy-on") (Ortho)—an anatomical landmark in operative procedures designed to reduce ulnar nerve compression which occurs as the ulnar nerve passes behind the medial epicondyle, between the heads of the flexor carpi ulnaris, or along Guyon's canal from the pisiform bone to the hook of the hamate.

Guyton-Park eye speculum.

GVHD (graft-versus-host disease) (or reaction). See *graft-versus-host disease.*

Gypsona—a rapid-setting cast material (Ortho).

gyromagnetic ratio—MRI term.

gyrus—a folding in the surface (cortex) of the cerebrum.

H, h

HA (hydroxyapatite).

Haab scleral resection knife (Oph).

Haag-Streit Goldmann perimeter.

Haag-Streit slit lamp (Oph).

habenula (''hah-ben'-u-lah'') (Neuro) —a small protuberance at the dorsal and posterior edge of the third ventricle, adjacent to the pineal body. It is part of the epithalamus.

Habitrol—see *Nicoderm.*

H-Ae interval (retrograde conduction)—a term used in electrophysiologic studies of supraventricular tachycardia (Cardio).

Haemonetics Cell Saver (Cardio)—a device used to collect a patient's blood for retransfusion at the end of an operative procedure.

Haemophilus ducreyi —the cause of soft chancres or chancroids on the genitalia of humans. Also called *Ducrey's bacillus.*

Haemophilus vaginalis—see *Gardnerella vaginalis.*

Haenig irrigating scissors.

Hafnia alvei (GI)—newer name for *Enterobacter hafnia*; associated with enteritis.

Hageman factor. See *coagulation factors, blood.*

Hagie pins (Ortho).

Haglund's deformity—causes traumatic inflammation of Achilles tendon and bursa.

hairy-cell leukemia (HCL). First described in 1958. On electron micrographs, the cells have projections radiating from their walls.

Hajek-Koffler sphenoid punch.

Hakim-Cordis pump (used in neurological surgery procedures).

Halbrecht's syndrome—ABO erythroblastosis.

Halcion (triazolam)—hypnotic for insomnia.

half and half nails—a dull-white proximal half of the fingernails meets a reddish-brown distal half. A sign of possible renal disease that may precede symptoms of renal disease.

half-hitch—a sailor's knot; also used in surgery.

Hall air drill.

Hall dermatome (Plas Surg). This is an oscillating blade type.

Hall neurosurgical craniotome.

Hall valvulotome (Cardio)—used to disrupt the valves in a vein and make the valve leaflets incompetent. This allows the vein to be used in distal saphenous vein bypass procedures.

Hall-Kaster mitral valve prosthesis.

Haller's layer—the vascular layer of the choroid of the eye.

Hallpike caloric stimulation test (ENT). See *caloric testing of vestibular function.*

Hallpike test. See *Dix-Hallpike test.*

Hall sternum saw (Thor Surg).

hallucinosis—a pathological entity characterized by hallucination. Types: alcoholic and drug-induced.

hallux abductovalgus (Pod)—the deformity which causes the great toe to be abducted and everted (abductovalgus) and usually is corrected surgically with a bunionectomy.

halobetasol propionate (Ultravate)—a topical corticosteroid (Derm).

halo traction—see *cervical support.*

Halstead-Wepman Aphasia Screening Test (Neuro).

Halsted hemostatic mosquito forceps (straight/curved) (Oph).

Halsted inguinal herniorrhaphy (*not* Halstead). Named for William Stewart Halsted, M.D., a famous surgeon and teacher.

Hamman's sign—a sign of pneumopericardium, an acute medical emergency. The physician hears a loud clicking or crunching sound in time with the heart beat.

Hamman-Rich syndrome—diffuse interstitial pulmonary fibrosis.

hammer toe (Ortho)—clawlike flexion contracture of the second and distal phalanges.

hammer toe repair—see *DuVries hammer toe repair.*

Hampton's hump—a pleurally-based, triangular lung infiltrate.

Hancock M.O. Bioprosthesis (Cardio)—a tissue valve for the small aortic root; used instead of a porcine valve.

"H&H"—slang for hemoglobin and hematocrit.

hand, Myobock. See *Utah artificial arm* and *Myobock hand.*

H&E stain (hematoxylin and eosin).

Handtrol electrosurgical pencil.

hanging panniculus (Plas Surg). See *apron.*

hangman's fracture—sometimes the result of injury to the neck in motorcycle or automobile accidents, in which there is rupture of the anterior and posterior longitudinal ligaments, leading to anterior luxation of C2 over C3, with crushing of the intervertebral disk.

Hansel's stain (Path)—used in microscopic examination of eosinophils.

HA-1A (Centoxin)—a human monoclonal antibody found to be effective against gram-negative sepsis (a virulent and deadly multisystem disease caused by the endotoxins released in the bloodstream by gram-negative bacteria). HA-1A binds to the endotoxins, inactivating them.

Hapset (Oral Surg)—HA (hydroxyapatite) bone graft plaster also used for periodontal defects and tooth extraction sites. The plaster itself absorbs, leaving only an HA scaffold for bony ingrowth.

haptens—the little loops on implant cataract lens through which the sutures are passed to keep the lens in place. Used interchangeably with *haptics.*

haptics—see *haptens.*

Harada, in *Vogt-Koyanagi-Harada disease.*

Hardy microbipolar forceps.

Hardy-Duddy weighted vaginal speculum (Gyn).

Hardy-Rand-Littler (HRL) **screening plates.**

Hardy-Sella punch (Oph, Plas Surg)—a small punch used to create an osteotomy in the lacrimal fossa.

harness—see *Pavlik harness.*

Harrington retractor (called "sweetheart," probably because the tip of the blade is somewhat heart-shaped) (Surg).

Harrington rod (Ortho)—used to correct scoliosis.

Harris broach (Ortho).

Harris HD hip prosthesis (Ortho).

Harrison-Nicolle polypropylene pegs—used in hand surgery.

Harrison's groove—a horizontal groove along the lower thorax; seen in children with rickets, or in people who have had rickets.

Hartmann hemostatic mosquito forceps (straight/curved) (Oph).

Hartmann's solution (Ringer's lactate)—a physiologic salt solution.

Hartzler Micro II balloon—used in coronary angioplasty (Cardio).

Harvard pump—an infusion device which continually injects medication at a preset rate.

harvest (Surg, Ortho)—to remove tissue or organs from a donor for transplantation; to take skin, bone, or cartilage from the patient for an autologous graft. See also *stem-cell marrow harvesting.*

Hasson graspers (Surg)—used in endoscopic procedures; made by Weck.

Hauser procedure (Ortho)—medial transplantation of the patellar tendon insertion, with reefing of the vastus medialis.

HAV (hepatitis A virus).

Haverhill fever (also, ratbite fever)—named for Haverhill, Massachusetts, where the first epidemic of this disease occurred. It is usually transmitted by the bite of an infected rat, but occasionally by the bite of an infected dog, cat, or squirrel. The responsible organism is *Streptobacillus moniliformis.* The symptoms include high fever; enlarged regional lymph nodes; red, painful, and swollen joints; and there may also be a rash and back pain. Responds to treatment with antibiotics.

haversian canal—a microscopic feature of bone.

Hawkins breast localization needle, with FlexStrand cable—used for marking nonpalpable lesions (Radiol). These needles are designated I, II, and III. Number III can be used to inject dye, or for aspiration. They come in 5, 7.5, 10, and 12.5 cm lengths.

HbAg, HB Ag ("H-bag")—hepatitis B antigen.

HBcAb—hepatitis B core antibody (not to be confused with HBcAg, which is hepatitis B core antigen).

HBeAb—hepatitis B "e" antibody (not to be confused with HBeAg, which is hepatitis B "e" antigen).

HBeAg—the soluble "e" antigen in hepatitis B antigen.

HBIG (hepatitis B immune globulin).

HBsAb—hepatitis B surface antibody (not to be confused with HBsAg, which is hepatitis B surface antigen).

HBsAg—hepatitis B surface antigen.

HBV (hepatitis B virus).

HC—see *4-HC.*

H-CAP (Oncol)—a standard chemotherapy protocol used to treat ovarian carcinoma. Consists of hexamethylmelamine, Cytoxan, Adriamycin, and Platinol.

hCG, HCG (human chorionic gonadotropin).

HCT, HCTZ (hydrochlorothiazide)—a diuretic.

HDL (high-density lipoprotein)—the so-called "good" cholesterol that protects from arteriosclerosis and heart attacks. It relates to risk factors for cardiovascular disease; HDL levels are high in those who exercise, run, walk, etc., and HDL is thought to reduce these risks. Cf. *LDL.*

HDPEB (high-dose PEB protocol)—chemotherapy protocol.

HDRV (human diploid cell strain rabies vaccine)—a rabies vaccine. See *RDRV.*

HD II total hip prosthesis. Also, HD 2.

HD-VAC (high-dose [methotrexate], vinblastine, Adriamycin, cisplatin)—chemotherapy protocol.

head, Zirconia orthopedic prosthetic.

headache
  ice cream
  thunderclap

headrest
  Light-Veley
  Mayfield-Kees
  Multipoise
  pin
  Veley

Healey, in *Rector-Gordon-Healey-Mendoza-Spitzer type IV renal tubular acidosis.*

Healon (sodium hyaluronate) (Oph)—a visco-elastic preparation used to protect eye tissues and cells during intraocular lens implantation.

Healon GV (Oph)—a solution that gently separates tissues and maintains a deep anterior chamber during capsulorhexis. GV stands for greater viscosity, an improvement in the solution over original Healon.

Healon Yellow (Oph)—Healon with added fluorescein; used for visualization of the eye.

heart
  artificial
  crisscross
  Symbion J-7-70 mL total artificial
  University of Akron artificial

heart block, Mobitz I and II AV.

Heartmate (Cardio)—battery-operated portable system to provide pumping assistance to the heart. A cannula is sewn into the left ventricle to reroute the patient's blood which is then circulated through a pneumatic pump and returned to the body via a cannula in the aorta.

Heart Rate, 1*2*3—trade name of a hand-held pulse rate monitor; it is so named because it displays the numbers 1*2*3 as it measures the time of the first three heart beats. On the fourth beat, the heart rate average is displayed.

HeatProbe (GI)—trade name of a water irrigation/lavage device by Olympus.

heave and lift—often used interchangeably; a diffuse lifting impulse along the left sternal heart border with each heartbeat.

heaves—see *dry heaves.*

heavy ion irradiation (Oph)—helium is usually used for this therapy.

heavy-metal screening—lab test for poisoning from heavy metallic elements such as arsenic, iron, lead, and mercury.

Hebra blade (Oph).

Hebra corneal curet (Oph).

Hebra fixation hook (Oph).

Hedspa—used in radionuclide bone imaging.

heel-to-shin test (Neuro). The patient is asked, while in the supine position,

heel-to-shin test *(cont.)* to place the heel of one foot on the knee of the other leg, and then to "run" the heel down the shin. This test is to be done bilaterally and provides (by the smoothness and coordination with which it is performed) an assessment of the patient's cerebellar function.

heel, SACH—for orthopedic appliance.

Heelbo decubitus heel/elbow protector.

heelstick hematocrit—blood obtained from the heel of premature infants for hematocrit test.

HEE syndrome—see *Gastaut syndrome.*

Heffington lumbar seat spinal surgery frame (Neuro, Ortho). This is a table on which the patient is placed, kneeling on a little shelf extending out from the end, with the chest flat on the table. This position helps to decrease epidural venous bleeding.

Heifitz clip (Neuro).

height—see *midparental height.*

Heimlich chest drainage valve.

Heimlich maneuver—a technique for removing foreign matter from the trachea of a choking victim.

Heineke-Mikulicz pyloroplasty.

Heinz body—seen in unstable hemoglobin disease (a congenital hemolytic anemia).

HeLa cells—cells from the first continuously cultured strain of human malignant tissue derived from the cervical carcinoma of Henrietta Lacks in Baltimore in 1951.

Helicobacter pylori (GI)—found in the duodenum and stomach of ulcer patients but not in patients who are free of ulcer disease. This bacterium may be the underlying cause of ulcers. Patients treated with Tagamet or Zantac may also now be treated with antibiotics for severe recurring ulcers.

heliotrope infraorbital discoloration—purplish discoloration under the eye (not ecchymosis).

Helistat (Surg)—absorbable collagen hemostatic sponge.

Heller-Belsey operation—for achalasia of esophagus.

Heller-Nissen operation—for achalasia of the esophagus.

HELLP syndrome (Obs)—a manifestation of preeclampsia. HELLP is an acronym for **h**emolysis, **e**levated **l**iver enzymes, and **l**ow **p**latelets.

Helmholtz coil—MRI term.

heloma durum—a callosity on the hand or the foot.

helper cell—also called helper/inducer cell and T-4 cell; these are the lymphocytes that the AIDS virus specifically attacks and converts into a tool for making additional virus, and this is done much more quickly than with other viruses.

helper/suppressor cell ratio—this ratio changes in AIDS and the change is diagnostic. It may be dictated as the ratio of T-helper to T-suppressor cells or of T-4 to T-8 cells, or you may hear that "the ratio of OKT4 to OKT8 is less than 1.0," OKT4 and OKT8 being monoclonal antibodies to T-4 and T-8. What all of these references are describing is the disappearance of functioning T-4 helper cells.

Hemabate (Ob-Gyn)—prostaglandin instilled into the uterus to initiate labor or to abort fetus.

Hemaflex sheath (Cardio)—a collagen hemostat product specifically designed to stop blood flow from vessels during cardiovascular surgery, as it is easy to wrap around vessels. Placed percutaneously in the femoral artery during PTCA.

hemangiopericytoma—rare neoplasm, vascular, usually benign.

Hemashield (Surg)—an enhanced graft with collagen which promotes intimal development and may reduce thrombogenicity.

hematocrit
dilutional
heelstick

hematopoiesis—the body's mechanism for replacing cells.

hematoporphyrin derivative (HpD)—given intravenously, this photosensitizing agent is absorbed only by malignant cells which can then be destroyed by laser surgery.

hemicolectomy (Duecollement maneuver).

Hemoccult II—a test for fecal occult blood.

Hemoclip—a ligating clip; it comes in titanium and also in tantalum.

HemoCue photometer—for a quick office test for hemoglobin determination done on a drop of blood.

Hemo-Dial dialysate additives.

hemodialysis system, Redy 2000.

hemodialyzer—apparatus used in the hemodialysis of kidney patients to remove toxic elements. There are three types of hemodialyzers: the coil, the hollow fiber, and the parallel plate.

hemofiltration (Nephrol)—a technique in hemodialysis where waste products of hemodialysis are removed from the blood along with plasma water by rapid ultrafiltration, and then the blood is reconstituted with a solution, either before or after hemodialysis. The technique appears to reduce side effects of dialysis and seems to assure better tolerance of fluid removal, particularly in patients with high vascular instability.

hemoglobin
glycosylated
pyridoxilated stroma-free (SFHb)
rHb1.1 (recombinant)

hemoglobulinuria, pyridoxilated stroma-free.

Hem-o-lok (only the initial letter is capitalized)—polymer ligating clip.

Hemopad—absorbable collagen hemostat, which comes as nonwoven pads that can be cut, folded, or wrapped around a bleeding site. It can be peeled away easily, but any remaining bits are soon absorbed by the tissues.

hemophilia A—factor VIII deficiency (classical hemophilia).

hemophilia B—factor IX deficiency. See *Christmas disease.*

Hemophilus—see *Haemophilus.*

Hemopump—a temporary external pump which completely supports circulation, used in the treatment of cardiogenic shock. This device is an improvement over the intra-aortic balloon pump which provides only 25% circulatory assistance.

hemorrhage
Duret
salmon-patch
splinter

hemostatic eraser—used for pinpoint hemostasis in anterior and posterior segment surgery (Oph).

Hemotene—absorbable collagen hemostat to control bleeding during surgery when sutures are not practical.

HeNe laser (**he**lium-**ne**on) (Oph)—has a visible low power red beam and is often used in conjunction with the carbon dioxide (CO_2) laser. The advantage of the HeNe is that the beam is visible and the surgeon can see its location.

Henning meniscal retractors used in knee surgery (Ortho).

Henoch-Schönlein purpura.

heparin lock—an intermittent infusion reservoir; permits periodic infusion of drugs without continuous fluid infusion; a heparin solution injected into the reservoir between infusions will keep the I.V. patent without the necessity of a continuous fluid drip. Although the heparin lock was first used for administration of heparin, it is also used for transfusion therapy and in the administration of a number of drugs, including chemotherapeutic agents, antibiotics, etc.

HepatAmine—a nutrient solution for patients with liver disease.

hepatic venous web disease (in patients with Budd-Chiari syndrome).

hepatic web dilation—to establish hepatic vein outflow (in hepatic venous web disease).

hepatitides (''heh-puh-tih'-tih-dees'')—plural form of hepatitis.

hepatitis—a viral disease which might be a cofactor in AIDS; it in itself can be fatal to an AIDS patient. Types:
A
B
C
chronic active
chronic persistent
D
delta
drug-induced
F
fulminant
HAV (A virus)
HBV (B virus)
NANB (non-A, non-B)
non-A
non-B
non-C

hepatitis *(cont.)*
peliosis
post-transfusion
viral

hepatitis B antigen (HbAg).

hepatitis C (GI)—the newer name for non-A, non-B hepatitis.

hepatitis F (GI)—the newer name for non-A, non-B, non-C hepatitis.

hepatization—transformation into a liver-like mass, as the solidified state of the lung in lobar pneumonia.

hepatojugular reflux (Cardio)—swelling of the jugular vein caused by applying pressure over the liver. This swelling indicates right heart insufficiency.

"hep lock" (medical slang for heparin lock). See *heparin lock.*

Heprofile ELISA (enzyme-linked immunosorbent assay) (Lab)—for hepatitis B.

Heptavax-B—trade name for a hepatitis B vaccine.

Heptran swab (Oph).

herald patch (Derm)—a single lesion that is seen before the eruption of pityriasis rosea.

Herculon suture—trade name for brand of synthetic suture material.

Herellea vaginicola.

Hering, nerve of—carotid sinus nerve.

hernia, Richter's.

Herp-Check (Lab)—an antibody test for herpes simplex virus which provides results in four hours rather than up to seven days as before.

herpes simplex virus (HSV)—can disseminate in AIDS.

herpes whitlow—herpesvirus infection, occurring in hospital workers and dentists, that can be transmitted through contact with the patient's oral mucous membrane or saliva. It

herpes whitlow *(cont.)* involves the folds of tissue around the fingernail and consists of pyogenic and vesicular paronychia. Related terms: paronychia, felon.

herpes zoster virus (HZV)—can disseminate in AIDS.

Herplex (idoxuridine).

Hertel rigid dilator stone forceps.

hertz (Hz)—a unit of frequency, equal to one cycle per second; measurement used in audiograms.

Hertzog intraocular lens.

Hespan (hetastarch)—plasma volume expander; used in treatment of shock (cheaper than albumin).

Hessburg trephine vacuum trephine. Also, Hessburg-Barron.

H&E stain—hematoxylin and eosin.

hetastarch (Hespan) **plasma volume expander.**

heterografts, bovine and porcine—used as valves in cardiac surgery; they are specially prepared so they are not rejected as foreign bodies.

Hewlett-Packard ear oximeter—used to record oxygen saturation continuously. See *ear oximeter.* (Note: Hewlett-Packard has a hyphen.)

Hexabrix (Vasc Surg)—contrast medium used in angiography.

Hexa-CAF—chemotherapeutic agent.

Hexalen (altretamine).

hexamethylmelamine (HMM, HXM, Hexastat) (Oncol)—an oral drug used in treatment of bronchogenic carcinoma and advanced ovarian cancer.

Hexastat (hexamethylmelamine).

Hexcel total condylar knee system—femoral and tibial components, and patellar dome.

Hexcelite (Ortho)—intermediate phase casting and thermoplastic light mesh immersed briefly in 80° C water and then wrapped around the extremity to be casted; hardens quickly.

Heyer-Schulte breast implant.

Heyer-Schulte tissue expander. See *expander.*

"H. flu"—slang for *Haemophilus influenzae.*

5-HIAA (hydroxyindoleacetic acid)—a substance found in the urine of patients with carcinoid tumors of intestine.

hGH (human growth hormone). See *Protropin.*

HIB disease—*Haemophilus influenzae* type B, a leading cause of bacterial meningitis.

HIB polysaccharide vaccine—used to treat HIB disease in children. See *HIB disease.*

Hibiclens—an antiseptic, antimicrobial skin cleanser (chlorhexidine gluconate). Used the same way that hexachlorophene and povidone-iodine are used in preoperative preparation and wound cleansing. Cf. *Hibitane, Hibistat.*

Hibistat—used for hand scrub and as a germicidal hand rinse in surgery (chlorhexidine gluconate). Cf. *Hibitane, Hibiclens.*

Hibitane tincture—used in preparing the patient's skin for an injection (chlorhexidine gluconate). Cf. *Hibiclens, Hibistat.*

Hickman catheter—an indwelling right atrial catheter used in treatment of patients receiving bone marrow transplants, and those whose medical care requires frequent access to their circulation, e.g., drawing blood, administering blood, for total parenteral nutrition. Also used for withdrawing blood for plasmapheresis, and for central venous pressure mon-

Hickman *(cont.)* itoring. Its use eliminates the need for frequent venipuncture. It is a modification of the Broviac catheter.

HIDA scan (''high-dah'') (hepatoiminodiacetic acid)—a technetium scan (also given as TcHIDA, or technetium-HIDA) for biliary imaging into liver and gallbladder. See *PIPIDA.*

Hieshima coaxial catheter—used in some interventional procedures in radiology (Dr. Grant B. Hieshima).

HIF (higher integrative functions) (Neuro, Psych).

Higgins technique for ureterointestinal anastomosis.

high-density linear array—term used in B-scan, Doppler, and color Doppler imaging (Radiol). See *B-scan.*

high-density lipoprotein (HDL)—see *HDL.*

higher integrative functions (HIF).

high field strength scanner (Radiol)—MRI device using a static magnetic field of maximal intensity.

high myope (Oph)—one who has a high degree of myopia (nearsightedness).

Hildebrandt uterine hemostatic forceps—has a split in the jaws of the forceps that permits suturing with the forceps in place and then removing the forceps without disturbing the sutures.

Hiles intraocular lens.

Hilgenreiner line—between the inferior edges of the triradiate cartilage and the line tangential to the medial ossified edge of the proximal metaphysis of the femur.

Hilger facial nerve stimulator—used for clinical evaluation of the facial nerve, clinical testing of muscle tissue viability, and for nerve identification and testing during surgery.

Hill cluster harvest technique—micrograft technique.

Hill-Sachs lesion, deformity (Ortho). Note: *Not* Hill-Sach's.

HIM (health information management) —formerly known as medical record management.

hinge, Kinematic rotating.

hippocampus (Greek *hippokampos,* sea horse)—area of cortex in bottom of inferior (temporal) horn of the lateral ventricle; it has the appearance of a seahorse, thus the name.

Hippocrates manipulation (Ortho)—for anterior dislocation of the shoulder joint. The physician exerts traction on the patient's arm, and at the same time places his heel (with the shoe removed first!) in the patient's axilla to give countertraction, thus forcing the head of the humerus from beneath the acromion.

hippocratic wreath—seen in men with male pattern baldness, the rim of hair surrounding the bald area.

hip replacement
Kirschner Medical ''Dimension''
SAF (self-articulating femoral)

hip spica cast (Ortho)—used after surgery for correction of congenital hip dysplasia.

Hirano inclusion body (in dementia).

Hirschberg measurement of esotropia.

Hirschman intraocular implant lens.

Hirschsprung's disease—congenital megacolon (giant colon).

Hismanal (astemizole)—antihistamine, for nasal congestion (ENT).

Hi Speed Pulse Lavage by Micro-Aire for debridement of bone surfaces during knee and hip replacements.

His-Purkinje conduction (''hiss purkin' gee'') (Cardio), as in bundle of His and Purkinje fibers.

Histoacryl glue (cyanoacrylate)—a tissue adhesive made in Germany. It is used to seal some perforating-type corneal wounds as may be seen in stromal herpetic keratitis.

Histoplasma—the fungus which causes histoplasmosis. Disseminated histoplasmosis was recently added to the growing list of once very rare (in disseminated form) infections which are now often seen in AIDS.

Histoplasma capsulatum polysaccharide antigen (HPA). Detection of HPA is a rapid method for detecting histoplasmosis.

HI titer (hemagglutination inhibition)—a rubella screening test.

HIV (human immunodeficiency virus)—the official name for the AIDS virus, changed because of the unwieldiness of the earlier terms and the debate over who discovered the virus first. HIV is a retrovirus, of the cytopathic lentivirus group.

HIV AC-le—AIDS vaccine by Bristol-Myers; currently undergoing clinical trials.

HIVAGEN—lab test for HIV.

HIV-associated thrombocytopenia treated with high-dose intravenous immune globulin therapy.

HIVID (ddc, dideoxycytidine)—used to treat patients with AIDS and ARC.

HKAFO (hip-knee-ankle-foot orthosis) (Ortho)—for ambulation in children with cerebral palsy and myelomeningocele. Orthosis in three forms: parapodium, reciprocating gait, and swivel walker.

HLA (human lymphocyte antigen)—a designation used in tissue typing for organ transplants.

HLA-A—one of four major loci of HLA (human lymphocyte antigen) which defines immunologic identity. Products of these loci are identified serologically. Used in tissue typing for transplantation. Also, *HLA-B, HLA-C, HLA-D.*

HLA-B, HLA-C, HLA-D—see *HLA-A.*

HLP (hyperlipoproteinemia).

HMD (oxymetholone).

HMG (human menopausal gonadotropin)—used in treatment of some types of infertility.

HMG-CoA reductase inhibitors (Cardio)—a class of drugs used to decrease hypercholesterolemia and hypertriglyceridemia. Examples: simvastatin (Zocor) and pravastatin (Pravachol).

HMM, HXM (hemamethylmelamine)—see *altretamine.*

HOCM (hypertrophic obstructive cardiomyopathy).

Hodge intestinal decompression tube.

Hoehne's sign (Ob-Gyn)—failure to respond to oxytocic drugs, a sign of uterine rupture.

Hoek-Bowen cement removal system by Micro-Aire (Ortho).

Hoen ventricular needle (Neuro).

Hoffa's tendon shortening (Ortho). Gathering stitches are run up a portion of the tendon, and then the suture is tightened to the appropriate length.

Hoffer intraocular implant lens.

Hoffman-Clayton procedure (Pod)—podiatric procedure to treat rheumatoid arthritis.

Hoffmann external fixation device (Ortho). Developed by a Swiss surgeon, Dr. Raoul Hoffmann.

Hoffmann reflex (Neuro)—twitching of the thumb when the middle finger is snapped.

Hofmeister gastroenterostomy.

Hofmeister-Shoemaker gastrojejunostomy.

Hohmann retractor (Pod). Also, Mini-Hohmann.

Holladay formula (Oph)—a formula for calculating the depth of the anterior chamber of the eye.

Hollande's solution—used as a fixative for some types of pathology specimens.

Hollenhorst plaques—yellow-orange cholesterol plaques which, when seen on examination of the optic fundi, indicate the presence of atherosclerosis. "His optic fundi were closely inspected and were benign for Hollenhorst plaques, for papilledema and hemorrhage."

hollow fiber dialyzer—see *hemodialyzer.*

holmium:YAG laser (Surg)—a laser used in endoscopic laser cholecystectomy and in angioplasty.

Holter
- shunt
- monitor
- tubing
- valve

Holtzman rats—a strain of rats used in laboratories.

Homans' sign—forced dorsiflexion of the foot causes discomfort behind the knee in thrombosis in the leg.

home O_2 (oxygen), as in "The patient was discharged on home O_2." In dictation it sounds like *homo-2.*

Homer-Wright rosette—sometimes seen on histologic examination of medulloblastomas.

Honan balloon—used in phakoemulsification of cataracts (Oph). "After ascertaining adequate akinesia and anesthesia, and after the Honan balloon was set at 30 mm of mercury for 15 minutes, the left face was prepared and draped in the usual sterile ophthalmic fashion."

Honan manometer—used in lowering intraocular pressure.

H_1 receptors (ENT)—histamine receptors in the respiratory tract which are blocked by antihistamines.

honeycomb mucosa (GI)—seen in the jejunum of patients with celiac disease.

honk, precordial—an abnormal heart sound.

hood O_2 (Peds)—humidified oxygen administered in a clear hard plastic container encasing the baby's head with an opening for the neck. Due to small air leaks around the neck it can attain only about 40% oxygen concentration.

Hood stoma stent (ENT)—a device which utilizes a valve to allow a patient with a tracheostomy to speak without first having to put a finger over the stoma.

hook
- boat
- Bonn micro iris
- Dohlman incus
- Hebra fixation
- Neivert polyp
- Praeger iris
- Sinskey
- Speare dural
- von Graefe muscle

hook wire, Sadowsky.

Hopkins rod lens telescope.

Hopkins 70° rigid telescope (ENT)—used in laryngoscopy.

hordeolum—acute inflammation of a sebaceous gland of the eyelid. See *stye (sty).*

Hormodendrum—an inhalant antigen.

hormone
- Biotropin (human growth hormone)
- follicle-stimulating (FSH)
- Genentech biosynthetic human growth (Protropin)

hormone *(cont.)*
gonadotropin-releasing (GnRH)
human growth hormone (Biotropin)
Humatrope human growth
hypothalamic luteinizing hormone-releasing
long-acting thyroid-stimulating (LATS)
luteinizing hormone-releasing (LHRH).
parathyroid (parathormone)
Protropin human growth

Horn endo-otoprobe (ENT)—a laser probe used in ear surgery.

Hoskins nylon suture laser lens (Oph) —used to cut subconjunctival nylon sutures in postoperative situations such as trabeculectomies, sutures in cataract wounds causing astigmatism, and flap sutures that are too tight to permit filtration. This is a noninvasive procedure.

Hot/Ice System III (Ortho)—for controlled cold therapy following orthopedic procedures.

hot potato voice (ENT)—a hollow voice caused by edema or paralysis of the soft palate; most commonly observed in severe pharyngitis or peritonsillar abscess.

Houget'a inguinal hernia repair.

Hough hoe ("huff") (ENT)—elevator with an angled tip and handle.

House and Pulec otic-perotic shunt (ENT)—for treatment of progressive endolymphatic hydrops (Ménière's disease).

housemaid's knee—older term for prepatellar bursitis, seen in patients who repeatedly traumatize the bursa by kneeling.

Hounsfield unit—density measurement indicative of calcium (on CT scan).

Houston Halo (Ortho)—used to treat cervical disorders.

Howell biopsy aspiration needle (GI).

Howmedica instruments; prostheses.

HPA axis suppression (hypothalamic-pituitary-adrenal)—a syndrome which occurs following systemic absorption of significant amounts of topically applied corticosteroids. This may occur from prolonged use or extensive use (over a large body area) of topical corticosteroids. Symptoms include Cushing's syndrome and elevated blood glucose levels.

HPA (*Histoplasma capsulatum* polysaccharide antigen).

HPA-23 (antimoniotungstate)—a drug used to treat AIDS.

HPC guide wire (hydrophilic) (GI)—a flexible guide wire used to cannulate the biliary duct. Produces less trauma than other methods, in the presence of tight strictures.

HpD—see *hematoporphyrin derivative.*

HPS (hematoxylin, phloxine, and safranin)—histochemical stains (Path).

HPV (human papillomavirus)—cause of genital warts, a sexually transmitted disease and a risk factor for cancer of the cervix.

H reflex study—electrodiagnostic test. Through an electrically induced spinal reflex, a determination can be made as to the presence of unilateral S1 radiculopathy.

HRL screening plates (Hardy–Rand–Littler) (Oph). These test charts are composed of dots of different colors; geometric figures can be seen among the dots. The charts are used to test color vision.

Hruby lens ("ruby") (Oph)—slit-lamp biomicroscopy.

HSSG (hysterosalpingosonography).

HSV (herpesvirus; herpes simplex virus).

HTLV-III (human T-cell lymphotropic virus)—name given to the virus isolated by Robert Gallo, the American researcher who thought he was the first to isolate the AIDS virus. The researchers at the Pasteur Institute in Paris were actually the first by a considerable margin. HIV (human immunodeficiency virus, now the official name for the AIDS virus), is one of the lentiviruses. See *HIV.*

HT receptor blockers—see *5-HT receptor blockers.*

H_2 blockers (GI)—a class of drugs that block H_2 receptors in the stomach to stop release of histamine which stimulates gastric acid secretion; e.g., cimetidine (Tagamet) and ranitidine (Zantac).

Hubbard hydrotherapy tank—including treatment for psoriasis.

Hubbell intraocular implant lens.

Huber needle—a specially designed needle for use with ports. The sharply angled bevel leaves a line-like tear (in the rubber-covered entry site) which self-seals easily. Comes in straight or 90° angle design, the latter being used for continuous infusion because it will lie flat when taped to the skin.

Hudson-Stahli line—a linear subepithelial deposit of iron pigment on the surface of the cornea (Oph).

"huff" hoe—see *Hough hoe.*

Hughston knee evaluation (or score) (Ortho)—divides the patient's clinical performance into three categories: subjective, functional, and objective, yielding a combined score.

Hughston view (Radiol, Ortho)—x-ray view of the flexed knee to demonstrate subluxation of the patella or fracture of the femoral condyle.

HUI uterine injector from Unimar (Gyn).

human chorionic gonadotropin (hCG or HCG).

human diploid cell strain rabies vaccine (HDRV).

human growth hormone (hGH).

human immunodeficiency virus (HIV).

human insulin. See *Humulin.* Cf. *semisynthetic human insulin.*

human lymphocyte antigen (HLA).

human menopausal gonadotropin (HMG).

human papillomavirus (HPV)—cause of genital warts, a sexually transmitted disease and a risk factor for cancer of the cervix.

Human Surf (Neonat)—natural surfactant obtained from amniotic fluid. Used to treat the lack of surfactant in premature infants which causes hyaline membrane disease.

human T-cell lymphotropic virus (HTLV-III).

Humatrope—human growth hormone, manufactured by recombinant DNA technology. It is used in treating children with growth hormone deficiencies. See *Protropin.*

humeral (Ortho)—pertaining to the humerus bone. Cf. *humoral, humorous.*

humerus (Ortho)—the long arm bone between the shoulder joint and the elbow joint. Cf. *humeral, humoral, humorous.*

HUMI uterine manipulator/injector (Ob-Gyn)—marketed by Unimar.

humoral—pertaining to the immunity provided by antibodies in the blood. Cf. *humeral, humorous.*

humorous—funny or witty in character. Cf. *humerus.*

hump
buffalo
dowager's
Hampton's

Humulin—a human insulin (of recombinant DNA origin).

Hunner's interstitial cystitis (*not* Hunter) (Urol)—a severe, chronic inflammation of mucosa and muscularis of the urinary bladder, associated with ulcers of the bladder. Also, *Hunner's ulcer.*

Hunner's ulcer (Urol)—see *Hunner's interstitial cystitis.*

Hunt, in *Tolosa-Hunt syndrome.*

Hunt and Hess neurological classification to predict the prognosis in patients with subarachnoid hemorrhage, grades 1-4.

Hunter open cord tendon implant—for hand tendon reconstruction (Hand Surg).

Hunter's canal (canalis adductorius)—contains the femoral vessels and saphenous nerve.

Hunter-Sessions balloon—used in inferior vena cava to intercept a venous embolus.

Hunter tendon rod insertion (Cardio)—a treatment for deep venous insufficiency (DVI) of the lower extremities. DVI causes symptoms of chronic edema and pain because the valves in the veins of the lower leg are incompetent. An incision is made at the back of the leg in the popliteal fossa. The Hunter tendon rod (made of Dacron) is sewn to the gracilis tendon at the side of the leg, woven through the popliteal artery and vein deep inside the leg, sutured to the biceps tendon on the other side of the leg, and drawn up snugly as a sling. This device then acts as a substitute valve by periodically occluding the popliteal vein as it passes tightly across it. When the patient stands or sits, the popliteal vein remains unoccluded. However, when the knee is actively flexed and the gracilis and biceps muscles retract, the popliteal vein is occluded to prevent venous reflux and venous stasis in the leg. Results are said to be superior to those obtained with other techniques.

Hurst mercury dilators; bougies.

Hutchinson's teeth—older term for one of the manifestations of congenital syphilis, now rare; the teeth are broad at the base and the biting surface is narrow and notched. Also, hutchinsonian molars.

HVS (hyperventilation syndrome).

hyaloid corpuscle—see *Mittendorf's dot.*

hycamptamine (Oncol)—see *topotecan.*

hydrazine sulfate (HDZ) (Oncol)—a drug to promote weight gain and appetite in patients with incurable colorectal carcinoma.

hydrocephalus, in *normal pressure hydrocephalus.*

Hydrocollator (Phys Ther)—The trade name for a silica gel pack used in applying localized heat. The silica gel is encased in a canvas bag. The pack is immersed in water and thermostatically heated to 140 to 160° F. The pack is then wrapped in several layers of terry cloth before applying to the area to be heated. The pack maintains its heat for approximately 20 to 30 minutes—which gives it an advantage over the hot water bottle.

Hydrocurve contact lenses.

Hydron Burn Bandage—a synthetic dressing for burns.

hydrophilic—water-loving. Used in medicine to refer to stains. Cf. *lipophilic.*

Hydro-Splint II (Ortho)—used to immobilize fractures of upper or lower extremities. It is not only a splint, but also a cold (or warm) compress, and provides soft tissue compression for chronic or acute swelling.

hydroxyapatite (or hydroxylapatite)—dense ceramic material manufactured from coral found in the ocean; it is porous, like human bone. Used as an adjunct to bone grafting in cranial defects, to restore normal contour (Neuro). In ophthalmology, it can be formed into a sphere and used as an ocular implant after enucleation of the eye. Note: Both spellings are used, although the first is preferred. Also, Biomatrix ocular implant, Durapatite, Interpore.

hydroxylapatite—see *hydroxyapatite.*

hydroxyindoleacetic acid (5-HIAA).

Hyfrecator—trade name of a desiccator-fulgurator-coagulator manufactured by Birtcher.

hygroma—fluid-filled cystic mass, often seen in the necks of children.

hymenal ring *(not* hymeneal, as it is often mispronounced).

hyper-, prefix meaning excessive, above, beyond. Cf. *hypo-.*

hyperbaric oxygen (high pressure)—used in treatment of cyanide poisoning, exceptionally high blood loss anemia, decompression sickness, and as adjunctive therapy in osteomyelitis, radiation injury, acute cerebral edema, and injury to the head and spinal cord.

hypericin (VIMRxyn)—a drug used to treat patients with AIDS. (Mfr., VIMRx Pharmaceuticals.)

hyperlipoproteinemia (HLP).

hyperopia—farsightedness.

hyperreninemia—a condition of elevated levels of renin in the blood, which may lead to aldosteronism and hypertension.

hypertelorism—abnormally increased distance between two organs, as in Crouzon's disease.

hyperthermia, whole body—used in the therapy regimen of patients with certain types of tumors, some bone metastases, and Ewing's sarcoma. These cancer cells are particularly sensitive to heat; therefore, heat increases the effectiveness of chemotherapy and radiotherapy. When the patient's body is heated to 108° F. *after* irradiation, the cancer cells cannot readily repair themselves. When the patient is given hyperthermia *before* chemotherapy is introduced, the cancer cells are more susceptible to the effects of chemotherapy agents.

hypertrophic obstructive cardiomyopathy (HOCM).

hypertrophy, asymmetric septal (ASH).

hypertylosis of the palms—see *tylosis* (Derm).

hypesthesia—diminished sensitivity to stimulation, feeling, sensation or perception. Also, *hypoesthesia.*

hypnosis—focused open neurosensory induction of hypnosis, a self-hypnotic method using vision, hearing, and kinesthetic sensations.

hypnotic—a drug used to induce sleep.

hypo-, prefix meaning deficient, decrease, under, beneath, below. Cf. *hyper-.*

hypoaeration (Radiol)—on chest x-ray, abnormal reduction in the amount of air in lung tissue.

hypoechoic ("hi-po-e-ko'-ic")—a term used in ultrasonography, when only

hypoechoic *(cont.)*
few echoes are given off as the ultrasound waves bounce off structures or tissues at which they are directed. "The patient had a hypoechoic area in the right lobe of the prostate."

hypokinesis (Radiol)—abnormal reduction of mobility or motility; reduced contractile movement in one or both cardiac ventricles.

hypophysectomy kit, Zervas (Neuro)—for stereotactic procedures.

hypophysis—pituitary gland (hypophysis cerebri); pharyngeal hypophysis (a mass in the wall of the pharynx similar in appearance to the hypophysis). Cf. *apophysis, epiphysis, hypothesis.*

hypothalamic-pituitary-adrenal axis (HPA).

hypothalamus—the portion of the brain that controls the autonomic mechanism.

hypothermia blanket—used for cooling patients to 28 to 30° C for open heart and brain surgery; reduces the need for the normal amount of oxygen.

hypothesis—a theory that appears to explain certain phenomena and is used as the basis of experimentation and reasoning to prove the theory. Cf. *apophysis, epiphysis, hypophysis.*

hysterosalpingosonography (HSSG) (Ob-Gyn)—a diagnostic ultrasound technique used to assess uterine cavity defects and patency of the fallopian tubes.

hysteroscope
Baggish contact panoramic
Baloser

Hysteroser (Gyn)—trade name for a contact hysteroscopy system used for uterine examination, to localize intrauterine devices (IUDs), in evaluation for ectopic pregnancy, polyps, hyperplasia, carcinoma, uterine synechiae. It is also used for examination of the endocervical canal.

Hy-Tape—waterproof, medicated tape safe for direct use on skin and especially used by ostomy patients.

Hytrin (terazosin).

HZV (herpes zoster virus).

I, i

IABP (intra-aortic balloon pump)—used with Fogarty embolectomy catheter in removing pulmonary emboli.

Ialo photocoagulation—of the whole retina (Oph).

I&D (incision and drainage). Cf. *IND.*

I&O, I/O (intake and output)—intake of liquid (intravenous, per mouth, per tube) and output (urine, tube, drain) plus insensible output, in a 24-hour period. Measured in cubic centimeters or milliliters. "The patient's I&O was monitored." See *INO; insensible output.*

I-beam—see *Jergesen I-beam.*

ibotenic acid—one of the poisons from the deadly mushroom *Amanita muscaria.*

ICA—see *islet cell antibodies.*

ice cream headache—probably needs no explanation; most of us have had that sensation on biting into extremely cold ice cream.

ICE (ifosfamide, carboplatin, etoposide)—a chemotherapy protocol used to treat small-cell lung carcinoma, and Hodgkin's and non-Hodgkin's lymphomas.

ICE disorders—immunoglobulin-complexed enzyme disorders.

ICE syndrome—irido-corneal-endothelial syndrome (Oph).

ICLH apparatus (Ortho), Imperial College, London Hospital.

ICP catheter (intracranial pressure)—used with Tele-Sensor monitor after brain surgery (Neuro). See *Cosman ICP Tele-Sensor.*

ICRF-187 (Oncol)—a drug used to prevent cardiotoxicity in pediatric patients with sarcoma receiving Adriamycin chemotherapy.

ICS—intracellular-like, calcium bearing crystalloid solution. See *cardioplegic solution.*

Idamycin (idarubicin).

idarubicin (Idamycin) (Oncol)—one of the special antibiotics (derived from the funguslike bacterium *Streptomyces*) used as a chemotherapy agent for the treatment of acute myeloid leukemia in adults.

ideation (noun)—the process of forming ideas or images (Psych). "He has no suicidal or homicidal ideation."

idée fixe ("ee-day'-feeks")—an obsessively fixed idea (Psych).

idiojunctional rhythm, junctional or nodal rhythm (Cardio). When effective electrical impulses are no longer generated by the sinoatrial (SA) node, the atrioventricular (AV) node (located near the junction of atria and ventricles) becomes the pacemaker for the heart.

idiopathic hypertrophic subaortic stenosis (IHSS).

idiopathic thrombocytopenic purpura (ITP).

IDIS angiography system (intraoperative digital subtraction).

idoxuridine (IUDR, Herplex, Stoxil)—used to treat herpes simplex virus infections.

I/E ratio (inspiratory/expiratory ratio), as in "Lungs: Normal I/E ratio, and no rales, rhonchi, or wheezes."

IFA test—indirect fluorescent antibody test for *Legionella pneumophila.* See also *DFA.*

IFN-A (interferon alfa).

ifosfamide (Ifex)—related chemically to Cytoxan, this drug is used to treat advanced testicular cancer.

IgG, platelet-associated (PAIgG).

IgG 2A monoclonal antibody (Immurait) (Oncol)—labeled with iodine-131. A drug used to treat B-cell lymphoma and leukemias.

Iglesias fiberoptic resectoscope.

IgM-RF antibody (rheumatoid factor).

IHSS (idiopathic hypertrophic subaortic stenosis). Now called ASH (asymmetric septal hypertrophy).

ILA surgical stapler.

ileal conduit (*not* ileoconduit or ileo conduit) (Urol, Surg)—a segment of ileum formed into a new bladder in patients who have undergone total cystectomy. The ends of the ureters are then anastomosed to the new ileal "bladder."

ileocystoplasty
Camey
LeDuc-Camey

ileostomy
Brooke
Kock

ileum—the part of the small intestine located between the jejunum and the large intestine. Cf. *ilium.*

ileus (Radiol)—small-bowel obstruction due to failure of peristalsis.

iliopsoas test. On abdominal examination, if pain is elicited when the patient flexes his thigh against pressure of the examiner's hand, there is an inflammatory process in contact with the iliopsoas muscle.

ilium—the superior portion of the hip bone. Cf. *ileum.*

Ilizarov limb lengthening procedure ("eh-liz'-a-rov") (Ortho).

Ilizarov system (Ortho)—to facilitate limb lengthening, fracture fixation, and nonunion of long bones.

illicit—unlawful, improper, not permitted, as "The patient denies use of illicit drugs." Cf. *elicit.*

illness, food-borne (FBI).

Illumina PROSeries—laparoscopy system.

illusion—an unreal or misleading image or perception, as "He was suffering from the illusion that there were insects crawling over him." Cf. *allusion, elusion.*

IL-1—see *interleukin-1.*

IL-2—see *interleukin-2.*
IL-3—see *interleukin-3.*
ILUS catheter (intraluminal ultrasound) (GI).
IMA (inferior mesenteric artery).
IMAB (internal mammary artery bypass).
image, imaging
antifibrin antibody
axial
echo planar
line
magnetic resonance
phase
planar spin
point
proton density
Purkinje's
sequential plane
sequential point
simultaneous volume
spin-echo
three-dimensional Fourier transform
two-dimensional Fourier transform
volume
image acquisition time—MRI term.
imaging agent—see *medication; radioisotope; technetium.*
IMED infusion device—for intravenous fluids.
IMEX scleral implants—solid silicone, sponge silicone, and Miragel buckling components (Oph). See *Miragel.*
Imitrex (sumatriptan).
immersion foot—the third stage of trauma due to exposure to cold; first stage—frostbite; second stage—trench foot.
imminent—about to occur in the near future; immediately threatening. Cf. *eminence.*
immobilize—prevent from moving. Cf. *mobilize.*
Immther (Oncol)—used to treat metastatic colorectal carcinoma.
immune globulins. See *antibody molecules.*
immune system modulator (Imreg-1).
immunity, cell-mediated (CMI).
immunofixation in agar (Agar-IF) of blood serum.
immunoperoxidase stain. Example of usage: "Immunoperoxidase stains were performed in formalin-fixed, paraffin-embedded sections, using the peroxidase-antiperoxidase (PAP) technique."
immunoreactive parathyroid hormone (iPTH) (lowercase *i*).
immunovar (British name for *isoprinosine*)—a drug used to treat AIDS.
ImmuRAID (CEA-Tc 99m)—an agent used in antibody imaging (Radiol). See *RAID.*
Immurait (IgG 2A monoclonal antibody).
Impact enteral formula—for advanced nutritional support.
impactor—see *vertebral body impactor.*
IMP-Capello arm support—provides stability and access to the patient's arm to monitor I.V., blood pressure, etc.; made by Innovative Medical Products (IMP).
impedance plethysmography (IPG).
impingement (Radiol)—contact or pressure, generally abnormal, between two structures.
implant—metal orthopedic implants are used mainly for total joint replacement, Silastic silicone rubber implants are used in plastic surgery, and silicone orthopedic implants are used for hand and foot. See *orthosis; prosthesis.* Examples of implants:
Arenberg-Denver inner-ear valve
Biocell RTV breast
Biocoral
Biodel
Biomatrix ocular

implant *(cont.)*
Coburn Mark IX eye
cochlear
Custodis
Durapapite
gentamicin
Gliadel
Heyer-Schulte breast
hydroxyapatite
IMEX scleral
Interpore
islet cell
McCutchen
McGhan breast
Mentor two-piece penile
methyl methacrylate beads
Miragel
Muhlberger orbital
Nexus
Septacin
Shepard intraocular lens
silicone
TheraSeed
vagal nerve

Implast bone cement (Ortho).

Implens (Sheets) **intraocular implant lens.**

impulse, apical—MRI term.

Imreg-1, Imreg-2 (immune system modulator)—used to treat AIDS, ARC, and Kaposi's sarcoma.

Imudon—see *pegademase bovine.*

Imuthiol (diethyldithiocarbamate)—a drug used to treat patients with AIDS and ARC.

IMV (intermittent mandatory ventilation) (Pulm)—used in weaning a patient from long-term ventilator use. While the patient remains on the ventilator, the number of mandatory breaths is gradually reduced. In between the mandatory breaths, the system allows the patient to breathe independently. With this method, the muscles used in breathing are gradually strengthened until the patient can breathe independently.

inactivation technique, psoralen.

incentive spirometry (Pulm).

incidence—in medicine, the number of new cases of a disease that occur in a given population in a certain period of time. Cf. *incidents.*

incidents—events, happenings, occurrences. Cf. *incidence.*

incipient—just beginning to appear; initial or early stage.

incision—a cut or a wound made by a sharp instrument. Cf. *excision.*
Types of incisions:
bayonet
Bevan
Bruner
Bruser
Cherney
chevron
Cohen uterine
cross-shaped
cross-tunneling
cruciate
curvilinear
intercartilaginous
J-shaped
Kocher collar (thyroidectomy)
Kocher's (biliary tract)
LaRoque herniorrhaphy
lazy H
lazy Z
L-curved
Lynch
modified Bruner
muscle-splitting
relaxing
relief
Rethi
Rockey-Davis
saber-cut
scoring

incision *(cont.)*
S-flap
Sloan
smiling
split
transverse
T-shaped
T-tube
U-shaped
Wilde
Y
Yorke-Mason
Z-plasty

incisura dextra of Gans (GI)—deep groove on the inferior surface of the liver near the bed of the gallbladder.

inclusion body
Hirano
Lafora
Lewy
lyssa
Negri
Pick

Incomplete Sentence Blank Test (ISB) (Psych)—mental status examination.

increment—amount by which a dose or value is increased, as "Steroids were increased in weekly increments of 5 mg to a maximum dose of 25 mg."

IND (investigational new drug)—a drug which may be used in clinical testing by licensed researchers with the permission of the FDA, but not yet approved by the FDA for marketing. Cf. *I&D.*

indecainide (Decabid) (Cardio)—a drug used to treat arrhythmias.

index
AHI (apnea/hypopnea)
Broders'
fetal-pelvic
Fick cardiac
foam stability
FTI (free thyroxine)

index *(cont.)*
Gravindex
Mengert's pelvimetry
penile-brachial pressure (PBPI)
SISI (short increment sensitivity)

Indiana pouch—a continent urinary diversion used in patients who require cystectomy, for carcinoma or because of trauma; patients who have a neurogenic bladder, bladder dysfunction or congenital anomaly. Other procedures that are used to accomplish continent urinary diversion: Camey ileocystoplasty, Kock pouch, Mainz pouch urinary reservoir.

Indiana reamer (Ortho).

indirect fluorescent antibody test (IFA).

indium-111-labeled human nonspecific immunoglobulin G (^{111}In-IgG)—a radiopharmaceutical for imaging focal inflammation in febrile granulocytopenic patients.

indium-111 scintigraphy scan (^{111}In) (Radiol).

indocyanine green dye—for detection of intracardial shunt.

inducer cell—a name for the T-4 helper lymphocyte, the specific target of the AIDS virus; also called the helper/inducer cell; it plays an important role in activating other parts of the immune system.

induration, brawny.

Inerpan (Derm)—a special dressing for burn patients that requires less frequent changing. This decreases pain for the patient and allows the donor site to heal more completely.

in extremis—at the point of death.

Infasurg (Neonat)—natural surfactant obtained from a saline lavage of cows' lungs. Used to treat the lack

Infasurg *(cont.)* of surfactant in premature infants causing hyaline membrane disease.

inferior mesenteric artery (IMA).

inflamed (one *m*, but note *inflammation, inflammatory*).

inflammation—classic signs of inflammation are rubor (redness), calor (heat), dolor (pain), tumor (swelling), and loss of function.

influenza vaccine—Researchers at the University of Pittsburgh School of Medicine have developed a unique application for an influenza vaccine that is administered as a nasal spray offering protection against flu. The flu vaccine has the ability to *immediately* block the growth of influenza viruses that cause disease. This is in addition to, and apart from, its ability to induce antibody formation. It is an attenuated live influenza virus but one which can block the growth of other influenza viruses. Although other vaccines against the flu require two weeks to adequately stimulate the body's antibody defenses to produce immunity, this flu vaccine provides almost instantaneous protection—a real plus when a flu epidemic strikes. Of note, influenza is still the sixth leading cause of death in this country.

infra-, prefix meaning *under, beneath, below.* Cf. *inter-, intra-, inner-.*

infranate—material that settles to the bottom of a liquid. Cf. *supernate.*

Infumorph—solution of morphine sulfate given by the intrathecal or epidural route.

Infusaid—an implantable drug infusion pump.

Infuse-a-port—implantable vascular access system. Used for administration of chemotherapeutic agent via cephalic vein (or possibly other veins).

infusion—the slow therapeutic introduction of fluid other than blood into a vein. Cf. *effusion.*

Ingram catheter.

Ingram regimen for psoriasis—similar to Goeckerman regimen (Derm). See *Goeckerman regimen.*

inhalant antigens (major outdoor allergens). Examples of fungi: *Alternaria, Cladosporium, Hormodendrum.*

Inhibace (cilazapril).

inhibitor—see *HMG-CoA reductase.*

injector—see *HUMI uterine.*

ink-potassium hydroxide test (Oph). "Ink-potassium hydroxide preparation of corneal scrapings showed *Acanthamoeba* cysts in the corneal stroma." India ink (or writing ink) is used in this test. The principle involved is similar to that of the Schiller test for cancer of the cervix—a negative stain. The ink is not absorbed by *Acanthamoeba* cysts, and they appear as light structures on a dark background of the ink. See *Schiller test.*

inlay graft—a bone graft, not to be confused with onlay graft. Both are used in craniofacial surgery. Skin can also be used as an inlay graft. Note that this term is not hyphenated.

Innovator Holter system (Cardio).

INO (intranuclear ophthalmoplegia). Cf. *I&O.*

inosine pranobex (Isoprinosine).

inosiplex (Isoprinosine) (Oncol)—a drug used to treat AIDS.

Inro surgical nail—for nail bed injuries that cause or require avulsion of the nail.

Insall/Burstein system—total knee replacement.

insensible fluid output—fluid loss that cannot be measured, such as by respiration and through the skin, without visible perspiration—as differen-

insensible *(cont.)* tiated from measurable fluid output such as urine.

insidious—gradual or subtle development.

in situ—in the natural or normal place; confined to the site of origin without invasion of neighboring tissues; e.g., carcinoma in situ.

Inspiron (Pulm, Rehab)—small inspiratory training device to strengthen the muscles used in breathing.

inspissated—a thickened or dried out secretion within a duct or cavity.

instill—administration of a liquid, drop by drop. Do not confuse with "install," although some dictators use these words interchangeably.

instrument—see *device* or type of instrument, e.g., *clamp, forceps.*

Insuflon —indwelling device for delivering insulin. It consists of a small needle inserted subcutaneously and allowed to remain in place for up to one week. The needle is connected to a small catheter which is easily accessible on the surface of the skin. The patient injects the insulin dose into the catheter. Insuflon eliminates multiple injections for patients whose diabetes requires one or more shots each day.

insulin
- Actrapid
- beef
- beef-pork
- bonito fish
- human
- Humulin
- Humulin 70/30
- Humulin BR
- Humulin L
- Humulin N
- Humulin R

insulin *(cont.)*
- Humulin U
- INH
- Insultard NPH
- Lente Iletin I
- Lente Iletin II
- Mixtard 70/30
- Monotard
- Novolin L
- Novolin N
- Novolin R
- Novolin 70/30
- NPH Iletin I
- NPH Iletin II
- pork
- protamine zinc insulin (PZI)
- Regular Iletin I
- Regular Iletin II
- Semilente Iletin I
- Ultralente Iletin I
- Velosulin

insulinotardic—when insulin comes out too slowly and in insufficient quantity.

insulin pump—see *pump.*

intake and output (I&O). See *I&O.*

intentional transoperative hemodilution—a blood transfusion method. When a patient is prepared for surgery, up to 3 units of blood are taken from the patient and stored in regular blood donor bags. Blood expanders are then administered to the patient to restore the blood volume. Thus, during surgery, the patient loses only *diluted* blood. Then, near the end of the operative procedure, the previously removed blood is infused. This reduces the need for blood transfusion, with all its attendant risks.

inter-—a prefix meaning *between.* Cf. *intra-.*

intercartilaginous incision (ENT, Plas Surg)—used in rhinoplasties.

Interceed Adhesion Barrier—a pliable, biodegradable cellulose fabric that is used to prevent adhesions between tissues and organs following surgery, and specifically to prevent or reduce the possibility of pelvic adhesions. The knitted absorbable fabric becomes a gelatinous coating (over the organs just under the incision) which is absorbed in less than a month. Also known as Interceed (TC7) Absorbable Adhesion Barrier.

interferometer. See *Takata laser interferometer.*

interferon—glycoproteins produced by some cells in response to viral infections, which also seem to have antitumor properties. See *IL-2.*

interferon alfa-nl (Wellferon)—a drug used to treat Kaposi's sarcoma in AIDS patients.

interferon alfa-n3 (Alferon LDO, Alferon N)—interferon that is not manufactured using recombinant DNA techniques but is derived from human WBCs. It is indicated for the treatment of genital warts (external condylomata acuminata) by intradermal injection. Alferon LDO is used to treat patients with AIDS and ARC. Note the spelling *alfa,* not *alpha.*

interferon alfa-2a (Roferon-A)—a drug used to treat various leukemias, carcinomas, AIDS, and Kaposi's sarcoma.

interferon alfa-2b (Intron A)—a drug used for various leukemias, carcinomas, hepatitis, and patients with AIDS and ARC.

interferon, human recombinant beta (Betaseron)—used to treat CMV retinitis in AIDS patients.

interleukin-1 (IL-1), or **lymphocyte activating factor** (LAF)—a monokine released (in vitro) by cultured macrophages. It may affect the systemic response to inflammation by inducing fever and by stimulating the release of acute-phase reactants.

interleukin-2, PEG—a drug used to treat AIDS.

interleukin-2, recombinant (IL-2, Proleukin, teceleukin)—a drug used to treat patients with AIDS and ARC, renal cell carcinoma, and malignant melanoma.

interleukin-3 (IL-3)—a drug used to treat HIV-positive patients.

internal mammary artery bypass (IMAB).

International 10-20 system—for placing electrodes on the scalp when performing electroencephalograms. The electrodes are placed in predetermined positions that are 10 to 20 percent of the distance between certain pairs of skull reference points.

International System of Measuring Units (SI, the initials for *Système International d'Unités* in French, but SI is used internationally). In the U.S., the American Medical Association and the College of American Pathologists are sponsoring its use. We are already using *gray* (Gy) as the unit of measuring absorbed radiation dose, equal to 100 rads; *becquerel* (Bq) as the unit of radioactivity; *joule* (J) as the unit of energy; *hertz* (Hz) as the unit of frequency equal to 1 cycle per second.

Interpore—a form of hydroxyapatite. See *hydroxyapatite.*

interpulse time—MRI term.

interrupted near-far, far-near sutures.

interstitial markings (Radiol)—the radiographic appearance of lung tissue, as opposed to the appearance of air contained in the lung.

interval
Ae-H
H-Ae
Q-Tc

in-the-ear (ITE) **hearing aid.**

intra-—a prefix meaning *within.* Cf. *inter-.*

intra-aortic balloon pumping (IABP) —effective for short-term support of cardiac patients. (Dictionaries retain a hyphen between the two *a*'s in intra-abdominal, intra-aortic, and intra-atrial, although some publications omit the hyphen.) Cf. *intra-atrial baffle.*

intra-atrial baffle—used in repair of atrial septal defect.

Intracath catheter.

intracellular-like, calcium bearing crystalloid solution (ICS).

intracranial pressure (ICP) **catheter; monitor.**

IntraDop (Surg)—intraoperative Doppler probe used for blood vessel identification during laparoscopic surgery.

intralocular—within the locules of a structure. Cf. *intraocular.*

Intran disposable intrauterine pressure measurement catheter (Obs).

intranuclear ophthalmoplegia (INO).

intraocular—within the eye. Cf. *intralocular.*

Intra-Op autotransfusion—a system by Davol for collecting and reinfusing autologous blood during surgery.

intraoperative digital subtraction angiography (IDIS system) (Radiol).

intraperitoneal hyperthermic perfusion (IPHP).

intraretinal microangiopathy (IRMA).

intraretinal microvascular abnormalities (IRMA).

IntraSite gel (Surg)—premixed interactive wound dressings.

intrauterine growth retardation (IUGR).

intrauterine pregnancy (IUP).

intravascular oxygenator (IVOX)—artificial lung. See *IVOX.*

intravenous drug abuse (IVDA).

intravenous fluorescein angiography (IVFA).

intravenous pyelogram (IVP) (Radiol) —evaluation of the urinary system by introduction of contrast material into a vein, and by x-ray films observing the concentration of the contrast material in the renal pelves, renal calices, ureters, and urinary bladder. This procedure demonstrates the presence of tumors, stones, or structural abnormalities.

Intravent tissue expander (Plas Surg).

Intrel II spinal cord stimulation system (Neuro)—to control chronic pain.

Intrepid PTCA catheter (percutaneous transluminal coronary angioplasty) (Cardio).

introducer
Check-Flo
Desilets-Hoffman
Littleford/Spector
LPS Peel-away
Micropuncture Peel-Away
Nottingham
permanent lead
Razi cannula
Tuohy-Bost

Intron A—see *interferon alfa-2b.*

intubation—see *CAGEIN.*

invasive procedure—defined by the Centers for Disease Control as surgical entry into tissues, cavities, or

invasive procedure *(cont.)* organs, or repair of major traumatic injuries associated with any of the following: 1) an operating or delivery room, emergency department or outpatient setting, including both physicians' and dentists' offices; 2) cardiac catheterization and angiographic procedures; 3) a vaginal or cesarean delivery or other invasive obstetric procedure during which bleeding may occur; or 4) the manipulation, cutting, or removal of any oral or perioral tissues, including tooth structure, during which bleeding occurs or the potential for bleeding exists.

inventory
Beck Depression
Myers-Briggs Personality
Strong-Campbell Vocational Interest (SCVII)

inversion-recovery technique—MRI term.

inversion time (TI)—MRI term.

in vitro (L., in glass)—in the laboratory in glass dishes. Cell growth can be observed in vitro in scientific investigation in the laboratory. Cf. *in vivo.* See *GIFT; LAK; ZIFT.*

in vivo (L., *vivus,* living)—within the living body. Cf. *in vitro.*

INVOS 2100—a new early warning test for breast cancer, using optical spectroscopy to detect growths before mammography.

Ioban antimicrobial incise drape *(not* loban)—an iodine drape.

Iodamoeba buetschlii—an intestinal protozoan parasite.

iodinated contrast medium (Radiol)—a contrast medium containing iodine rather than a metallic salt; used in angiography, intravenous pyelography, oral cholecystography, and other studies.

iodine-131-MIBG, iodine-123-MIBG (I-131-MIBG, I-123-MIBG; ^{131}I-MIBG, ^{123}I-MIBG) (Radiol)—radioactive imaging agents used in CT scan and scintigram to demonstrate the primary tumor of neuroblastoma and metastasis. MIBG (metaiodobenzylguanidine). ^{131}I-MIBG theoretically has the possibility of delivering to the primary and metastatic sites of neuroblastoma a fatal dose of radiation, doses easily tolerated by the whole body. Synthetic MIBG is a guanethidine derivative similar to norepinephrine.

iodoform gauze.

iodophor—an iodine compound used in preoperative skin preparation and postoperative skin closure for protection against infection by controlling skin bacteria. Cf. *iodoform gauze.*

IOL (intraocular lenses).

Iolab intraocular lenses.

Iolab Slimfit lens (Oph)—a three-piece intraocular lens made of PMMA; it has flexible haptics.

I/1 size test object (Oph). Roman numeral I relates to luminescence, I to V, Arabic numeral 1 relates to size in millimeters, 1 to 5.

I-131 and I-132—radioactive iodine with atomic weights 131 and 132. Also written ^{131}I, ^{132}I.

IOP (intraocular pressure) (Oph)—the pressure of aqueous humor within the eye, as measured with a tonometer. IOP above 20 or 21 indicates the presence of glaucoma.

Ionescu tri-leaflet valve (Cardio).

Ionescu-Shiley pericardial xenograft; valve (Cardio).

iontophoresis—a process of administering narcotics for pain relief. An electric current is used to transport the drug through the skin. Cf. *electrophoresis.*

iopentol—a nonionic contrast medium (Radiol).

iophendylate (Radiol)—a diagnostic aid and radiopaque medium. Also *Ethodian, Neurotrast.*

Iopidine (apraclonidine).

IORT (Oncol)—intraoperative radiotherapy.

Iowa trumpet—guiding instrument used in the administration of a pudendal block.

IPG (impedance plethysmography)—a noninvasive test to determine the presence and degree of deep vein obstruction in venous thrombosis. It evaluates patency of the veins by measuring venous volume changes.

IPHP (intraperitoneal hyperthermic perfusion).

iproplatin (Oncol)—an antineoplastic agent, a second-generation platinum compound, with fewer renal side effects than cisplatin (its parent drug).

IPSID (immunoproliferative small-intestinal disease)—most prevalent in developing countries.

ipsilateral—on the same side.

iPTH (immunoreactive parathyroid hormone) (yes, lowercase *i*).

iridectomy—excision of a portion of the iris, either surgically or through laser photocoagulation.

irides—plural of iris (Oph).

iridencleisis (*not* iridenclysis)—an operative procedure that creates a permanent drain which filters the aqueous from the anterior chamber to the subconjunctival tissue. The procedure is performed to reduce intraocular pressure.

iridis—see *rubeosis iridis.*

irido-corneal-endothelial syndrome (ICE).

iridium-192 (Iriditope)—a radioactive agent used in scans.

iris bombé (''bom-bay'')—curving or swelling outward.

iritis—an acute or chronic inflammation of the iris.

IRMA (intraretinal microangiopathy).

IRMA (intraretinal microvascular abnormalities).

irradiation—see *heavy ion irradiation.*

irregularly irregular cardiac rhythm (Cardio)—abnormal cardiac rhythm without any discernible pattern, beats occurring at random intervals.

irrigation/lavage device, HeatProbe.

irrigator, Vozzle Vacu-Irrigator.

IRS (impaired regeneration syndrome).

ISCs (irreversible sickled [red] cells).

iscador—a drug used to treat patients with AIDS and ARC.

ISG (immune serum globulin).

Ishihara plates (Oph)—test for color vision.

island of Reil—structure in the brain.

islet cell (*not* eyelet)—the cells that compose the islets of Langerhans in the pancreas.

islet cell antibodies (ICA)—a screening test for persons at high risk for developing type I (insulin dependent) diabetes mellitus. High levels of ICA indicate that the person's immune system is attacking the insulin-secreting islets of Langerhans in the pancreas.

islet cell implant—technique of injecting islet cells from a cadaver into the portal vein of patients with diabetes. The islet cells migrate to the pancreas, where they begin to produce insulin.

Ismo (isosorbide mononitrate) (Cardio)—used to prevent anginal attacks.

isobutyl 2-cyanoacrylate—a substance used to occlude an unresectable aortic aneurysm after axillofemoral grafting.

isoechoic (''i-so-eh-ko'-ic'')—refers to the even distribution of echoes in ultrasonography as the ultrasound waves bounce off structures or tissue. ''The seminal vesicles were small and isoechoic.''

isoenzymes—see *CPK isoenzymes.*

isolated heat perfusion of an extremity (Vasc Surg)—therapy for malignant melanoma of the extremities. The vessels of the extremity are cannulated and the cannulae attached to the cardiopulmonary bypass machine. The temperature of the limb is elevated and perfusion carried out with melphalan included in the perfusate. The limb temperature may be elevated to about 40° C. The extremity vessels are washed out and perfused with fresh blood.

isoprinosine (inosine pranobex, inosiplex methisoprinol)—a drug used to treat HIV-positive patients and those with ARC.

Isospora—the protozoan parasite causing isosporiasis, which can cause an unusually virulent diarrhea in AIDS patients.

isosulfan blue—see *Lymphazurin.*

isotretinoin (13-cis-retinoic acid, 13-CRA, Accutane) (Oncol, Derm)—a chemotherapy drug used to treat mycosis fungoides and cutaneous T-cell lymphoma. Also commonly known as a dermatology drug used to treat severe recalcitrant cystic acne.

isovaleric acidemia—an inborn error of metabolism in which there is marked elevation in the isovaleric acid levels in the serum because of an inability to metabolize protein-rich foods. Manifested by severe metabolic acidosis and coma, slight intention tremor, slight psychomotor retardation, retinal vessel tortuosity, nonspecific mottling of the retina, and a locker room odor of the body, urine, and breath of patients with this entity. Also called locker room syndrome.

Isovis—a wound protector used to isolate contaminating viscera from incision, subcutaneous tissues, and wound cavity.

IsoVue, IsoVue M (iopamidol, injectable) (Radiol)—a nonionic contrast agent used in intra-arterial digital subtraction angiography and in other special radiological procedures.

isoxicam (Maxicam)—a nonsteroidal anti-inflammatory drug for arthritis.

isradipine (DynaCirc) (Cardio)—a calcium channel blocker used to treat hypertension. Relaxes the smooth muscle of blood vessels to lower blood pressure.

ISS (Injury Severity Scale)—a system used to describe multiple trauma injuries.

ITE hearing aid (ITE, in-the-ear).

ITP (idiopathic thrombocytopenic purpura).

itraconazole (Sporanox)—an antifungal used to treat histoplasmosis, blastomycosis, aspergillosis, and cryptococcal meningitis in AIDS patients.

it's, its. How to use *it's* and *its* correctly seems to present problems for many people; I see them misused all too often. Put as simply as I can, *it's* is a contraction of *it is;* use of the apostrophe indicates that a letter has been omitted. Its meaning changes when the apostrophe is omitted; it's then the possessive form, *its.* It might be helpful, when you use the word *it's,* to read the sentence aloud and substitute ''it is''; you will then hear whether the sentence says what you mean to say.

IUdR (idoxuridine)—a halogenated thymidine analogue, a radiosensitizer. Cf. *BUdR, FUdR.*

IUGR (intrauterine growth retardation) (Obs).

IUP (intrauterine pregnancy).

IVAC electronic thermometer. IVAC is the manufacturer.

IVAC volumetric infusion pump—a positive pressure infusion device for delivery of intravenous solutions or drugs. IVAC is the manufacturer.

IVB (intraventricular block).

IVC (inferior vena cava).

IVDA (intravenous drug abuse).

I.V. drip—intravenous administration of drugs in which the drug is mixed with the fluid in the I.V. bag or bottle and administered over several hours as the I.V. runs in slowly. Cf. *I.V. push.*

Ivemark's syndrome—splenic agenesis syndrome.

IVF (in vitro fertilization) (Ob-Gyn)—used for women with blocked fallopian tubes, to achieve pregnancy. The woman's eggs are placed in a dish with sperm from either her husband or a donor. The embryos are then placed into the uterus. Success rate is currently estimated at about 11%. See *GIFT; ZIFT.*

IVFA (intravenous fluorescein angiography) (Oph).

IVOX (intravascular oxygenator) (Pulm)—an artificial lung designed for temporary use in patients whose respiratory failure is caused by infection or trauma. It consists of a number of very thin 24-inch hollow tubes which are inserted together through the femoral vein into the vena cava. The tubes are then connected to a catheter which supplies oxygen. The oxygen diffuses through the tubes into the bloodstream. The IVOX helps reduce demands on the patient's lungs temporarily until they can again function fully.

I.V. piggyback. See *piggyback.*

I.V. port. See *port.*

I.V. push—a method of administering drugs in which the entire dose of a drug is given intravenously by manually injecting it directly into a port in the I.V. line. The therapeutic effect is felt immediately. This method is often used in emergency situations. Cf. *I.V. drip.*

Ivy bleeding time.

Ivy mastoid rongeur (ENT).

Ixodes dammini—a species of tick, the carrier of Lyme disease.

Ixodes pacificus—western black-legged tick, implicated as a carrier in tularemia on the West Coast. Cf. *erythema migrans; Ixodes dammini; Lyme disease.*

J, j

Jabaley-Stille Super Cut Scissors.

jacket
  Bair Hugger
  Biliblanket Phototherapy
  Kydex body
  orthoplast
  Royalite body

jackknife position—The patient lies on his stomach with shoulders elevated and thighs at right angles to the abdomen. Used for rectal and coccygeal procedures. Also, *Kraske's position.*

Jackson's epilepsy (Neuro), but jacksonian epilepsy.

Jackson's sign—the wheezing produced by foreign bodies lodged in the bronchus or trachea, similar to that of asthma, audible without a stethoscope.

jacksonian march (Neuro)—progression of a jacksonian seizure from one muscle group to adjacent areas or to a generalized motor seizure.

jacksonian seizure—focal seizure (also rolandic). Usually starts as a spasm in the face, a hand, or a foot, and then spreads to other muscles. Note that *jacksonian* is an adjectival form and therefore is not capitalized, as in rolandic epilepsy, sylvian fissure, eustachian tube, graafian follicle, glaserian fissure, addisonian type of anemia, draconian laws, euclidian geometry.

Jackson-Pratt catheter; drain.

jackstone calculus—a kidney stone shaped like the 6-pointed metal jacks that children play with.

Jacquemier's sign (Obs)—the bluish-violet color seen in the vagina and cervix at 8 to 12 weeks of pregnancy. Also known as Chadwick's sign.

Jacobson's organ—an obscure structure in the nose of all mammals except porpoises, with its own nerve supply. It is thought to be important in chemoreception to pheromones.

Jaeger eye chart, in which findings on examination are given as J and a number, indicating the line on the chart with the smallest letters the patient can see.

Jaeger keratome (Oph).

Jaffe intraocular implant lens (Oph).

Jaffee capsulorhexis forceps (Oph)—forceps with blunt tips to hold the capsular bag and to tear a continuous curvilinear capsulorhexis.

Jahnke anastomosis clamp (Surg).

Jako facial nerve monitor (ENT)—for middle ear and mastoid surgery; it enables the surgeon to judge the depth of the nerve beneath the exposed tissue bed.

Jako laryngoscope (ENT).

jamais vu (Fr., "never seen")—the incorrect feeling that one has never seen or experienced a certain thing before, in contrast to *déjà vu,* "already seen," the incorrect feeling that one has seen or experienced something before.

Jamar dynamometer (Ortho, Neuro)—a device used to measure hand strength by calibrating the hand grip. Three readings are made for each hand, measured in pounds. Usually higher readings are seen on tests of the dominant hand, unless there has been an injury on that side.

Jamar grip test —using the Jamar dynamometer.

James fibers (Cardio)—in AV nodal area of the heart.

Jameson calipers (Plas Surg)—used to measure the lid crease in blepharoplasty.

Jamshidi biopsy needle.

Janeway lesions—erythematous macules that may be seen on the palms and soles in infective endocarditis.

Jannetta retractor (Neuro).

Jansen-Middleton septum forceps.

Javid shunt.

Jedmed/DGH A-scan (Oph).

Jelco catheter—an I.V. catheter.

Jenckel cholecystoduodenostomy (GI).

Jendrassik's maneuver.

Jenner's stain.

Jergesen I-beam; tube (Ortho).

jerk
- ankle (AJ)
- biceps (BJ)
- knee (KJ)

jet lesion (Path)—usually an autopsy finding. A valvular or septal cardiac defect allows a strong jet of blood, over time, to produce an area of endocardial fibrosis or even an endocardial pocket.

Jevity isotonic liquid nutrition—for supplemental feeding tube nutritional support.

Jewett brace (Ortho)—used for spondylitis, spinal fusion, compression fractures.

Jewett's classification of bladder carcinoma:
- O noninfiltrating (in situ)
- A infiltrating submucosa
- B invading muscle
- C involvement of surrounding tissue
- D distant involvement

jittery (Peds)—describes involuntary jerky muscle movements of extremities of babies with hypoglycemia or drug addiction.

JL4 catheter (Cardio)—Judkins left 4 cm curve catheter.

JL5 catheter (Cardio)—Judkins left 5 cm curve catheter.

Jobst stockings (Vasc Surg).

Joe's hoe—a retractor (also known as the Weinberg retractor) (Surg).

Joffroy's sign—in exophthalmos, when the patient attempts to look upward and there is no wrinkling of the forehead.

joint
- Gaffney
- Gillette
- Oklahoma ankle
- Select

joint mice (Ortho)—loose fragments of cartilage or other material within the synovial capsule of a joint.

joint position sense (JPS).

joker—operating room slang for an instrument; in different services it could refer to different instruments.

Jonas modification of the Norwood procedure for hypoplastic left-sided heart syndrome. See *Gill/Jonas; Fontan; Sade.*

Jones criteria, revised—used as a guide in the diagnosis of rheumatic fever. If there has been an earlier strep infection, the presence of one major and two minor manifestations, or of two major manifestations of the disease, makes the diagnosis of rheumatic fever likely. Minor manifestations: history of rheumatic fever or evidence of preexisting rheumatic heart disease; fever; arthralgias; abnormal erythrocyte sedimentation rate (ESR) or C-reactive protein, or EKG changes. Major manifestations: subcutaneous nodules; carditis; chorea; polyarthritis; erythema marginatum.

Jonnson's maneuver—a modified Valsalva maneuver; produces maximal distention of the hypopharynx by holding the patient's nose and mouth closed while he makes forcible expiratory efforts. Note spelling: Jonnson.

Josephs-Diamond-Blackfan syndrome—see *Blackfan-Diamond syndrome.*

joule ("jewel")—unit of electric power (Cardio), as in "The heart was defibrillated with a single shock of 40 joules." Named for J. P. Joule, an English physicist. Abbreviated *J.*

J point (Cardio)—on an EKG tracing, the junction between the end of the QRS complex and the beginning of the ST segment.

JPS (joint position sense) (Neuro).

Judd-Masson bladder retractor (Urol).

Judd postoperative ventral hernia repair (Surg).

Judet hip prosthesis ("joo-day") (Ortho)—a prosthesis which does not require the use of cement; the femoral and acetabular components are made to fit tightly.

Judkins selective coronary arteriography (*not* Judkin's). Also, see *Dotter-Judkins technique.*

jugulodigastric nodes—deep cervical nodes in the area of the jugular trunk and the digastric muscle.

Jung-Schaffer intraocular lens.

juxtaposition—see *apposition.*

J-Vac closed wound drainage system—consists of a Blake silicone drain and a J-Vac suction reservoir.

JVP (jugular venous pressure).

J-wire—used in a procedure to support extracorporeal membrane oxygenation (ECMO) in infants with severe pulmonary insufficiency and pulmonary hypertension. "The chest tube catheter was then withdrawn, and we then used a J-wire which we passed down the jugular vein into the inferior vena cava. With this, we were able to slip the venous cannula over the J-wire into the right atrium, and the J-wire was then removed."

K, k

K (kelvin)—see *kelvin.*

KAFO (knee-ankle-foot orthosis) (Ortho).

kallikrein-kinin (KK) **system.** You may be hearing about this with reference to its possible mediator function in vasogenic brain edema.

Kaltostat (Surg)—wound packing material which is highly absorbent.

Kanavel brain-exploring cannula.

Kaplan–Meier survival curves, used in the prognosis of cancer.

Kaposi's sarcoma (KS) (''kap'o-sheez'') —the most common cancer associated with AIDS. Prior to the AIDS epidemic, Kaposi's sarcoma was a relatively benign and rare affliction, and the change in this disease was one of the first clues that an epidemic of contagious destruction of the immune system had begun.

Kapp-Beck serration.

Karaya powder (marketed by Sween).

Karickhoff laser lens (Oph)—used for panretinal photocoagulation.

Karl Storz Calcutript (Urol)—for use with the Karl Storz ureteropyeloscope in upper urinary tract procedures.

Karl Storz flexible ureteropyeloscope (Urol)—used to visualize the upper urinary tract and perform retrograde intrarenal surgery.

Karnofsky rating scale of performance status of patients with malignant neoplasms.

100—normal, no complaint or evidence of disease
90—normal activity, with minor symptoms
80—normal activity, with effort, and some symptoms
70—cares for self, unable to do normal activity
60—requires occasional assistance
50—requires considerable assistance and care
40—disabled, requires special care and assistance
30—severely disabled; requires supportive measures
20—very sick
10—moribund

Karnofsky status—tumor grading. See *Karnofsky rating scale.*

karyotype—chromosomal composition, e.g., the human cell normally has 46 chromosomes in its karyotype.

Kasabach-Merritt syndrome—occurs in infants and is marked by giant hemangiomas of the skin and spleen associated with thrombocytopenic purpura and afibrinogenemia (Peds).

Kasai peritoneal venous shunt—for biliary atresia in infants, to deal with accumulated ascitic fluid.

Kaster mitral valve prosthesis. Also, Hall-Kaster.

Katena trephine.

Katzin corneal transplant scissors.

Kaufman vitrector (Oph).

Kawasaki disease (Peds)—mucocutaneous lymph node syndrome; usually occurs in infants and small children.

Kaycel towels—absorbent sterile towels used in the operating room as a drape. They have adhesive areas for sealing at the wound site and also for holding the drape in place. Cf. *Kay Ciel, KCl.*

Kay Ciel (''kay-see-el'') (Urol)—trade name for potassium chloride given to patients on diuretic therapy. It is often not recognized as a trade name drug and is mistakenly transcribed as KCl (the abbreviation for the chemical name *potassium chloride*).

Kayser-Fleischer ring (Oph)—seen in the cornea of patients with Wilson's hepaticolenticular degeneration, a completely or partially pigmented ring which is green, and which encircles the cornea near the limbus.

Kazanjian shears (Plas Surg).

Kaznelson's syndrome—see *Blackfan-Diamond syndrome.*

K-blade (Oph)—a microsurgery blade for intraocular procedures manufactured by Katena Products, Inc.

KCl—chemical symbol for potassium chloride. Cf. *Kay Ciel, Kaycel.*

KDF-2.3 intrauterine catheter—trade name for catheter used for artificial insemination.

Kearney side-notch intraocular lens.

Kearns-Sayre syndrome (Oph)—progressive ophthalmoplegia, with pigmentary retinopathy, ptosis, and heart block. Also, Kearns-Sayre-Shy syndrome, ophthalmoplegic plus, oculocraniosomatic neuromuscular disease, mitochondrial cytopathy.

Keates intraocular implant lens.

Kech and Kelly osteotomy (Pod)—surgery for Haglund's foot deformity.

keel—see *McNaught keel.*

Keeler cryophake unit (Oph).

Keeler indirect ophthalmoscope.

Kegel exercises (developed by Arnold H. Kegel, M.D.) (Ob-Gyn, Urol)—exercises to strengthen the pelvic/vaginal muscles, for control of stress incontinence.

Keith's bundle (Cardio)—a bundle of fibers located in the right atrial wall of the heart, between the openings of the venae cavae. Also called sinoatrial bundle.

Keith-Wagener (K-W) **classification of hypertensive retinopathy,** Roman numerals I through IV. (Not to be confused with *Kimmelstiel-Wilson disease,* also abbreviated K-W.)

Kell—blood antibody type; factor in agglutination. Also *Duffy, Kidd, Lewis, Lutheran.*

Kellan cannula (Oph)—used for intraocular hydrodelineation and hydrodissection.

Kellan hydrodissection cannula (Oph)—used during cataract surgery.

Keller arthroplasty; bunionectomy.

Kelman air cystitome (Oph).

Kelman intraocular implant lens.

Kelman-McPherson angled forceps (Oph).

Kelman phacoemulsification (Oph)—used in cataract extraction.

kelvin (K). The kelvin is a unit of absolute temperature in the International System (SI) on a scale in which the zero point corresponds to absolute zero. When using the Kelvin scale, you do not use a degree sign—just the numerals followed by K. To convert temperatures from the Kelvin scale to the Celsius system, add 273.16. Named for Lord Kelvin, a British physicist. (Note that the unit *kelvin* is lowercase, and *Kelvin scale* is capitalized.)

Ken nail (Ortho)—used in hip fracture repair.

Kent bundle—atrioventricular bundle in the heart. See *AV bundle.*

Keofeed feeding tube—used in nasogastric feeding.

keratic precipitates *or* **keratoprecipitates** (KPs) (Oph).

keratin—a highly insoluble protein (scleroprotein) in epidermis, hair, nails, and part of the teeth. Cf. *carotene, creatine, creatinine.*

keratin whorls *(not* whirls)—layers of squamous cells spiraled onto each other, producing a spherical body rich in the protein keratin.

keratitic precipitates, keratic precipitates, keratoprecipitates (KPs) (Oph).

keratoconus—a conical protrusion of the center of the cornea, without inflammation. Occurs most often in pubescent females.

keratome—see *Jaeger keratome.*

keratometer—see *Terry keratometer.*

keratoprecipitates, keratic precipitates, keratitic precipitates (KPs) (Oph).

keratoscope, van Loonen operating.

keratosis—production of keratin, producing a horny growth such as a wart or callosity. See *solar keratosis.*

keratotomy, radial.

Kerley's A lines (Radiol) (*not* curly)—centrally located horizontal linear densities seen on chest x-ray. Also, *Kerley's B lines* and *Kerley's C lines.*

Kerley's B lines (Radiol) (*not* curly)—horizontal linear densities seen on chest x-ray; located at the base of the lungs. Also known as *costophrenic septal lines.* Cf. *Kerley's A lines* and *Kerley's C lines.*

Kerley's C lines (Radiol) (*not* curly)—fine linear shadows seen on x-ray, interlaced through the lung, giving a spiderweb appearance. Cf. *Kerley's A lines* and *Kerley's B lines.*

Kerlix bandage.

Kernig sign (Neuro).

Kernohan grading of malignant astrocytoma of the spinal cord, given in Roman numerals (Neuro).

Kernohan notch—indentation and necrosis of the brain caused by pressure on the brain by the free edge of the tentorium cerebelli; this is sometimes associated with tentorial herniation.

Kessler suture.

Kestenbach-Anderson eye procedure (Oph).

Kestenbaum operation—for nystagmic torticollis (Oph).

ketorolac tromethamine (Toradol)—a nonsteroidal anti-inflammatory drug available in oral and injectable forms. It inhibits the synthesis of prostaglandins to control inflammation and pain and to reduce fever.

ketotifen (Zaditen) (Pulm)—an oral drug used to prevent attacks of bronchial asthma.

Kevorkian-Younge uterine biopsy forceps.
Khodadad clip (Neuro).
kHz (kilohertz).
kick counts (Obs)—If there are enough kicks by the fetus, this is an indication of a healthy baby. It gives a picture of the activity of the fetus.
Kidd—blood antibody type; factor in agglutination. Also, Duffy, Kell, Lewis, Lutheran.
Kidney Internal Splint/Stent catheter. See *KISS.*
Kiel classification—of non-Hodgkin's lymphoma.
Kielland forceps (Ob-Gyn). Also, Kjelland, although Kielland is preferred.
Kienböck's disease—lunatomalacia (refers to the lunate bone in the wrist). Thought to be caused by vascular interruption or by fracture of the lunate bone.
Kifa catheter.
Killian-Lynch laryngoscope (ENT).
Killip wire—inserted to give the heart a shock during cardiac arrest.
kilohertz (kHz).
kilopascal (kPa)—a blood gas pressure measurement, equaling 1000 pascals; an SI unit of measurement.
Kimmelstiel-Wilson disease. (Not to be confused with *Keith-Wagener,* for both are often given as "K-W.")
Kim-Ray Greenfield caval filter (Thor Surg)—a metallic filter inserted into the inferior vena cava for prevention of pulmonary embolism; transvenous insertion is the approach used. See *Mobin-Uddin umbrella filter,* which is not synonymous.
Kinematic rotating hinge—knee prosthesis.
KineTec hip CPM machine (continuous passive motion) (Ortho).
KinetiX (capital X) **ventilation monitor**—hand-held, compact monitor, used when single expired breath or maximum voluntary ventilation tests are needed.
King-Armstrong unit—measurement of alkaline phosphatase. See also *Bodansky unit, Bessey-Lowry unit.*
Kinsey atherectomy catheter (Cardio).
Kinyoun stain—for acid-fast bacilli.
Kiricuta reconstructive breast operation.
Kirklin fence (Thor Surg)—area of mediastinal pleura used to retract the lung in thoracic surgery.
Kirschner Medical "Dimension" hip replacement system (Ortho).
Ki-67 (Oncol)—an immunophenotypic marker on the cells of patients with multiple myeloma; it is being evaluated for its correlation with relapses and overall survival.
KISS (Kidney Internal Splint / Stent)—a catheter believed to provide more reliable urinary drainage after pyeloplasty in children. The KISS catheter prevents occlusion because the segment of the tube draining the ureter/pelvis is constructed as a trough. The catheter is passed in a retrograde manner through the renal cortex using the trocar tip, and the trough is positioned in the pelvis/ureter. After pyeloplasty, the catheter drains externally for 24 hours, and after a week is clamped and removed.
Kistner tracheostomy tube (ENT).
Kitner dissector—see *Küttner.*
KJ (knee jerk) (Neuro).
Kjelland forceps. Cf. *Kielland forceps.*
KK system (kallikrein-kinin).
Klagsbrun technique—to harvest chondrocytes which are used to provide

Klagsbrun *(cont.)*
a template for new cartilage formation in vivo.

Klatskin needle—used for liver biopsy.

***Klebsiella pneumoniae,* Friedländer's bacillus**—a component of the normal flora of the oropharynx and GI tract in patients with functioning immune systems, but in AIDS it can cause a fatal sepsis.

Klebsiella oxytoca—newer name for *K. pneumoniae.*

kleeblattschädel—German, "cloverleaf skull."

Kleihauer-Betke test (K-B test)—used in assessing hemolysis.

Kleihauer test—of fetal-maternal hemoglobin.

Klein punch (Oph).

Kleinsasser anterior commissure laryngoscope (ENT).

Klein-Tolentino ring (Oph). Also, Tolentino ring.

Klemme laminectomy retractor (Neuro).

Klinefelter's XXY syndrome.

Kling—adhesive dressing.

Klonopin (clonazepam)—newer name for Clonopin. The name of this drug was changed to avoid confusion with the medication *clonidine.*

Knapt scissors (ENT).

knee jerk (KJ) (Neuro).

knee—see *housemaid's knee.*

knife
A-OK ShortCut
Barkan goniotomy
bladebreaker
Castroviejo
Edgeahead phaco slit
Foerster capsulotomy
Freedom
Gamma radiosurgical
Haab scleral resection
Lebsche
Moebius cataract

knife *(cont.)*
Neoflex bendable
NeoKnife
Paufique
roentgen radiosurgical
Scheie goniopuncture
Sharpoint microsurgical
ShortCut
Stecher arachnoid
Tiemann Meals tenolysis

Knolle posterior capsule polisher ("kun-o-lee").

knot
clove-hitch
friction
half-hitch
square
surgeon's
syncytial

Knowles pin (Ortho).

Kocher collar incision—used in thyroidectomy.

Kocher incision—approach to biliary tract.

Kocher-McFarland hip arthroplasty.

Koch-Mason dressing.

Koch nucleus hydrolysis needle (Oph) —used during cataract surgery.

Koch's node—see *sinoatrial node.*

Koch phaco manipulator/splitter (Oph) —used during phacoemulsification to push and fracture the nucleus during cataract surgery.

Koch technique (Oph)—a technique for intraocular lens insertion using a 4-5 mm incision and closure with the suture knots buried.

Kock ("coke") **pouch; continent ileostomy; reservoir ileostomy**—an artificial bladder created from a section of intestine.

Kock pouch modified procedure (Urol) —to enable women who are postcystectomy to urinate through the rectum. The Kock pouch is connected to the kidneys via the ureters and

Kock pouch modified *(cont.)* then surgically attached to the sigmoid colon just above the rectum. Urine collects in the pouch and subsequently is eliminated through the rectum. Backflow is prevented by two valves. In a similar procedure for men, a Kock pouch is connected to the urethra, permitting normal elimination.

Kodak Ektascan laser printer—for digital imaging (Radiol).

Koebner phenomenon (koebnerization) —psoriasis at the site of an injury.

Koenig MPJ implant and arthroplasty (Pod)—two-component system for replacement of the first MPJ (metatarsophalangeal joint).

Koeppe lens (Oph).

Koerber-Salus-Elschnig syndrome (Oph).

Koffler sphenoid punch—see *Hajek-Koffler sphenoid punch.*

KOH mount (potassium hydroxide)—a test used in diagnosing cutaneous fungal disease. Scrapings are taken from the skin in the affected area. A few drops of 15% to 20% potassium hydroxide (KOH) are added to the scrapings on a slide. The slide is then heated over a flame several times and can then be examined for fungal organisms.

Köhler lines (Ortho)—used to grade hip protrusion.

Kohn, pores of. See *pores of Kohn.*

koilocytotic—characteristic of a wart cell.

Kold Kap—plastic bag with a frozen gel, applied to scalp of patient undergoing chemotherapy to decrease hair loss. Also, ChemoCap.

König disease (Ortho)—osteochondritis dissecans *(not* dessicans) of the knee.

Kono procedure—patch enlargement of ascending aorta.

Konton catheter (Cardio)—used to position intra-aortic balloon pump.

Kontrast U—a radiopaque medium (Radiol). May be used in myelography and also in x-raying the urinary tract.

Koplik's spots—an indication of measles; tiny gray-white spots with a rim of erythema, appearing on the buccal mucosa before the skin rash of measles appears.

Korotkoff sounds—the sounds heard through the sphygmomanometer which, properly calibrated, indicate blood pressure. "The first and fifth phase Korotkoff sounds were taken as systolic and diastolic pressures, respectively."

Kostmann's infantile agranulocytosis.

kPa (kilopascal)—a blood gas pressure measure, equaling 1000 pascals; an SI unit of measure.

KPs (keratoprecipitates, keratic precipitates, or keratitic precipitates) (Oph) —large white keratic precipitates that resemble drops of solidified mutton fat; they are seen on corneal endothelium.

Kraff intraocular implant lens.

Kraff nucleus splitter (Oph)—fine forceps with serrated tips used to grasp and fracture the nucleus during cataract surgery.

Kraff-Utrata tear capsulotomy forceps (Oph)—used to make the circular tear in the anterior capsule when performing capsulorhexis.

Krakow's point—orthopedic landmark in the knee.

Kraske's position in surgery—the jackknife position used for rectal and coccygeal procedures.

Krasnov implant cataract lens.

Kratz intraocular implant lens.

Kratz scratcher—posterior capsule polisher (Oph).

kraurosis vulvae (Ob-Gyn)—progressive atrophy of the vulva in postmenopausal women.

Kreiselman unit—apparatus used in resuscitation of newborn infants; provides oxygen, heat, suction, etc.

Kreuscher bunionectomy (Pod).

Krimsky measurement—of exotropia.

Krukenberg's spindle (Oph)—an opacity on the posterior surface of the cornea which is vertical, spindle-shaped, and brownish-red in color.

Krukenberg's tumor (Ob-Gyn)—carcinoma of the ovary, usually metastatic from cancer of the intestinal tract, stomach, or breast.

Krumeich—see *BKS-1000.*

Krupin-Denver eye valve—surgically implanted for control of glaucoma (made by Storz).

Kruskal-Wallis test—for acoustic neuroma.

krypton, inhalation of—in positron scanning technique for measuring cerebral blood flow.

krypton (red) laser photocoagulation (Oph)—used in treating choroidal neovascular membrane, and pigment epithelial detachment.

KS—see *Kaposi's sarcoma.*

KTP laser (potassium-titanyl-phosphate) —used in laparoscopic laser cholecystectomy.

K-Tube—trade name for a silicone jejunostomy tube designed to facilitate easy surgical placement for use in enteral nutritional support in patients who are in bed or are ambulatory.

KUB (kidneys, ureters, and urinary bladder) (Radiol).

Kugelberg-Welander disease—juvenile hereditary motor neuron disease.

Kulchitsky cells (Radiol).

Kun colocolpopoiesis—see *colocolpo-neopoiesis.*

Kuntscher nail; reamer; rod (Ortho).

Kupffer cell—a type of phagocytic cell found in the liver.

Kurtzke disability score (''kerts-key'') (Neuro)—used in evaluating patients with multiple sclerosis. Composed of two sections, one of functional systems—pyramidal functions, cerebellar functions, brain stem functions, sensory functions, bowel and bladder functions, visual functions, mental functions, and other functions; and a disability status scale from 0 to 10.

Kushner-Tandatnick endometrial biopsy curet (Gyn).

Kussmaul's respiration—extremely severe dyspnea with increased respiratory rate, increased deep breathing, labored, panting breathing, as seen in diabetic ketoacidosis and renal failure. See *air hunger.*

Küttner blunt dissecting instrument (Surg)—dissecting sponge with a radiopaque tip used in laparoscopic cholecystectomy, laparoscopy, pelviscopy, and lymphatic dissection.

Küttner dissector (Surg)—either a ''pusher'' or ''peanut'' type; used as an aid in performing a laparoscopic cholecystectomy.

K value for glucose assimilation in diabetes. Not to be confused with ''K,'' the chemical symbol for potassium.

Kveim reaction; test—for sarcoidosis.

KVO-type I.V. (keep vein open)—an intravenous infusion given as slowly as possible to keep the blood from clotting in the needle, but not to give the patient any fluid volume. Also, *TKO-type I.V.* (to keep open).

K-W disease
Keith-Wagener
Kimmelstiel-Wilson

Kwitko intraocular implant lens.

Kydex body jacket; brace (Ortho).

kyphectomy, Sharrard-type.

kyphosis—see *Scheuermann juvenile kyphosis.*

kyphoscoliosis (Radiol).

kyphotic pelvis (Radiol).

L, l

LAAM (L-alpha-acetyl-methadol)—a drug used to treat heroin addiction.

LABA (laser-assisted balloon angioplasty).

Labbé, vein of ("lab-bay").

label (Radiol)—to render a substance radioactive by incorporating a radionuclide in it; also, to cause a tissue or organ to take up radioactive material. Cf. *sensitize; tag.*

la belle indifférence—seen in certain patients with strokes or conversion disorders who show an inappropriate lack of concern about their disabilities.

labial (adj., lips)—(1) referring to the labia majora and labia minora, the fleshy structures in the genital area just anterior to the vagina (Gyn); (2) the surface of the incisor and canine teeth directly opposite the lips (Dental). Cf. *labile.*

labile (Cardio, Psych)—an adjective describing a condition or emotion easily or spontaneously changed; unstable. Examples: labile hypertension, labile affect.

labor (Obs)—see *arrest of labor; stages of labor.*

Lachman test (Ortho)—used to determine the presence of a tear in the anterior cruciate ligament.

lactamase—see *beta-lactamase.*

lactated Ringer's solution—a physiologic salt solution used for irrigation in surgery. *Lactated* does *not* refer to milk, but to lactic acid solution (of negatively-charged ions).

lactoferrin—a protein found in a number of human secretions (bile, saliva, milk, tears). It is an iron-binding protein, and has been found to retard fungal and bacterial growth, possibly by depriving these organisms of iron.

LAD artery (left anterior descending).

ladakamycin—older name for *azacitidine.*

Ladd procedure (Surg)—for correction of malrotation of the bowel (freeing up the duodenum and Ladd's bands, and bringing up the small bowel over to the right side of the abdomen and leaving the colon on the left side of the abdomen, thus broadening the base of the mesentery).

Laerdal resuscitator (Pulm).

Laerdal valve (Pulm)—a right-angled non-rebreathing valve.

LAF (lymphocyte activating factor)—see *interleukin-1.*

Lafora body (inclusion body in myoclonus epilepsy).

LAG (lymphangiogram).

lagophthalmos—incomplete closure of the palpebral fissure when an attempt is made to shut the eyelids. May be caused by involvement of the facial nerve. It results in exposure and injury to the bulbar conjunctiva and cornea.

Laing concentric hip cup (Ortho).

LAK cells—lymphokine-activated killer cells capable of killing tumor cells in vitro. LAK cells are produced by incubation of peripheral blood lymphocytes (PBLs) with interleukin-2 for three days. Although LAK cells are capable of killing a great many autologous and allogenic tumor cells, they do not affect normal cells. LAK cells are used in treatment of gliomas and some other types of cancers, sometimes in combination with interleukin-2.

LAL test (Limulus amoebocyte lysate)—pregnancy test. Also known as Bang's horseshoe-crab blood test, a replacement for the rabbit test for pregnancy.

Laminaria (Gyn)—a genus of seaweed (kelp). The dried *Laminaria digitata* is often used in induced abortion, since, as it absorbs fluids, it expands, thus dilating the cervix. See *Dilapan; laminaria.*

laminaria (L., *lamina,* a blade) (Gyn)—a sterile applicator made of kelp, used to dilate the cervix. See *Dilapan; Laminaria.*

Lamprene (clofazimine)—a drug used to treat leprosy, now used to treat MAC infection in AIDS patients.

lancinating pain—stabbing, piercing.

Landolt pituitary speculum (Neuro).

Landolt ring (Oph)—a device for testing vision. It is like a letter C with a very small opening. The opening is moved up, down, and to each side and is used to test vision in the same way as the E chart.

Landry-Guillain-Barré-Strohl syndrome (Neuro)—acute idiopathic polyneuritis. See *Guillain-Barré syndrome.*

Landry Vein Light Venoscope—a fiberoptic illumination device. It has two arms, separated by a few inches, which, when pressed to the skin of the patient, transilluminate the skin and reveal the location of veins. It facilitates the visualization of veins which are deep seated or difficult to find so that an intravenous line can be quickly inserted.

Landsmeer's ligament—a deep fascial band in the hand (Ortho). Reference is made to this structure in operative procedures for correction of Dupuytren's contracture.

Lange skin-fold calipers—used to measure fat in certain areas of the body in diet and weight assessment.

Lange tendon lengthening and repair (Ortho).

Lanz low-pressure cuff endotracheal tube.

lap—brief form for laparotomy. See *lap tape.*

laparoscope—see *Valleylab.*

laparoscopic laser cholecystectomy—elective gallbladder surgery with laser and laparoscope. Must be done immediately after the presence of gallstones is determined, for once the gallbladder is acutely inflamed, this procedure is not an option, and a

laparoscopic laser *(cont.)* traditional cholecystectomy is necessary. Laparoscopic laser cholecystectomy requires only four small punctures about the navel, each about the diameter of a pencil. The procedure is performed under general anesthesia, but the patient's abdomen does not have to be opened, muscles are not cut, and only an overnight hospital stay is required.

laparotomy—see *second-look.*

Laplacian mapping—see *body surface Laplacian mapping.*

lap tape (or sponge)—a large laparotomy sponge used in major abdominal (laparotomy) surgery. A small one is called "appy" tape (for appendectomy) (Surg, Ob-Gyn). "The wound was packed with a moist lap tape."

LAP test—leucine aminopeptidase test performed on patients with high alkaline phosphatase. Normal is 15-33 IU/liter.

LAP test—leukocyte alkaline phosphatase test for chronic myelogenous leukemia. Result is given as a score, with normal being greater than 20.

Lapwall—trade name of a laparotomy sponge and wound protector.

large-loop excision of the transformation zone (LLETZ).

large vestibular aqueduct syndrome.

Larmor equation; frequency—terms used in MRI.

LaRoque herniorrhaphy incision.

laryngoscope
- Benjamin pediatric
- Benjamin binocular slimline
- Bizzari-Giuffrida
- Dedo-Pilling
- Jako
- Killian-Lynch

laryngoscope *(cont.)*
- Kleinsasser
- Lindholm
- Olympus ENF-P2
- Ossoff-Karlen
- Shapshay/Healy
- Weerda distending operating

LAS (lymphadenopathy syndrome)—considered by some to be a prodrome to development of AIDS.

Lasègue's sign ("la-segz")—straight leg raising test. A positive Lasègue's sign is indicative of nerve root irritation or possible low back pathology.

laser (**l**ight **a**mplification by **s**timulated **e**mission of **r**adiation)—used in many procedures. See individual entries:
- argon
- argon/krypton
- ArthroProbe
- CHRYS CO_2
- ClearView CO_2
- CO_2
- dye
- Gherini-Kauffman endo-otoprobe
- green
- helium-neon (HeNe)
- HeNe (helium-neon)
- holmium:YAG
- krypton
- krypton photocoagulation
- KTP (potassium-titanyl-phosphate)
- Microlase transpupillary diode
- Nd:holmium:YAG
- Nd:YAG
- OcuLight SL diode
- potassium-titanyl-phosphate (KTP)
- Pulsolith lithotriptor
- red
- ruby
- Sharplan 733 CO_2
- THC:YAG
- thulium/holmium:YAG
- VersaPulse holmium

laser *(cont.)*
Visulas Nd:YAG
Xanar 20 Ambulase CO_2
YAG (yttrium-aluminum-garnet)

laser-assisted balloon angioplasty (LABA) (Cardio)—a thermal laser delivery system that creates a small channel in the artery (particularly the femoral artery), followed by balloon angioplasty to dilate the residual stenosis, thereby allowing sufficient blood flow for symptom relief.

Laserflo blood perfusion monitor (BPM)—for evaluating or monitoring in situ microvascular circulation invasively or noninvasively.

laser image custom arthroplasty (LICA).

laser nucleotomy (Neuro)—a surgical technique for correction of a herniated disk. Under local anesthesia, the VersaPulse holmium laser is inserted into the nucleus pulposus of the disk, and a portion of the disk vaporized.

LaserSonics EndoBlade—for laparoscopic use (Surg).

LaserSonics Nd:YAG LaserBlade scalpels (Gyn).

LaserSonics SurgiBlade—for colposcopic procedures.

laser speckle—used to assess degree of night myopia (Oph). When light from a laser is reflected from a granular surface, a speckled pattern is seen; and when a patient with night myopia looks at this pattern and moves his head, the speckles seem to move, and move opposite to the direction of head movement if the eye is myopic at that distance. Correcting the refractive error with lenses will neutralize the pattern's movement.

laser uterosacral nerve ablation (LUNA).

Lash hysterectomy technique.

L-asparaginase
Erwinia
E. coli.

Latarjet, Andre, a French anatomist. See *nerve of Latarjet.* Also, Latarjet's vein (vena prepylorica).

lateral mamillary nucleus of Rose (Neuro).

latissimus dorsi myocutaneous flap (Plas Surg)—a method of breast reconstruction utilizing the latissimus dorsi muscle, and skin transferred from the back. It can be combined with a breast implant to produce a larger breast mound.

LATS hormone (long-acting thyroid-stimulating).

lattice degeneration (retinal)—a sharply demarcated circumferential lesion that is located at, or somewhat anterior to, the equator, characterized by an interconnecting network of fine white lines, and may be associated with numerous round, punched-out areas of retinal thinning or actual retinal holes. May lead to retinal detachment.

Latzko vesicovaginal fistula repair.

Laufe aspirating curet (Gyn).

Laurence-Moon-Biedl syndrome—hereditary syndrome characterized by obesity, retinitis pigmentosa, mental retardation, polydactyly and hypogonadism. Other abnormalties may include ataxia, dwarfism, heart defects, and ocular complications.

LAV (lymphadenopathy-associated virus)—the name first given to the AIDS virus by its discoverers, the group working at the Pasteur Institute with Luc Montagnier. The name of the AIDS virus was subsequently changed to HIV (human immunodeficiency virus) for political reasons.

LAV *(cont.)*
Normally in science the privilege of naming goes along with discovery, so this is an extraordinary exception.

LAV/HTLV-III—earlier compromise name used in journal articles published before the smoke surrounding the sequence of discovery of the AIDS virus cleared; now called HIV (human immunodeficiency virus), also as a compromise. See *HIV, LAV, HTLV-III.*

lavage
Easi-Lav
Hi Speed Pulse Lavage
Ortholav
Simpulse
Tum-E-Vac

lavage/irrigation device, HeatProbe.

lazy H incision (Surg).

lazy leukocyte syndrome (LLS).

lazy Z incision (Surg).

LCD (liquor carbonis detergens) (Derm).

LCF (left circumflex) **coronary artery.**

LCT (liquid crystal thermogram) (or thermography).

LDL (low-density lipoprotein).

LDR room—labor, delivery, and recovery room. The expectant mother goes through labor, delivery, and recovery in the same room.

lead, leads—on electrocardiogram.

lead line—a blue line which is observed on the gums in lead poisoning cases.

Leadbetter-Politano ureterovesicoplasty—submucosal tunnel technique.

Leber's disease (''lay-berz'')—hereditary optic atrophy occurring in young men between the ages of 20 and 30. The optic nerve degeneration is rapidly progressive, but finally stabilizes, and some vision remains.

Lebsche knife—a heavy knife with a curved end (to hook under the xiphoid process) and a T-shaped handle; used for splitting the sternum for quick entry into the thoracic cavity.

lecithin/sphingomyelin ratio—see *L/S ratio.*

Leder stain (chloracetate esterase)—used in identifying granulocytic sarcoma by differentiating that entity from lymphoma, Ewing's sarcoma, embryonal rhabdomyosarcoma, and undifferentiated carcinoma.

LeDuc-Camey ileocystoplasty (Urol)—antireflux implantation of the ureters, for patients with bladder cancer.

LEEP (loop electrosurgical excision procedure) (Ob-Gyn)—used to treat precancerous lesions of the cervix, in addition to laser and cryosurgery techniques. A wire loop through which radio waves are conducted is used to excise cervical tissue. Both cryosurgery and laser surgery destroy the precancerous tissue, but LEEP allows cervical specimens to be excised and examined by the pathologist.

LeFort I apertognathia repair.

LeFort II fracture—pyramidal fracture of the maxilla.

LeFort III fracture—craniofacial disjunction and transverse facial fracture.

LeFort urethral sound.

LeFort uterine prolapse repair.

left anterior descending (LAD) **artery.**

left circumflex (LCF) **coronary artery.**

left shift—see *shift to the left.*

legionnaires' disease—pulmonary form of legionellosis, resulting from infection with *Legionella pneumophila.* Called legionnaires' disease because of an outbreak at a 1976 convention

legionnaires' disease *(cont.)* of the American Legion in Philadelphia, when the causative agent was first identified. Patients with this disease have very high fevers, abdominal pain, headaches, and pneumonia. They may also have kidney, liver, and nervous system involvement. Halogen disinfectants and aerosol sprays are suspect in the etiology of legionnaires' disease.

Legionella pneumophila—gram-negative organism causing legionnaires' disease and Pontiac fever. Can be devastating in AIDS patients. Also:
L. bozemanii
L. dumoffii
L. feeleii
L. gormanii
L. jordanis
L. longbeachae (serogroups 1 and 2)
L. micdadei

leg positioner—see *Picket Fence.*

Leinbach prosthesis (Ortho).

Leishmania donovani (GI)—an opportunistic parasite found in the GI tract of patients with AIDS. It causes leishmaniasis.

Leiske intraocular lens (Oph).

Lejeune's syndrome—see *cri du chat.*

Leksell rongeur.

Leksell stereotaxic frame (Neuro)—used to place electrodes.

Lennox-Gastaut syndrome (Neuro)—mixed seizure disorder.

Lenox Hill brace *(not* Lennox)—knee orthosis (Ortho).

lens, lenses
AC-IOL
Acuvue disposable
Adaptar contact
Advent flexible
Alcon
Alpar

lens *(cont.)*
Anis Staple
Appolionio
Azar Tripod
Bagolini
Baron
Beale
Bietti
Binkhorst
Boyd
Bunker
Byron
Charles
Choyce
Cilco
Cilco MonoFlex PMMA
Cilco Slant haptics IOL
Clayman
Clayman-Kelman
Coburn intraocular
Darin
Dickerson
Drews
Dulaney
Dura-T
Eifrig
Ellingson
etafilcon A
Fechner
FormFlex
Foroblique
Fydorov
Galand disc
Galin
Gills
Gilmore
Goldmann
Gould
Greene
Hertzog
Hiles
Hirschman
Hoffer
Hopkins

lens *(cont.)*
Hoskins nylon suture laser
Hruby ("ruby")
Hubbell
Hydrocurve
Implens (Sheets)
Iolab
Iolab Slimfit
Jaffe
Jung-Schaffer
Karickhoff
Keates
Kelman
Koeppe
Kraff
Krasnov
Kratz
Kwitko
Leiske
Lieb-Guerry
Liteflex
Little
Machemer
Machemer infusion
Mainster retina laser
Manschot
McCannel
McGhan
McIntyre
Michelis
Monoflex
Optiflex
Osher
PC-IOL
Pearce Tripod
PhacoFlex
Platina clip
PMMA
Prokop
Ridley
"ruby" (Hruby)
Sauflon PW (lidofilcon B)
Schachar
Scharf

lens *(cont.)*
SeeQuence disposable
Severin
Shearing
Sheets (Implens)
Shepard
Simcoe
SingleStitch PhacoFlex
Sinskey
Slant
Smith
Soflens
Staar
Staar foldable IOL
Stein
Straatsma
Strampelli
Surgidev
Tennant
T lens
Volk Pan Retinal
Volk QuadrAspheric fundus
Worst
Worst gonioprism contact

lenses, intraocular (IOL). Styles:
anterior chamber IOL (secured in front of iris)
posterior chamber IOL (secured in back of iris)
iridocapsular/iris fixation lens or iris plane lens (sewn to iris)

lenses, soft contact—may be cleaned with ultraviolet light in the future. Because of the increase in serious eye infections due to incorrectly disinfected soft contact lenses, researchers at the University of Maryland School of Medicine are testing a new device which disinfects these with ultraviolet light, killing even the most resistant pathogens.

Lente insulin—a trade name for insulin zinc suspension. Marketed by Lilly and by Squibb/Novo.

lenticular nuclear sclerosis.
lentinan—a drug used to treat patients with AIDS and ARC.
lentivirus—a retrovirus.
Lepley-Ernst tube.
Lepper-Trier formula (Oph)—a formula for calculating the depth of the anterior chamber of the eye.
leptomeninges—inner two membranes covering the brain and spinal cord.
Leriche syndrome—intermittent claudication of the buttocks and inability to maintain an erection, due to insufficiency of the external iliac arteries.
LES incompetence (GI)—lower esophageal sphincter incompetence, which can cause severe esophagitis.
Lesch-Nyhan syndrome—hereditary hyperuricemia.
lesion
- Brown-Séquard
- bull's eye
- dendritic
- desmoid
- DREZ
- frondy
- herald patch
- Hill-Sachs
- Janeway
- jet
- phlyctenule
- pinguecula
- satellite
- shagreen
- SLAP
- target (of Lyme disease)

Lester Martin modification of the Duhamel procedure for Hirschsprung's disease.
Letterer-Siwe disease—a fulminant disease with multisystem manifestations, including skin, bone, pulmonary, central nervous system and endocrine features, and hepatosplenomegaly.
leucine aminopeptidase test (LAP).
Leucomax (GM-CSF, molgramostim)—used to treat Kaposi's sarcoma, AIDS, and CMV retinitis.
leucovorin rescue (Oncol)—used to decrease the toxicity of folic acid antagonist chemotherapy drugs such as methotrexate and fluorouracil. It rescues normal cells, but not malignant cells, from the toxic effects of the chemotherapy. Also known as citrovorum factor rescue and folinic acid rescue.
leukanakmesis (Path)—arrest of maturation of white cell series.
leukemia
- acute lymphoblastic (ALL)
- acute myeloblastic (AML)
- acute myelomonoblastic (AMMOL)
- acute monoblastic (AMOL)
- Burkitt-type acute lymphoblastic
- chronic lymphocytic (CLL)
- chronic myelocytic (CML)
- hairy-cell
- monoblastic
- null cell lymphoblastic

leukemia classification
- FAB, M1 (myeloblastic, with no differentiation)
- FAB, M2 (myeloblastic, with differentiation)
- FAB, M3 (promyelocytic)
- FAB, M5 (monocytic)
- FAB, M6 (erythroleukemia)

Leukine (GM-CSF, sargramostim)—used to treat Kaposi's sarcoma, AIDS, and CMV retinitis.
leukocyte alkaline phosphatase test (LAP).
leukocyte-poor red blood cells—red blood cells from which at least 70% of the leukocytes have been removed by a saline-washing process or by centrifuge. Used for patients who have had severe, febrile nonhemolytic reactions to blood transfusion.

leukoencephalopathy—see *progressive multifocal leukoencephalopathy.*

leukopoietin—see *sargramostim.*

leuko-poor red cells—see *leukocyte-poor red blood cells.*

Leukotrap RC (red cell) **storage system**—used to reduce transfusion reactions and HLA sensitization by removing the white cells prior to red cell storage.

Leukotrap red cell storage system—used to reduce transfusion reactions and HLA sensitization by removing the white cells prior to red cell storage.

leukovirus—an RNA virus causing leukemia and tumors.

levamisole (Ergamisol) (Oncol)—chemotherapy agent that increases T-cell response and also that of other cellular components in the blood (including neutrophils, monocytes, and antibodies) responsible for destroying cancerous cells. Given I.V. in combination with fluorouracil (Adrucil, 5-FU), for treating Dukes' stage C cancer of the colon.

LeVeen peritoneal shunt; valve—used in peritoneal venous shunt for portal venous drainage in Budd-Chiari syndrome.

level
butyrocholinesterase
cidal
phosphatidylglycerol
PLAP
p24 (or P24) antigen
renin
somatomedin
sweat chloride

Levin thermocouple cordotomy electrode (Neuro).

levonorgestrel—see *Norplant.*

Lewis blood antibody type—a factor in agglutination. Also *Duffy, Kell, Kidd, Lutheran.*

Lewis Pair-Pak needle (Oph)—a needle with a double-armed suture used in intraocular surgery.

Lewis-Tanner procedure (GI)—a subtotal esophagectomy and reconstruction.

Lewy inclusion body—in Parkinson's disease.

Leydig cells—endocrine cells of the testis, producing testosterone. When Leydig cells are found with Reinke crystals on testicular biopsy of prepubertal boys, they are indicative of precocious puberty.

Leyla retractor (Neuro).

Lezak's Malingering Test (Psych).

L-5HTP (L-5-hydroxytryptophan)—a drug for postanoxic intention myoclonus.

LFTs (liver function tests).

LGV (lymphogranuloma venereum).

Lhermitte-Duclos disease (dysplastic gangliocytoma of the cerebellum) (Neuro). This uncommon condition is seen usually in young and middle-aged adults. It is a benign mass lesion of the cerebellum, probably hamartomatous.

LHRH (luteinizing hormone-releasing hormone)—polypeptide hormone also known as GnRH (gonadotropin-releasing hormone). This hormone is currently being used in research on contraception, including contraceptives to be taken by males. It has been used in treatment of precocious puberty, delayed puberty, cryptorchidism, endometriosis, acute intermittent porphyria, and hormone-dependent tumors.

LICA (laser image custom arthroplasty).
lichen planus—a skin disorder.
Lich-Gregoire repair—used in kidney transplant surgery.
Lichtenstein hernia repair.
lid lag—abnormally sluggish movement of the upper eyelid over the eye in exophthalmos. Commonly seen in thyroid disease.
lidocaine (Xylocaine)—given I.V. to treat ventricular arrhythmias or injected as a local anesthetic. Also used topically during bowel surgery; it is applied to the cut edges of the colon to relax the colonic musculature, and allows the insertion of the EEA circular stapler for anastomosis.
lie (noun)—the relative position of the long axis of a fetus with respect to that of the mother: longitudinal or transverse.
Lieb–Guerry cataract implant lens (Oph).
Lifemed cannula.
lift—see *heave and lift.*
ligand (L., to bind) (Radiol)—organic molecules (chemical "superglue") used to bond therapeutic agents to monoclonal antibodies.
Liga surgical clips.
ligament
  ATFL (anterior talofibular)
  CFL (calcaneofibular)
  Cleland's
  Grayson's
  Landsmeer's
  natatory
  Toldt
  Whitnall's
ligator, in *Rudd-Clinic hemorrhoidal ligator.*
ligature carrier, Raz double-prong.
ligature—see *suture ligature.*
light amplification by stimulated emission of radiation (laser). See *laser.*
light reflex—constriction of the pupil in response to light striking the retina.
Light Talker—a computerized communication device (designed by Dr. Janice Light) which enables patients who are unable to speak (due to neurological or traumatic injuries) to convey messages. With a movement even as slight as raising an eyebrow, the patient can indicate a selection which is spoken by a speech synthesizer or printed out on paper.
Light-Veley headrest (Neuro).
Liliequist membrane (Neuro)—located near the pituitary gland and stalk.
limbal groove.
Limberg flap (Plas Surg).
limbus corneae—the edge of the cornea where it joins the sclera.
Limulus amoebocyte lysate test (LAL) —for pregnancy. Also called Bang's horseshoe-crab blood test, a replacement for the rabbit test.
Lincoff sponge.
Lindholm operating laryngoscope (ENT).
line, lines
  Beau's
  central venous pressure (CVP)
  gray
  Hilgenreiner
  Hudson-Stahli
  Kerley's A
  Kerley's B
  Kerley's C
  Köhler
  lead
  Lorentzian
  Mees'
  scorbutic white
  Toldt
  TPN (total parenteral nutrition)
  Vogt
  Zahn
line imaging—MRI term.

line of Zahn—a phenomenon due to the layering of fibrin and blood cells in a clot.

line scanning—MRI term.

line width—MRI term.

liner
Enduron acetabular
UHMWPe ball

lingoscope (ENT)—an endoscope (modified laryngoscope) used to facilitate visualization of the base of the tongue and excision of the lingual tonsils.

Link Stack Split Splint (Ortho)—finger splint with a split down the middle, for ease of application and removal.

Linn-Graefe iris forceps (Oph).

Linton tube.

LIP (lymphocytic interstitial pneumonitis).

lipectomy, suction-assisted.

lipid-associated sialic acid—a nonspecific tumor-associated marker seen on serum assays for the presence of gynecological malignancies.

Lipiodol (Radiol)—trade name of an iodized poppy seed oil used as a myelographic contrast medium.

lipoid nephrosis. See *nil disease.*

lipophilic—fat-loving. Cf. *hydrophilic.*

liposomes, encapsulated (Oncol)—particles of water surrounded by a membrane of phospholipids. They hold (or encapsulate) certain drugs such as amphotericin B (to treat severe systemic fungal infections without producing symptoms of drug toxicity), doxorubicin (to treat various types of cancer while reducing symptoms of cardiotoxicity and other side effects), and TLC G-65 (an antibiotic used to treat MAI infection).

liquefaciens
Enterobacter
Serratia

liquid crystal thermography (LCT).

Liquifilm sterile ophthalmic solution (Oph).

liquor carbonis detergens (LCD).

listing gait (Neuro)—leaning toward one side when walking.

Liteflex intraocular lens.

lithium carbonate—sometimes used in AIDS treatment for anemia, instead of for its effect against bipolar psychiatric disorders; it has what used to be considered a side effect of raising the white blood cell count.

Lithostar—a lithotriptor. In earlier lithotripsy treatment, the patient was immersed in water, and the shock waves that disintegrated the stones were conducted through the water. With the Lithostar, the patient is treated on a table and requires no anesthesia.

lithotripsy, extracorporeal shock-wave—procedure for treating upper urinary tract stones. See *lithotriptor.*

lithotriptor (or lithotripter)—an extracorporeal stone-disintegrating machine. It generates shock waves that are focused on the kidney stones to break them up. The patient is immersed in water while the shock waves are generated. The disintegrated stones are then passed in the urine over a several-day period. See *Pulsolith laser lithotripter; Lithostar.* Also, Dornier gallstone lithotriptor.

lithotrite (Urol)—an instrument used to grasp and crush large stones occurring in the bladder.

litmus test—for acidity and alkalinity. Cf. *Titmus test.*

Littauer scissors.

Little (a name, not a size) **intraocular lens implant.**

Littleford/Spector introducer (Cardio)—a device developed in 1977 that allows the rapid and atraumatic insertion of one or more permanent pacemaker electrodes into the heart using a peel-away sheath in the subclavian vein. Also known as subclavian peel-away sheath and permanent lead introducer. (Reference: Philip O. Littleford, M.D.)

Littler scissors.

Littre, glands of (Urol)—glands in the distal urethra of the male where gonococcal infection usually begins.

Litwak mitral valve scissors (Cardio).

liver flap—asterixis; a coarse flapping tremor of the hands, so called because it is often seen in hepatic failure.

liver function tests (LFTs).

liver palms—intense redness of the hypothenar and thenar eminences, suggestive of cirrhosis of the liver on physical examination.

liver span (the size of the liver)—the distance between the upper and lower limits of hepatic dullness, as determined by percussion. Normal range is 6 to 12 cm, depending upon the age, sex, and size of the patient.

LLETZ (large loop excision of the transformation zone) (Ob-Gyn)—an alternative to colposcopically directed punch biopsy for diagnosing cervical intraepithelial neoplasia (CIN). LLETZ is also used as an alternative to the carbon dioxide laser in the treatment of CIN.

L-leucovorin—drug used with the antibiotic Bactrim in treating AIDS patients who have *Pneumocystis carinii* pneumonia.

Llobera fixation forceps (Oph).

Lloyd-Davies scissors (GI).

LLS (lazy leukocyte syndrome).

LM-427—see *ansamycin.*

LMR (localized magnetic resonance)—MRI term.

loading dose—an initial dose of a medication, larger than the subsequent maintenance doses, given in order to achieve effective blood and tissue levels promptly.

loath (adj.)—reluctant, unwilling. "The patient is loath to undertake surgery at this time, so we will follow her closely for a while longer." Cf. *loathe.*

loathe (verb)—dislike intensely; hate; detest. Cf. *loath.*

locator—see *Berman locator.*

Locke clamp (Pod)—used in podiatric surgery to grasp the phalanx, metatarsal, or sesamoid.

locked-in syndrome (Neuro)—complete paralysis due to brain stem injury. The patient cannot communicate but is thought to remain fully conscious.

locker room syndrome—see *isovaleric acidemia.*

locking Wills-Oglesby catheter.

loculated effusion (Radiol)—on chest x-ray, a collection of fluid in the pleural space; its distribution is limited by adjacent normal or abnormal structures.

locus of HLA (human leukocyte antigen)—used in tissue typing for transplants. Each HLA locus (A, B, C, D, or DR) contains multiple alleles. Some 19 alleles have thus far been identified at locus A, 20 at locus B, 8 at locus C, 10 at locus D, and 10 at locus DR. These are written HLA-C8, HLA-DR2, etc. (no subscript or superscript).

Lodine (etodolac)—analgesic and anti-inflammatory drug.

Löffler's syndrome (also Loeffler)—chronic eosinophilic pneumonia.

logorrhea—extreme loquacity; a copious flow of talk, often incoherent.

Lone Star retractor (GI). Produced by Lone Star Medical Products of Houston, Texas, this self-retaining retractor encircles the anus and uses eight elastic holders, or stays, around the anal circumference (which gives the instrument a star-shaped appearance) to hold back all edges of the anal canal. Used to facilitate surgical access during a mucosal proctectomy and said to eliminate the need for anal dilatation and the use of a Gelpi retractor.

long-acting thyroid-stimulating hormone (LATS).

longitudinal magnetization; relaxation—MRI terms.

long TR/TE (also, "T2 weighted")—MRI term. TR (repetition time); TE (echo time).

long tract—the main spinal nerve fibers and their pathways connecting the spinal cord and the brain. See *long tract signs.*

long tract signs (Neuro)—seen in patients with upper neuron damage, include the upgoing great toe on the Babinski, twitching of the thumb on the Hoffmann, and twitching of the chin on the palmomental test.

lonidamine (AF 1890)—chemotherapy drug.

loop—oval, closed or nearly closed turn in a tube, suture, rope, or figure. Example: loop of bowel, sentinel loop. Cf. *loupe.*

loop electrosurgical excision procedure (LEEP).

loopogram—ileostogram.

Lo-Por vascular graft prosthesis.

Lorabid (loracarbef).

loracarbef (Lorabid)—an antibiotic drug used to treat ENT, pulmonary, skin, and urinary tract infections.

loratadine (Claritin) (ENT)—a long-acting, nonsedating antihistamine, taken orally once a day.

Lord total hip prosthesis (Ortho)—uses no cement; instead, its rough surface stimulates growth of new bone in the medullary canal, and the growth of new cancellous bone incorporates the prosthesis into the structure of the limb. Also known as the madreporic hip.

Lorentzian line—MRI term.

Losec (omeprazole)—former trade name which has been changed to Prilosec to avoid confusion with Lasix. See *omeprazole.*

Lotensin (benazepril).

Louis-Bar's syndrome—ataxia telangiectasia.

loupe ("loop")—convex lens in a short tube, used for magnifying or for concentrating light on an object. Used by ophthalmologists, microsurgeons, and jewelers. Cf. *loop.*

Lovibond's angle—the angle at which the fingernail meets the finger, normally, less than 180°, but exceeding this in clubbing of the fingers.

Low-Beers projection (Radiol).

low-density lipoprotein (LDL)—the so-called "bad" cholesterol linked with arteriosclerosis and myocardial infarctions. This is a plasma protein which carries cholesterol through the blood. At high levels, it increases risk of arteriosclerosis and heart attack. Cf. *high-density lipoprotein.*

low-dose screen-film technique (Radiol)—a radiographic technique designed to provide adequate imaging

low-dose technique *(cont.)* with less radiation than is used in conventional techniques.

low signal intensity—MRI term.

Lowe's syndrome—inborn error of metabolism resulting in mental retardation, cataracts and glaucoma, muscular dystrophy, and renal tubular defect for amino acids.

Lown and Woolf method—see *Compuscan Hittman computerized electrocardioscanner.*

Lown–Ganong–Levine syndrome—a combination of short P-R interval and short QRS complex demonstrated by electrocardiography, and including paroxysmal tachycardia.

L-PAM (L-phenylalanine mustard). See *melphalan.*

LPPS hydroxyapatite (Ortho)—for cementless fixation. LPPS (low-pressure plasma spray).

LSA_2L_2 chemotherapy regimen used in treatment of nonlocalized non-Hodgkin's lymphoma in children.

L–17M (Oncol)—a drug used to treat lymphoblastic lymphoma.

L–697,661—drug used to treat HIV infection, marketed by Merck.

L/S ratio (Neonat)—a test on amniotic fluid (by amniocentesis) to determine the maturity of the fetal lungs. Lecithin and sphingomyelin are the two phospholipids which comprise surfactant. Low levels of surfactant contribute to hyaline membrane disease in premature infants.

LSU reciprocation-gait orthosis (Louisiana State University)—a bracing device for use by paralytic patients or patients who would otherwise be confined to wheelchairs. It gives structural support to the trunk and lower extremities and consists of a system of cables and joint-locking devices.

LTC facility (long-term-care).

lucent defect (Radiol)—abnormal zone of decreased resistance to x-rays.

LUCs (large undifferentiated cells)—may be dictated in the differential leukocyte count.

Ludwig's angina—infection of the deep tissues of the neck and floor of the mouth. The resultant swelling can push the tongue up and back, interfering with breathing. Edema of the glottis can occur and the process can be fatal before fluctuation or redness of the neck occurs. Antibiotics have made this a rare condition.

Luedde exophthalmometer (Oph).

Luer-Lok catheter connection.

Luhr maxillofacial system.

Lukes-Collins classification—of non-Hodgkin's lymphoma.

Lumiwand—light used in eye examination.

LUNA (laser uterosacral nerve ablation) (Gyn).

Lund Browder burn diagram, modified—diagram of the anterior and posterior aspects of the human body, divided into segments; used in estimating the percentage of burned body tissue area. One of these diagrams is made at each surgery, to show the areas covered with skin, skin grafts, donor sites, biosynthetic grafts, or xenografts. These will provide a continuous picture of the progress of the coverage of the burn wounds. Note: No hyphen in *Lund Browder.*

Lunderquist guide wires *(not* Linderquist) (Urol)—used with a Chiba

Lunderquist *(cont.)*
needle for percutaneous stone manipulation, and in catheter cholangiography. Also, Chiba needle, fine needle, skinny needle.

Lunderquist-Ring torque guide—used in catheter cholangiography, and in maintaining long-term percutaneous antegrade biliary drainage.

Lundh meals.

Lundsgaard sclerotome (Oph).

lung disease
Bible printer's
cheese worker's
detergent worker's
farmer's
fish meal
furrier's
mushroom worker's
wood pulp worker's

lunger, chronic—see *chronic lunger.*

lunula (pl., lunulae)—a crescent-shaped light-colored area at the base of the fingernail. "Examination of the thumb reveals swelling and tenderness over the lunula and paronychial margin medially, with some pus seen under the nail."

lupus pernio (Derm)—seen in sarcoidosis as violaceous, shiny patches on the skin of the face, fingers, and toes.

Luque instrumentation (Ortho)—a method of fixation used in spinal fusion for scoliosis. Also, Luque rod.

Lusk instruments (ENT)—for pediatric endoscopic sinus surgery.

lutein—yellow pigment from the corpus luteum. Lutein change in the ovary is revealed by the amount of lutein remaining of an egg cell which secretes hormones to support a pregnancy.

luteinizing hormone-releasing hormone (LHRH). See *LHRH, GnRH.*

Lutrepulse (gonadorelin acetate).

Luxtec fiberoptic system—a fiberoptic light source for diagnostic and surgical visualization; used with arthroscopes and endoscopes.

Luys, nucleus of.

LVEDP (left ventricular end diastolic pressure).

lwoffi
Achromobacter
Acinetobacter
Moraxella

Lyme disease ("lime")—named for Old Lyme, Connecticut, where the disease was first recognized. This is a fairly new illness, transmitted by the bite of the deer tick. The infectious agent is the spirochete, *Borrelia burgdorferi.* The first manifestations of Lyme disease are a skin rash at the site of the bite, chills, fever, flu-like symptoms, drowsiness, fatigue, joint swelling, headache, which responds to antibiotics. There may be a second stage of the disease, with cardiac irregularities, meningitis symptoms, and, rarely, paralysis. There may also be third-stage symptoms of arthritis, and occasionally skin and neurologic manifestations.

lym-1 monoclonal antibody (Oncol)—labeled with iodine-131. Used to treat B-cell lymphoma.

lymphadenopathy-associated virus (LAV).

lymphadenopathy syndrome (LAS).

lymphapheresis—removal of peripheral blood lymphocytes; used on an experimental basis as pretreatment in rejection of liver transplants.

Lymphazurin (isosulfan blue)—a diagnostic aid for lymphangiography.

lymphedema praecox—the classic form of primary lymphedema, seen mostly in young women in their early twenties.

lymphocyte activating factor (LAF). See *interleukin-1.*

lymphocyte, tumor-infiltrating (TIL).

lymphocytic interstitial pneumonitis (LIP)—once a rare pulmonary disease, and now seen more frequently in AIDS patients.

lymphogranuloma venereum (LGV)—also called "the fifth venereal disease"; caused by a strain of *Chlamydia.*

lymphokines—a group of substances produced by various stimulated cells of the immune system, which include interferons and interleukin-2. Since these are products of the immune system itself which enhance its activity, research in the area shows great promise. See *interleukin-2.*

lymphoma
  Burkitt's
  Hodgkin's

lymphoma *(cont.)*
  non-Hodgkin's
  null-type non-Hodgkin's

Lynch incision (ENT).

LYOfoam dressing (Surg)—its gas-permeable design reduces wound maceration. Also, LYOfoam C and LYOfoam tracheostomy dressings.

lyophilized—freeze-dried, as in frozen corneal tissue used for lamellar keratoplasty.

Lysholm knee score (Ortho)—a subjective evaluation system with eight categories: instability, pain, locking, swelling, support, limp, stairs, and squatting.

lyssa inclusion body (lowercase *l*)—found in rabies. Also, Negri body.

lytic lesion (or osteolytic) (Radiol)—a disease or abnormality resulting from or consisting of focal breakdown of bone, with reduction in density.

M, m

MAA (macroaggregated albumin)—used in a technetium perfusion lung scan in nuclear medicine.

Maalox HRF (GI)—a specially formulated Maalox to relieve heartburn. HRF (heartburn relief formula).

Ma and Griffith end-to-end anastomosis (Ortho)—to repair a lacerated Achilles tendon.

MAb, MoAB, MOAB (monoclonal antibody).

MAC (Oncol)—a standard chemotherapy protocol used to treat metastatic gestational trophoblastic neoplasm. Consists of the drugs methotrexate, actinomycin D, and Cytoxan.

MAC collar (Miami Acute Care)—for cervical support.

MAC infection *(Mycobacterium avium* complex)—an infection frequently seen in AIDS patients. Also called Battey-avium complex.

machinery murmur (Cardio)—a rumbling cardiac murmur, continuous through systole and diastole with only slight variation in pitch and intensity, heard in patent ductus arteriosus.

Macewen's sign (Neuro) (pronounced "mak-u'-enz" and written with lowercase first *e*). Also called cracked pot sign.

Machemer calipers (Oph).

Machemer infusion contact lens (Oph).

Machemer VISC (vitreous infusion suction cutter) (Oph).

MACHO (methotrexate, asparaginase, Cytoxan, hydroxydaunomycin, Oncovin)—chemotherapy protocol.

Mackay-Marg tonometer (Oph)—used to measure intraocular pressure.

MACOP-B (Oncol)—a standard chemotherapy protocol used to treat adult non-Hodgkin's lymphoma. Consists of the drugs methotrexate, Adriamycin, Cytoxan, Oncovin, prednisone, and bleomycin.

macro-—a prefix meaning large or abnormally big in size. Cf. *micro-*.

macrolides—a class of antibiotics similar in effectiveness to penicillin and erythromycin but with fewer side effects. Particularly effective against *Mycoplasma pneumoniae* and resistant strains of *Haemophilus influ-*

macrolides *(cont.)* *enzae.* Examples: clarithromycin (Biaxin) and troleandomycin (Tao).

macroscopic magnetization vector.

macula—a spot or area which can be distinguished by color or other characteristic from surrounding tissue; often refers to the macula retinae.

macular fan; star (Oph)—a fan- or star-shaped folding or pleating of the retina due to edema.

macular rash (Derm).

Maddacrawler Crawler (Ortho). This device consists of an adjustable tubular frame with attached pad. It supports the abdomen of a child while the legs and arms are free to touch the floor and initiate movement. Assists crawling motions for children in therapy.

Madden technique—for repair of incisional hernia.

MADDOC (mechlorethamine, Adriamycin, dacarbazine, DDP [cisplatin], Oncovin, Cytoxan)—chemotherapy protocol used to treat neuroblastoma.

Maddox rod test—assesses the degree of muscle dysfunction (Oph).

Madigan prostatectomy (Urol)—a procedure in which adenomatous tissue is removed from outside the urethra which is preserved intact, so that the urinary tract is never entered.

madreporic coral (Madrepora group, genus *Porites*). Madreporic coral is used as a substitute for autologous bone in cranial reproduction, in bur holes, and even larger implants. A coral graft can be at least partially ossified, and with its use, incisions for harvesting rib or iliac crest grafts are unnecessary (thus obviating the pain and the risk of infection), and the operative procedure takes less time to perform. The coral is prepared for use by ultrasonic treatment and is then cut into cone-shaped plugs for bur holes, and in various-sized blocks which can be cut and shaped intraoperatively. See *Biocoral.*

madreporic hip prosthesis—see *Lord total hip prosthesis* and *madreporic coral.* Also called madreporic trochanterodiaphysary support system.

Madsen Tympan-O-Scope (ENT).

Madura foot—a rare fungal infection of the feet, seen in farm workers who work without shoes.

magnetic resonance imaging (MRI)—noninvasive radiologic procedure for imaging tissues of high fat and water content that cannot be seen with other radiologic techniques. An MRI image gives information about the chemical makeup of tissues, thus making it possible to distinguish normal, cancerous, atherosclerotic, and traumatized tissue masses in the image. It can measure vessel flow and does not involve ionizing radiation. Formerly called *nuclear magnetic resonance imaging* (NMR). Some MRI terms in dictation include:

acquisition time
adiabatic fast passage
analog to digital converter
angular frequency
angular momentum
antenna
array processor
artifact
Bloch equation
Boltzmann distribution
Carr-Purcell sequence
Carr-Purcell-Meiboom-Gill sequence
chemical shift
coherence
coil
continuous wave

magnetic resonance imaging *(cont.)*
crossed coil
cryomagnet
cryostat
demodulator
detector
diamagnetic
diffusion
digital to analog converter
echo, echoes
echo planar imaging
echo time (TE)
eddy currents; eddies
excitation
Faraday shield
fast-Fourier transform
ferromagnetic
field gradient
FID (free induction decay)
field lock
filling factor
filtered-back projection
flip angle
Fourier transform
free induction decay (FID)
free induction signal
frequency
gauss
Golay coil
gradient coil
gradient magnetic field
gyromagnetic ratio
Helmholtz coil
hertz (Hz)
homogeneity
image acquisition time
inductance
inhomogeneity
interface
interpulse time
inversion
inversion recovery
inversion time (TI)
kilohertz (kHz)
Larmor equation

magnetic resonance imaging *(cont.)*
Larmor frequency
lattice
line imaging
line scanning
line width
LMR (localized magnetic resonance)
longitudinal magnetization
longitudinal relaxation
Lorentzian line
macroscopic magnetization moment
macroscopic magnetization vector
magnetic dipole
magnetic field
magnetic gradient
magnetic induction
magnetic moment
magnetic resonance
magnetic resonance signal
magnetic susceptibility
magnetization
multiple line-scan imaging (MLSI)
multiple plane imaging
multiple sensitive point
nuclear magnetic resonance
nuclear signal
nuclear spin
nuclear spin quantum number
nucleon
nutation
orientation
coronal
sagittal
transverse
paramagnetic
partial saturation
permanent magnet
permeability
phantom
phase
phase sensitive detector
pixel (picture element)
planar spin imaging

magnetic resonance imaging *(cont.)*
point imaging
point scanning
precession
precessional frequency
proton
pulsed gradients
pulse length
pulse, radiofrequency
pulse width
pulse sequences
quadrature detector
quality factor
quenching
radian
radiofrequency (RF)
radiofrequency coil
radiofrequency pulse
readout delay
receiver
receiver coil
reconstruction
relaxation rate
relaxation time
repeated FID (free induction decay)
repetition time (TR)
rephasing gradient
resistive magnet
resolution, spatial
resonance
resonant frequency
RF (radiofrequency)
RF coil
RF pulse
rotating frame of reference
saddle coil
saturation recovery
saturation transfer
selective excitation
selective irradiation
sensitive plane
sensitive point
sensitive volume
sequence time

magnetic resonance imaging *(cont.)*
sequential plane imaging
sequential point imaging
shim coil
shimming
signal-to-noise ratio (SNR or S/N ratio)
simultaneous volume imaging
skin depth
SNR (signal-to-noise ratio)
S/N ratio (signal-to-noise)
solenoid coil
spectrometer
spectrum
spin
spin density
spin echo
spin-echo imaging
spin-lattice relaxation time
spin-spin relaxation time
spin-warp imaging
steady state free precession (SSFP)
superconducting magnet
surface coil MR
T1 (spin-lattice or longitudinal relaxation time)
T2 (spin-spin or transverse relaxation time)
TE (echo time)
tesla (T)
three-dimensional Fourier transform imaging
TI (inversion time)
TR (repetition time)
transverse magnetization
tuning
tunnel
two-dimensional Fourier transform imaging
vector
volume imaging
voxel (volume element)
zeugmatography, Fourier transformation

magnetic resonance spectroscopy (MRS)—a noninvasive technique to study the body chemistry, using magnetism and radio waves, no radiation or needles. The patient is placed within a large circular magnet (as in magnetic resonance imaging), and radio waves are beamed toward the patient. The body's atoms are excited by these waves, and the radio frequency of each chemical is interpreted by computer, which thus maps out the chemical components of each area. Chemical changes caused by heart attack or stroke can be detected quickly. The MRS may prove useful in studying changes in muscle of patients with multiple sclerosis, and could lead to new forms of therapy.

magnetic stimulation—a treatment for nonunion of fractures. It has been shown that electric, or magnetic, currents stimulate more rapid regrowth of bone in cases of failure of healing in fractures of long bones. This is a noninvasive means of treatment and may avoid the necessity of resorting to surgery and possible bone grafting. See *EBI bone healing system* and *OrthoGen/OsteoGen.*

Magnevist (gadopentetate dimeglumine)—injectable contrast medium for magnetic resonance imaging.

Magnum guide wire (Cardio)—used during coronary angioplasty.

Magnuson-Stack shoulder arthrotomy (Ortho).

MAGPI operation (Urol)—an acronym for **m**eatal **a**dvancement, **g**landuloplasty, **p**enoscrotal junction meatotomy, a procedure to correct hypospadias. It's pronounced "magpie," like the bird.

Magrina-Bookwalter vaginal retractor (Ob-Gyn, Surg)—provides exposure of the vagina for surgical procedures; it can expand for use in multiple surgical fields. See *Bookwalter retractor system.*

Mahaim bundle in the heart (Cardio)—a term in electrophysiologic studies of supraventricular tachycardia.

Mahurkar catheter. See *Quinton Mahurkar dual-lumen catheter.*

MAI infection (*Mycobacterium avium-intracellulare*)—a TB variant once considered not to be a pathogen in humans, but now appearing as disseminated tuberculosis in AIDS patients. "The patient was referred for ongoing management of HIV-related issues, including MAI bacteremia." Cf. *MAC infection* (*Mycobacterium avium* complex).

Maico-MA 20 audiometer—used to perform bedside audiography.

main d'accoucheur ("obstetrician's hand")—the position in tetany that the hand assumes after a positive Trousseau's sign (carpopedal spasm). See *Trousseau's sign.*

Mainster retina laser lens (Oph)—for panretinal photocoagulation and focal laser therapy.

maintain—to control or limit the effects of an illness or abnormal state with diet, medicine, or other means.

Mainz pouch urinary reservoir (Urol)—a urinary pouch made from a combination of cecum and ileum. Pronounced "mintz" with a long *i.*

MAK-6 (**m**onoclonal **a**nti-cyto**k**eratin) (Path)—cocktail that identifies normal and malignant cells of epithelial origin to facilitate identification of poorly differentiated epithelial malignancies.

maladie-de-Roger (Fr., "ro-zhay") (Roger's disease)—congenital defect of the interventricular septum of the heart.

malaria—infectious febrile disease characterized by periodic paroxysms of fever, chills, and sweating. It is caused by four species of protozoa of the genus *Plasmodium (P. vivax, P. falciparum, P. malariae,* and *P. ovale),* parasitic in the red blood cells, and transmitted to the bloodstream of humans by the bite of *Anopheles* mosquitoes. Cf. *miliaria.*

Malassezia furfur—a fungus causing tinea versicolor.

male pattern baldness (Derm)—characteristic thinning of hair along the temples, front, and back of the head in men. Also called male pattern alopecia.

malformation
arteriovenous (AVM)
atrioventricular (AVM)

Malgaigne's fracture—bilateral vertical pelvic fracture.

Malis angled-up bipolar forceps (Neuro).

Malis CMC-II bipolar coagulator (Neuro). Used with Malis irrigation forceps, and irrigation module, for irrigation, coagulation, and cutting.

Malis irrigation forceps (Neuro).

malleable retractor (Surg).

malleolus—the rounded lateral projections of the bone at the ankle. See *malleus.*

mallet toe (Ortho)—flexion contracture of the distal joints of the second, third, fourth, and fifth toes.

malleus (ENT)—the outermost of the three small bones in the ear. Cf. *malleolus.*

malleus nipper (ENT)—a surgical instrument used in ear surgery.

Mallinckrodt feeding tube.

Mallinckrodt Laser-Flex tube—stainless steel, laser-resistant endotracheal tube.

Mallory-Azan stain—a special stain for collagen fiber.

Mallory's PTAH (phosphotungstic acid-hematoxylin) (Path). See *PTAH.*

Mallory-Weiss tear—tear in the mucosa at the cardioesophageal junction, generally caused by retching or vomiting, resulting in upper GI bleed.

Maloney endo-otoprobe (ENT)—laser probe used in ear surgery.

Maloney esophageal dilator.

malpighian corpuscles—urine-forming units in renal cortex of kidneys; aggregations of lymphoid tissue in white pulp of spleen.

mammaplasty—see *mammoplasty.*

mammoplasty (Plas Surg)—plastic augmentation or reduction reconstruction of the breast. Also spelled *mammaplasty.*

m-AMSA (amsacrine) (Oncol)—a drug used in treatment of acute adult leukemia.

Mancini plates—referred to in quantitation of immunoglobulins, as: "Mancini plates showed IgA 72 g/L, IgG 2.5 g/L."

mandrin, wire—a probe, stylet, or guide for a catheter. Examples:
coudé curve
Guyon-Benique curve
malleable tip
Van Buren curve

maneuver
Adson
Bruhat
Credé
Duecollement
Gowers'
Heimlich
Houget's
Jendrassik's
Jonnson's
Mattox
Mauriceau-Smellie-Veit

maneuver *(cont.)*
McMurray's
Nylen-Bárány
Phalen's
Queckenstedt
Roos
Sellick
Smellie-Veit
Valsalva
manic-depressive—see *bipolar affective disorder* (Psych).
manifest refraction (Oph).
manipulation, Hippocrates.
manipulator, Grieshaber.
manipulator/injector, HUMI uterine.
manipulator/splitter, Koch phaco.
manometer
Dinamap ultrasound blood pressure
Honan
Manschot intraocular implant lens (Oph).
Mantoux test—an intradermal tuberculin test. Read at 48 to 72 hours after injection, induration of more than 10 mm in diameter at the injection site is considered positive.
MAP (mean arterial pressure).
maple bark stripper's disease—extrinsic allergic alveolitis caused by exposure to moldy maple bark.
maple-syrup urine disease (MSUD)—caused by a defect in metabolism of the keto-acid analogues of leucine, isoleucine, and valine. The maple-syrup odor in the urine is caused by the presence of these compounds.
mapping, body surface Laplacian.
Maquet technique ("muh-kay'") (Ortho)—advancement of the tibial tuberosity by elevation of the tibial crest.
Marathon guiding catheter (Cardio)—used during coronary angioplasty.
march fracture (not an eponym)—a fracture of the shaft of the second or third metatarsal bone without a history of injury.
march—see *jacksonian march.*
Marchiafava-Bignami disease—uncommon demyelination of the corpus callosum.
Marcus Gunn syndrome ("jaw winking") (Oph)—unilateral ptosis of the eyelid, with association of movements of the affected upper eyelid with those of the jaw. Named for Robert Marcus Gunn, an English ophthalmologist. Note: There is no hyphen in the name.
Marie's ataxia—a hereditary disease of the nervous system.
Marinol (dronarinol)—an antiemetic drug given with chemotherapy; also used to treat loss of appetite in AIDS patients. The active ingredient is derived from the marijuana plant.
Marinesco-Radovici, palmomental reflex of. See *palmomental reflex.*
marital—pertaining to marriage, as in "marital relationship" or "marital introitus." Cf. *martial.* These are often confused. It is, of course, entirely possible that both adjectives could apply to the same relationship.
marker
AFP (alpha-fetoprotein)
ALZ-50 (Alzheimer's disease)
CA 15-3 tumor
CA 19-9 tumor
CA 72-4 tumor
cathepsin D
CEA (carcinoembryonic antigen)
D'Assumpcao rhytidoplasty
DNA polymerase-alpha
DSM
Freeman cookie cutter areola

marker *(cont.)*
Friedlander
Friedlander arcuate
Friedlander transverse incision
G6PD cell
Ki-67
P-glycoprotein gene
PLAP serum
PSA (prostate specific antigen)
sigmaS
Storz radial incision
Thornton 360° arcuate
tripe palm
tumor

Mark II Chandler retractor (Ortho)—used to retract soft tissue away from bone during hip and knee surgery.

Marlex—synthetic graft material (used in hernioplasties and in other abdominal surgery where the tissues need reinforcement).

MARSA (methicillin-aminoglycoside-resistant *Staphylococcus aureus)*—a strain of *S. aureus* which is resistant to methicillin and the aminoglycoside class of antibiotics (gentamicin, kanamycin, tobramycin). See *MRSA.*

Marshall and Tanner pubertal staging. See *Tanner Developmental Scale.*

martial—pertaining to war or battle. Cf. *marital.*

Martin, in *Lester Martin modification.*

Martorell hypertensive ulcer.

Mascot indirect ophthalmoscope (Oph).

mask facies—the expressionless appearance of the face seen in patients with Parkinson's disease.

Masket technique (Oph)—a technique for intraocular lens insertion using a 4-7 mm incision with closure involving multiple small, interlaced stitches with the suture knots buried.

Mason abdominotranssphincteric resection (Surg).

Mason vertical-banded gastroplasty.

mass effect (Radiol)—the radiographic appearance created by an abnormal mass in or adjacent to the area of study.

mass lesion (Radiol)—anything that occupies space within the body and is not normal tissue.

massage
Ohashiatsu
Shiatsu

mast cell—a type of inflammatory cell which releases histamine and is important in allergic reactions.

mastectomy, Auchincloss modified radial.

Master Flow Pumpette—a disposable I.V. pump that maintains I.V. flow rate under changing conditions, i.e., bed height, patient position, and fluctuations in venous pressure.

Master's two-step test—a timed stress test in which the patient climbs and descends two 9-inch steps a given number of times; indicates the degree of decreased coronary artery blood flow and the consequent degree of ischemic heart disease.

MAST trousers (military anti-shock treatment) (or trousers). The whole suit can be worn, or the trousers alone, as indicated.

maternal serum alpha-fetoprotein (MSAFP) (Ob-Gyn)—screening performed to identify presence of twins, erroneously-dated pregnancies, fetal demise, and to identify fetal anomalies such as spina bifida and abdominal wall defects.

matricectomy ("may-tris-sec'tum-ee") —excision of nail matrix (nail plate) for chronic nail disease or deformity.

Matsner median episiotomy and repair (Ob-Gyn).

Mattox aorta clamp.

Mattox maneuver (Surg)—extensive mobilization of the left colon, left kidney, spleen and tail of the pancreas, and stomach, and reflecting these structures to the midline, in exposure of the suprarenal aorta. Used in treating patients with vascular injuries (hematoma or active hemorrhage) from penetrating abdominal wounds.

mature cataract (Oph)—a cataract in which the lens is completely opaque or ripe or surgery.

maturity onset diabetes of the young (MODY).

Mauriceau-Smellie-Veit maneuver (Ob-Gyn)—method of delivery of the aftercoming head, with the infant resting on the physician's forearm. Also, Smellie-Veit, Smellie method, Mauriceau method.

MaxCast—a fiberglass casting tape consisting of a knitted fiberglass fabric impregnated with a water-activated polyurethane resin (Ortho). Cf. *Fractura Flex, Gypsona.*

Max Fine tying forceps (Oph). Named for Max Fine, M.D., an ophthalmic surgeon.

Max Force catheter (GI)—balloon catheter used to dilate biliary stenosis.

Maxicam (isoxicam) (Ortho)—nonsteroidal anti-inflammatory used for arthritis.

Maxima II TENS unit—see *TENS.*

maximum predicted heart rate (MPHR).

Maxon polyglyconate monofilament suture.

Mayer's view.

Mayfield-Kees headrest (Neuro).

Mayo-Gibbon heart-lung machine—artificial cardiopulmonary support in extracorporeal membrane oxygenation (ECMO).

Mayo stand (Surg)—operating room equipment.

MAZE (m-AMSA, azacitidine, etoposide)—chemotherapy protocol used to treat acute myeloid leukemia.

Mazicon (flumazenil).

mazindol (Sanorex)—a drug used to treat Duchenne muscular dystrophy.

M-BACOD (methotrexate, bleomycin, Adriamycin, Cytoxan, Oncovin, dexamethasone)—chemotherapy protocol for treatment of lymphoma.

M-BACOS (methotrexate, bleomycin, Adriamycin, Cytoxan, Oncovin, Solu-Medrol)—chemotherapy protocol used to treat advanced lymphomas.

MB bands of CPK. The number of these bands relates to the amount of myocardial damage in myocardial infarction, or suspected myocardial infarction.

MCA (middle cerebral artery).

MCAG (multiple colloid adenomatous goiter).

MCC gene (mutated in colon cancer) (Oncol). Researchers at the Johns Hopkins Medical Institute have discovered genes which normally act to suppress the formation of malignant tumors in the body. When damaged, these tumor-suppressing genes are unable to function and cancer can develop. Damage to four different genes has been linked to the development of colon cancer: the MCC gene on chromosome 5, the p53 gene, the DCC gene, and the RAS oncogene. The MCC gene seems to be involved with the regulation of growth in normal and cancer cells and may suggest a way in which a new class of chemotherapy drugs might be developed.

McCannel intraocular implant lens (Oph).

McCarey-Kaufman (M-K) **medium**—used to store excised cornea with scleral rim attached. This preserves the corneal endothelium for grafting purposes.

M-component—See *M-protein.*

McCort's sign—one of the radiologic criteria of the presence of ascites.

McCutchen implant (Ortho)—press-fit titanium femoral implant with longitudinal grooves that enhance rotational stability; made by Dow Corning Wright.

McDonald procedure (Gyn)—cervical cerclage.

McElroy curet (Ortho).

McFadden clip (Neuro).

McFarland, in *Kocher-McFarland approach in hip arthroplasty.*

MCFSR (mean circumferential fiber shortening rate) (Cardio).

McGaw volumetric pump—used for continuous nasogastric feedings.

McGee platinum/stainless steel piston (ENT)—used in ear reconstruction.

McGhan breast implant (Plas Surg).

McGhan intraocular lens (Oph).

McGill pain questionnaire—method used in pain management programs to rate pain.

McGoon coronary perfusion catheter (Cardio).

McHardy, in *Brown-McHardy pneumatic dilator.*

McIntire aspiration-irrigation system (Oph).

McIntosh double-lumen catheter (Vasc Surg).

McIntyre intraocular implant lens (Oph).

McIvor mouth gag (ENT)—used in tonsillectomies.

McKee-Farrar
acetabular cup
hip prosthesis
total hip arthroplasty

McKeever Vitallium cap prosthesis (Ortho)—patellar prosthesis. There is also a recent polyethylene modification of this prosthesis.

McKrae strain—herpes simplex virus.

McLeod blood phenotype—reported in patients with chronic granulomatous disease (CGD).

McMurray's maneuver (Ortho). To demonstrate, flex the knee and turn the foot out and feel knee cartilage; flex the knee and turn the foot in and feel knee cartilage. This is to feel for a clicking which indicates a torn knee cartilage.

McMurray sign (Ortho).

McNaught keel—laryngeal prosthesis.

McNeill-Goldmann blepharostat—a fixation ring (Oph).

McNemar's test—test for the presence of ascites.

McPherson lens forceps (Oph).

McPherson-Vannas iris scissors (Oph).

MCTC (metrizamide CT cisternogram) (Neuro).

MCTD (mixed connective tissue disease).

MCT oil (medium-chain triglyceride)—source of extra calories, given in formula to premature infants (Peds).

MCV (methotrexate, cisplatin, vinblastine)—chemotherapy protocol used to treat bladder carcinoma.

McVay hernia repair.

MDAC (multiple dose activated charcoal) for drug overdose.

MDLO (metoclopramide, dexamethasone, lorazepam, ondansetron) (Oncol)—a protocol of drugs used to prevent vomiting in patients receiving

MDLO *(cont.)*
cisplatin chemotherapy. Consists of a gastric stimulant, a steroid, an antianxiety agent, and a centrally acting antiemetic.

MDR (multidrug resistance) to chemotherapy agents.

MDR-TB (Pulm)—multidrug-resistant tuberculosis.

MEA (multiple endocrine adenopathies, or abnormalities).

Meadox Microvel arterial graft material (Vasc Surg)—double velour knitted Dacron.

meal—see *Lundh meal.*

measurement. See also *unit* and *unit of measurement.*
- Hirschberg
- Krimsky
- OFC (ocipitofrontal circumference)
- SNA and SNB orthodontic
- torr
- Van Herick

meat wrapper's asthma—from inhalation of the isocyanate fumes caused by heat used in cutting and sealing plastic wrapping for meat.

Mebadin (dehydroemetine).

meconium stain (Ob/Gyn)—fecal material produced by the fetus, which stains the placenta and membranes when decreased oxygen is present.

median furrow of the prostate (Urol).

median sternotomy *(not* medium sternotomy)—a midline incision into the sternum. See *mediastinotomy* and *mediastinum. (Not* mediosternotomy or medial sternotomy.)

mediastinoscope, Carlens' fiberoptic.

mediastinotomy—incision into the mediastinum; may be an anterior mediastinotomy or cervical mediastinotomy; may also be a dorsal or posterior mediastinotomy. Cf. *median sternotomy.*

mediastinum—group of tissues and organs separating the sternum in front and the vertebral column behind, containing the heart and large vessels, trachea, esophagus, thymus, lymph nodes, and other structures and tissues. It is divided into anterior, middle, posterior, and superior regions.

medication—a quick-reference list of pharmaceuticals defined in main entries throughout the book, including AIDS drugs, chemicals, chemotherapy drugs and protocols, classes of drugs, contrast media, investigational drugs, natural substances, prescription and over-the-counter drugs, monoclonal antibodies, radioisotopes, and solutions.
- ABCD (amphotericin B colloidal dispersion)
- ABLC (amphotericin B lipid complex)
- ABPP (bropirimine)
- Abrodil (methiodal sodium)
- ABVD chemotherapy protocol
- ABVE chemotherapy protocol
- Accupril (quinapril)
- Accutane (isotretinoin)
- ACE chemotherapy protocol
- acebutolol (Sectral)
- acecainide (Napa)
- acemannan (Carrisyn)
- acetylsalicylic acid (ASA, aspirin)
- acivicin (AT-125)
- Aclacinomycin (aclarubicin)
- aclarubicin (Aclacinomycin)
- ACNU (nimustine)
- ACOP chemotherapy protocol
- acridinyl anisidide (amsacrine)
- Actigall (ursodiol)
- actinomycin-D (ACT-D, dactinomycin)
- activated charcoal

medication *(cont.)*
acycloguanosine (acyclovir, Zovirax)
acyclovir (Zovirax)
Adagen (pegademase bovine, PEG-ADA)
ADE chemotherapy protocol
Adenocard (adenosine)
adenine arabinoside (Ara-A)
adrenergic antagonist
adrenergic receptor
ADR-529
Adriamycin (doxorubicin, hydroxy-daunomycin)
Adrucil (fluorouracil)
Aeropent (aerosolized pentamidine)
aerosolized pentamidine (Aeropent, NebuPent)
AF 1890 (lonidamine)
AFM chemotherapy protocol
aggregated human IgG (AHuG)
agonist drug
AGT (aminoglutethimide)
AHG (antihemophilic globulin)
AL-721
Aldredase (tolrestat)
alfa interferon (interferon alfa)
alfacalcidol (One-Alpha)
Alferon LDO (interferon alfa-n3)
Alferon N (interferon alfa-n3)
alglucerase (Ceredase)
Alkaban-AQ (vinblastine)
Alkeran (melphalan)
Allergan 211 (idoxuridine)
allopurinol (Zyloprim)
all-trans-retinoic acid (tretinoin)
allylamine class of drugs
Alpha Chymar (alpha-chymotrypsin)
$alpha_1$-proteinase inhibitor
alpha-chymotrypsin (Alpha Chymar)
alpha interferon (IFN-A, interferon alfa)
alpha-TGI (teroxirone)
AlphaNine
$alpha_1$-antitrypsin

medication *(cont.)*
alpha 2 interferon (IFN-alpha 2)
Alredase (tolrestat)
Altace (ramipril)
altretamine (Hexalen, Hexastat)
amethopterin (methotrexate)
amifostine (ethiofos)
amiloride (Midamor)
Amin-Aid enteral nutrition
aminoglutethimide (AGT, Cytadren, Elipten)
aminopyridine (4-aminopyridine)
aminothiadiazole (ATDA)
amiodarone
amiodipine (Norvasc)
Amipaque
AML-2-23 monoclonal antibody
AMMEN-0E5 monoclonal antibody
amonafide
amoxapine (Asendin)
amphotericin B colloid dispersion (ABCD)
amphotericin B lipid complex (ABLC)
Ampligen (polyribonucleotide)
AMSA (methanesulfon-m-anisidide)
amsacrine (AMSA, m-AMSA, Amsidyl)
Amsidyl (amsacrine)
Amvisc (sodium hyaluronate)
Anadrol-50 (oxymetholone)
Anafranil (clomipramine)
anagrelide
anandron (ANAN)
Ancobon (flucytosine)
Android-F (fluoxymesterone)
anistreplase (APSAC, Eminase)
ansamycin (LM-427, Mycobutin, rifabutin)
Antabuse
antagonist drug
anthracenedione class of drugs
anti-B4/blocked ricin immunoconjugate monoclonal antibody
anti-CD3 monoclonal antibody

medication *(cont.)*
anti-CEA monoclonal antibody
anti-EGFR monoclonal antibody
anti-endotoxin monoclonal antibody
antiepilepsirine
anti-ganglioside GD2 monoclonal antibody
anti-ganglioside monoclonal antibody
anti-GD2 monoclonal antibody
anti-GD3 R24 monoclonal antibody
anti-glioma monoclonal antibody
antihemophilic globulin (AHG)
Antilirium (physostigmine salicylate)
antimoniotungstate (HPA-23)
anti-TAC-H monoclonal antibody
anti-TAC-72 monoclonal antibody
anti-T3 monoclonal antibody
antithrombin III (ATnativ)
antithymocyte globulin (ATG)
anti-transferrin receptor monoclonal antibody
antitussive class of drugs
anxiolytic class of drugs
AOPA chemotherapy protocol
AOPE chemotherapy protocol
APC chemotherapy protocol
APD (aminohydroxypropylidene, disodium pamidronate)
APE chemotherapy protocol
APO chemotherapy protocol
APSAC (anisoylated plasminogen streptokinase activator complex; anistreplase)
Ara-A (adenine arabinoside, vidarabine)
Ara-AC (fazarabine)
Ara-C (cytarabine)
Arduan (pipecuronium)
Aredia (pamidronate disodium)
Arvin
ASA (acetylsalicylic acid, aspirin)
Asacol (mesalamine)

medication *(cont.)*
Asendin (amoxapine)
A-SHAP chemotherapy protocol
ASN (L-asparaginase)
AS-101
asparaginase (L-asparaginase)
aspirin (ASA, acetylsalicylic acid)
astemizole (Hismanal)
ATDA (aminothiadiazole)
ATG (antithymocyte globulin)
AT-125 (acivicin)
A33 monoclonal antibody
ATnativ (antithrombin III)
Autoplex
Avitene
Avlosulfon (dapsone)
azacitidine (azacytidine)
azacytidine (5-azacytidine, azacitidine)
azalide class of drugs
azathioprine (AZTP)
AZC (azacitidine)
AzdU (azidouridine)
azidothymidine (AZT, compound S, Retrovir, zidovudine)
azidouridine (AzdU)
aziridinylbenzoquinone (AZQ)
azithromycin (Zithromax)
Azmacort
AZQ (aziridinylbenzoquinone, diaziquone)
AZT (azidothymidine)
AZTP (azathioprine)
Azulfidine
bacitracin
BACT chemotherapy protocol
balanced electrolyte solution (BES)
balanced salt solution (BSS)
Baypress (nitrendipine)
BBVP-M chemotherapy protocol
BCD chemotherapy protocol
BCG (bacillus Calmette-Guérin vaccine; Tice)
BCNU or BiCNU (carmustine)

medication *(cont.)*
BEAC chemotherapy protocol
Belganyl (suramin)
BEMP chemotherapy protocol
benazepril (Lotensin)
benzodiazepine class of drugs
BEP chemotherapy protocol
bepridil (Vascor)
beractant (Survanta)
Berotec (fenoterol)
BES (balanced electrolyte solution)
Betadine Helafoam solution
beta-endorphin
Betapace (sotalol)
Betaseron (recombinant human interferon beta)
bethanidine
Biaxin (clarithromycin)
Bicarbolyte
B-IFN (beta-interferon)
Biodel
Biotropin (human growth hormone)
BIP chemotherapy protocol
bisphosphonate APD
bitolterol (Tornalate)
Blenoxane (bleomycin sulfate)
bleomycin sulfate (Blenoxane)
BMY-28090 (elsamitrucin)
Bonefos
BOP chemotherapy protocol
botulinum toxin type A (Oculinum, Ortholinum)
Bouin's solution
brequinar sodium (DuP 785)
bromodeoxyuridine (BUdR, broxuridine)
Brompton solution
Bronkaid
Bronkosol
bropirimine (ABPP)
broxuridine (bromodeoxyuridine)
B72.3 monoclonal antibody
BSO (buthionine sulfoximine)
BSRL (buserelin)

medication *(cont.)*
BSS (balanced salt solution)
BSS Plus
Bucrylate
BUdR (bromodeoxyuridine, broxuridine)
Burow's solution
buserelin (BSRL)
BuSpar (buspirone)
buspirone (BuSpar)
busulfan (MeliBu, Myleran)
buthionine sulfoximine (BSO)
butorphanol tartrate (Stadol NS)
butyl-DNJ (deoxynojirmycin)
BW 301U (piritrexim)
BW A770U (crisnatol mesylate)
CAC chemotherapy protocol
CACP (cisplatin)
CAD chemotherapy protocol
CAE chemotherapy protocol
CAF chemotherapy protocol
caffeine
CAFTH chemotherapy protocol
Calan (verapamil)
calcium acetate (PhosLo)
calcium channel blockers
calcium entry blockers
CALF chemotherapy protocol
CALF-E chemotherapy protocol
calusterone
CAP chemotherapy protocol
CAPPr chemotherapy protocol
Capulets
caracemide
Carafate (sucralfate)
carbacephem class of drugs
carbetimer
carboplatin (Paraplatin)
carbovir
Cardiolite (^{99m}Tc sestamibi)
cardioplegic solution
CardioTek (^{99m}Tc teboroxime)
Cardizem CD
Cardizem SR

medication *(cont.)*
Cardura (doxazosin mesylate)
carmustine (BCNU, BiCNU)
carprofen (Rimadyl)
Carrisyn (acemannan)
Casodex
C-asparaginase (Crasnitin)
Catapres (clonidine)
cathepsin D
CAV chemotherapy protocol
CAVP16 chemotherapy protocol
CB10-277
CBV chemotherapy protocol
CC49 monoclonal antibody
CCNU (CeeNu, lomustine)
CDA (chenodeoxycholic acid)
CDDP (cisplatin)
CDE chemotherapy protocol
CD4, recombinant soluble human (Receptin)
CD4-IgG
CD5+ monoclonal antibody
CD5-T lymphocyte immunotoxin
CEAker
CEA-Tc 99m (^{99m}Tc CEA)
CEB chemotherapy protocol
CECA chemotherapy protocol
CeeNu (lomustine)
CEF chemotherapy protocol
cefmetazole (Zefazone)
cefprozil (Cefzil)
ceftazidime (Ceptaz, Fortaz, Tazidime)
Cefzil (cefprozil)
celiprolol (Selecor)
CEM chemotherapy protocol
Centovir (C-58 monoclonal antibody)
Centoxin (HA-1A) monoclonal antibody
CEP chemotherapy protocol
cephalosporin class of drugs
Ceptaz (ceftazidime)
Ceredase (alglucerase)

medication *(cont.)*
Cerubidine (daunorubicin HCl)
cesium chloride
cetiedil citrate
cetirizine (Reactine)
CF (citrovorum factor; leucovorin)
C-58 monoclonal antibody (Centovir)
CGP 19835A
Chemet (succimer)
ChemoCap
Chenix (chenodiol)
chenodeoxycholic acid (CDA)
chenodiol (Chenix)
Chibroxin (norfloxacin)
chimeric monoclonal antibody
CHIP (iproplatin)
chlorambucil (CLB, Leukeran)
chlorotrianisene (TACE)
ChlVPP chemotherapy protocol
CHOD chemotherapy protocol
CHOP chemotherapy protocol
CHOP-BLEO chemotherapy protocol
CHOPE chemotherapy protocol
chromic phosphate (P-32)
cifenline succinate (Cipralan)
cilazapril (Inhibace)
Ciloxan (ciprofloxacin)
cimetidine (Tagamet)
Cipralan (cifenline succinate)
ciprofloxacin (Ciloxan)
CISCA chemotherapy protocol
cis-retinoic acid (isotretinoin)
cisplatin (Platinol)
cis-platinum (cisplatin)
citrovorum factor (CF, leucovorin)
clarithromycin (Biaxin)
Claritin (loratadine)
clindamycin
Clinoril (sulindac)
clobazam (Frisium)
clofazimine (Lamprene)
clomipramine (Anafranil)

medication *(cont.)*
clonidine (Catapres)
clozapine (Clozaril)
Clozaril (clozapine)
CL 286558
CMF chemotherapy protocol
CMFP chemotherapy protocol
CMFPT chemotherapy protocol
CMFPTH chemotherapy protocol
CMFVP chemotherapy protocol
CMH chemotherapy protocol
CMOPP chemotherapy protocol
CMV chemotherapy protocol
CMV monoclonal antibody
CNOP chemotherapy protocol
COAP chemotherapy protocol
COF/COM chemotherapy protocol
Cognex (tacrine)
Colbenemid (probenecid-colchicine)
colchicine
colfosceril palmitate (Exosurf Pediatric)
Collins' solution
colloid solution
COL-1 monoclonal antibody
Colyte
compound Q (GLQ223, trichosanthin)
compound S (azidothymidine, zidovudine)
Comprecin (enoxacin)
conjugated estrogens
Conray
COPBLAM chemotherapy protocol
COP-BLEO chemotherapy protocol
COPE chemotherapy protocol
Corgard (nadolol)
Cosmegen (dactinomycin)
CPA (cyclophosphamide, Cytoxan)
CPB chemotherapy protocol
CPC chemotherapy protocol
CPM (cyclophosphamide, Cytoxan)
Crasnitin (C-asparaginase)
CRF-187

medication *(cont.)*
crisnatol mesylate (BW A770U)
Cronassial
crystalloid solution
CTCb chemotherapy protocol
C219 monoclonal antibody
Cutivate (fluticasone propionate)
CVAD chemotherapy protocol
CVD chemotherapy protocol
CVP chemotherapy protocol
CVPP chemotherapy protocol
cyclocytidine
cyclophosphamide (Cytoxan, Neosar)
Cyclo-Prostin (epoprostenol)
CyHOP chemotherapy protocol
cyproterone acetate (CPTR)
Cytadren (aminoglutethimide)
cytarabine (Cytosar-U; Ara-C)
CytoGam (cytomegalovirus immune globulin)
cytokine class of drugs
cytomegalovirus immune globulin (CytoGam)
cytomegalovirus monoclonal antibody
CYT-103 monoclonal antibody
Cytosar-U (cytosine arabinoside, cytarabine)
cytosine arabinoside (cytarabine)
Cytovene (ganciclovir)
Cytoxan (cyclophosphamide)
CYVADIC chemotherapy protocol
dacarbazine (DTIC-Dome)
dactinomycin (actinomycin-D, Cosmegen)
Dakin's solution
Dalgan (dezocine)
DAP/TMP (dapsone plus trimethoprim)
dapiprazole (Rev-Eyes)
dapsone (Avlosulfon)
dapsone plus trimethoprim (DAP/TMP)

medication *(cont.)*
Daraprim (pyrimethamine)
DAT chemotherapy protocol
DATVP chemotherapy protocol
daunorubicin HCl (Cerubidine)
daunorubicin, liposomal (Daunoxome)
Daunoxome (liposomal daunorubicin)
DAVA (desacetyl vinblastine amide, vindesine)
DBD (dibromodulcitol)
DCF (2'-deoxycoformycin; pentostatin)
ddC (dideoxycytidine, HIVID)
ddI (didanosine, dideoxyinosine, Videx)
DDP (cisplatin)
Decabid (indecainide)
DECAL chemotherapy protocol
dehydroemetine (Mebadin)
Demser (metyrosine)
deoxy-D-glucose
deoxycoformycin (DCF, pentostatin)
deoxydoxorubin (IDX)
deoxynojirmycin (butyl-DNJ)
deoxyspergualin (DSG)
Depo-Provera (medroxyprogesterone)
Dermablend
DES (diethylstilbestrol)
desflurane
dexamethasone (DM)
dextran sulfate (Uendex)
Dey-Wash skin wound cleaner
dezocine (Dalgan)
DFMO (difluoromethylornithine, eflornithine, Ornidyl)
DFMO-MGBG chemotherapy protocol
d4T (didehydrodideoxythymidine, stavudine)
DFV chemotherapy protocol
DHAC (dihydro-5-azacytidine)

medication *(cont.)*
DHAD (mitoxantrone)
DHAP chemotherapy protocol
DHE (dihematoporphyrin ether)
DHE, DHE-45 (dihydroergotamine)
DHPG (dihydroxypropoxymethylguanine, ganciclovir)
DiaBeta (glyburide)
diaziquone (AZQ)
dibenzodiazepine class of drugs
dibromodulcitol (DBD, mitolactol)
didanosine (ddI, Videx)
didemnin B
dideoxycytidine (ddC, HIVID)
dideoxyinosine (ddI, didanosine, Videx)
Didronel (etidronate)
diethyldithiocarbamate (Imuthiol)
diethylstilbestrol (DES, Stilbestrol)
Diflucan (fluconazole)
difluorodeoxycytidine (gemcitabine)
difluoromethylornithine (DFMO, eflornithine)
Digibind (digoxin immune Fab)
Digidote (digoxin immune Fab)
digoxin immune Fab (Digibind, Digidote)
dihematoporphyrin ether (DHE)
dihydroergotamine (DHE, DHE-45)
dihydroxypropoxymethylguanine (DHPG, ganciclovir)
Dilapan
dilevalol (Unicard)
dimercaptosuccinic acid (DMSA)
Dimer-X
dimethylbusulfan
dinitrochlorobenzene (DNCB)
Dipentum (olsalazine)
dipyridamole (Persantine)
disodium pamidronate (Aredia)
Diulo (methyl metolazone)
DMARDs (disease-modifying antirheumatic drugs)
DMSA (dimercaptosuccinic acid)

medication *(cont.)*
DNCB (dinitrochlorobenzene)
DNJ (N-butyl-deoxynojirmycin)
domperidone (Motilium)
Doral (quazepam)
dothiepin (Prothiaden)
doxacurium chloride (Nuromax)
doxorubicin (Adriamycin, Rubrex)
doxozosin mesylate (Cardura)
doxycycline (Monodox, Vibramycin)
D6.12 monoclonal antibody
dromperidone (Motilium)
dronarinol (Marinol)
DSM (degradable starch microspheres)
DST (donor-specific transfusion)
DTC (diethyldithiocarbamate, Imuthiol)
DTIC-Dome (dacarbazine)
DTPA
DuP 785 (brequinar sodium)
DuP 937
Duragesic (fentanyl)
Duralutin (hydroxyprogesterone)
Duraprep surgical solution
DVP chemotherapy protocol
DVPL-ASP chemotherapy protocol
DynaCirc (isradipine)
Dysport (*Clostridium botulinum* toxin type A)
EA (ethacrynic acid)
EAP chemotherapy protocol
echinomycin
ECMV chemotherapy protocol
E. coli L-asparaginase
ECS (extracellular-like, calcium-free solution)
EDAM (10-EDAM)
EDAP chemotherapy protocol
E5 monoclonal antibody
eflornithine (DFMO, Ornidyl)
Einhorn chemotherapy regimen
Eldisine (vindesine)

medication *(cont.)*
elemental diet
ELF chemotherapy protocol
Elipten (aminoglutethimide)
EL10
elsamitrucin (BMY-28090)
Elspar (L-asparaginase)
Emcyt (estramustine phosphate sodium)
Eminase (anistreplase, APSAC)
E-MVAC chemotherapy protocol
enalapril maleate (Vasotec)
encainide (Enkaid)
encapsulated liposomes
Endosol
enisoprost
Enkaid (encainide)
Enlon-Plus
enoxacin (Comprecin, Penetrax)
Ensure enteral nutrition
Ensure Plus enteral nutrition
epi-ADR, epi-Adriamycin (epirubicin)
epidermal growth factor
epinephrine
epirubicin (EPI, epi-Adriamycin)
EPO (synthetic erythropoietin)
EPOCH chemotherapy protocol
epoetin alfa (EPO, erythropoietin, Epogen, Procrit)
Epogen (epoetin alfa)
epoprostenol (Flolan, Cyclo-Prostin)
Eppy (epinephrine borate)
Eprex (erythropoietin)
Ergamisol (levamisole)
Erwinia L-asparaginase
ERYC
Ery-Tab
erythropoietin, recombinant human (Eprex, Marogen)
estazolam (ProSom)
esterified estrogens
estradiol
Estradurin (polyestradiol)

medication *(cont.)*
estramustine phosphate sodium (Emcyt)
Estratab (esterified estrogen)
etanidazole (SR-2508)
ethacrynic acid (EA)
ethambutol (Myambutol)
ethanolamine oleate (Ethamolin)
ethinyl estradiol
Ethiodane
Ethiodol
ethiofos (amifostine, Ethyol, gammaphos, WR-2721)
Ethmozine (moricizine)
Ethodian (iophendylate)
Ethyol (ethiofos)
etidronate (Didronel)
etodolac (Lodine, Ultradol)
etoglucid
etoposide (VePesid, VP-16)
Eucerin
Eulexin (flutamide)
EVA chemotherapy protocol
Evac-Q-Kwik
EVAL (ethylene vinyl alcohol)
Exosurf Pediatric (colfosceril palmitate)
extracellular-like, calcium-free solution (ECS)
FAC chemotherapy protocol
FAC-M chemotherapy protocol
FAM chemotherapy protocol
FAM-CF chemotherapy protocol
FAME chemotherapy protocol
FAMP (fludarabine monophosphate)
FAMTX chemotherapy protocol
Fansidar (sulfadoxine-pyrimethamine)
FAP chemotherapy protocol
fazarabine (Ara-AC)
FCAP chemotherapy protocol
FEC chemotherapy protocol
FED chemotherapy protocol
felodipine (Plendil)

medication *(cont.)*
Feminone (ethinyl estradiol)
fenoterol (Berotec)
fenretinide
fentanyl (Duragesic)
fentanyl citrate tablet
FIAC (fiacitabine)
FIAU (fialuridine)
fibroblast growth factor (FGF)
Fibrogammin (factor XIII)
filgrastim (Neupogen)
finasteride (MK-906)
5-ASA (mesalamine)
5-azacytidine (azacytidine, azacitidine)
5-fluorouracil (5-FU)
5-FU (5-fluorouracil)
566C80
528-IgG2a monoclonal antibody
FK-506
FK-565
FLAC chemotherapy protocol
FLAP chemotherapy protocol
Flarex (fluorometholone acetate)
Flexeril
Flolan (epoprostenol)
Floxin (ofloxacin)
floxuridine (FUdR)
Floxyfral (fluvoxamine)
FLT (fluorothymidine)
fluconazole (Diflucan)
flucytosine (5-FC, Ancobon)
Fludara (fludarabine)
fludarabine (FAMP, Fludara)
fludarabine monophosphate (FAMP)
Flu-Glow
Flumadine (rimantadine)
flumazenil (Mazicon)
flumecinol (Zixoryn)
fluorodeoxyglucose (FDG)
Fluor-i-Strip
fluorodeoxyuridine (FUdR)
fluorometholone acetate (Flarex)
fluoroquinolone class of drugs

medication *(cont.)*
fluorosilicone oil
fluorothymidine (FLT)
fluorouracil (5-fluorouracil, 5-FU)
Fluosol
Fluosol-DA
fluoxetine (Prozac)
fluoxymesterone (FXM, Halotestin)
flupertine maleate
flurbiprofen sodium (Ocufen)
flutamide (Eulexin)
fluticasone propionate (Cutivate)
fluvoxamine (Floxyfral)
Folex (methotrexate)
folinic acid (leucovorin)
Fortaz (ceftazidime)
foscarnet (Foscavir, trisodium phosphonoformate)
Foscavir (foscarnet)
fosinopril (Monopril)
fotemustine (S 10036)
Fouchet's reagent
4-aminopyridine
4-aminosalicylic acid (Pamisyl, Rezipas)
4-HC (4-hydroperoxycyclophosphamide, Pergamid)
Fourneau 309 (suramin)
FNM chemotherapy protocol
Fourneau 309 (suramin)
FreAmine nutrient solution
Frisium (clobazam)
ftorafur
FUdR (floxuridine, fluorodeoxyuridine)
FUVAC chemotherapy protocol
gadolinium (Gd-DTPA)
gadopentetate dimeglumine (Magnevist)
gallium nitrate (Ganite)
Gamimune N (immunoglobulin)
gamma hydroxybutyrate (GHB)
gamma interferon (IFN-G)
gammaphos (ethiofos)

medication *(cont.)*
ganciclovir (Cytovene)
ganglioside GM1
Ganite (gallium nitrate)
Gastroccult
Gastrografin (meglumine diatrizoate)
Gastrozepine (pirenzepine)
G-CSF (granulocyte colony-stimulating factor; filgrastim)
Gd-DTPA (gadolinium diethylene-triamine-pentaacetate)
Gelfoam
gemcitabine (difluorodeoxycytidine)
Genoptic (gentamicin sulfate)
gentamicin liposome (TLC G-65)
gentamicin sulfate (Genoptic)
Geref (sermorelin acetate)
Germanin (suramin)
Gesterol (progesterone)
Gey's solution
GHB (gamma hydroxybutyrate)
Glandosane
Gliadel
GLQ223 (trichosanthin)
Glutose
glyburide (DiaBeta)
Glypressin (terlipressin)
GM-CSF (granulocyte/macrophage colony-stimulating factor; sargramostim)
GM1 monosialotetrahexosyl-ganglioside
GnRH (gonadotropin-releasing hormone)
Goeckerman psoriasis regimen
GoLytely
gonadorelin acetate (Lutrepulse)
gonatropin-releasing hormone (GnRH)
goserelin acetate (Zoladex)
gp120 AIDS vaccine
GR 63178A
G691
G250 monoclonal antibody

medication *(cont.)*
HA-1A monoclonal antibody (Centoxin)
Habitrol (nicotine patch)
Halcion (triazolam)
halobetasol propionate (Ultravate)
Halotestin (fluoxymesterone)
Hartmann's solution
HC (hydrocortisone)
H-CAP chemotherapy protocol
hCG or HCG (human chorionic gonadotropin)
HCT, HCTZ (hydrochlorothiazide)
HDARA-C (high dose Ara-C)
HDMTX (high dose methotrexate)
HDPEG chemotherapy protocol
HDRV (human diploid cell strain rabies vaccine)
HD37 monoclonal antibody
HD-VAC chemotherapy protocol
HDZ (hydrazine sulfate)
Healon (sodium hyaluronate)
Healon GV
Healon Yellow
Hedspa
Helistat
Hemabate
Hemaflex sheath
Hemashield
hematoporphyrin derivative (HpD)
Hemoccult II
Hemopad
Hemotene
HepatAmine solution
hepatoporphyrin derivative (HpD)
hepsulfam
Heptavax-B vaccine
Herp-Check
Herplex Liquifilm (idoxuridine)
Hexabrix
Hexa-CAF
Hexalen (altretamine)
hexamethylene bisacetamide (HMBA)

medication *(cont.)*
hexamethylmelamine (altretamine, Hexalen, Hexastat)
Hexastat (altretamine)
Hibiclens
Hibistat
Hibitane tincture
HIB polysaccharide vaccine
Hismanal (astemizole)
histrelin acetate (Supprelin)
HIVID (dideoxycytidine, ddC)
HMBA (hexamethylene bisacetamide)
HMD (oxymetholone)
HMG-CoA reductase inhibitor class of drugs
HMG (human menopausal gonadotropin)
Hollande's solution
homoharringtonine (HHT)
HPA-23 (antimoniotungstate)
HpD (hepatoporphyrin derivative)
H_2 blocker class of drugs
human diploid cell strain rabies vaccine (HDRV)
human growth hormone (hGH)
humanized monoclonal antibody
human menopausal gonadotropin (HMG)
human recombinant beta interferon
Human Surf
Humatrope
Humulin
hycamptamine (topotecan)
hydrazine sulfate (HDZ)
Hydrea (hydroxyurea)
hydrochlorothiazide (HCT, HCTZ)
Hydrocollator
hydrocortisone (HC)
hydroxydaunomycin (Adriamycin)
hydroxyurea (Hydrea)
hypericin (VIMRxyn)
Hytrin (terazosin)
ICE chemotherapy protocol

medication *(cont.)*
ICRF-187
ICS solution
Idamycin (idarubicin)
idarubicin (Idamycin)
IDMTX (intermediate dose methotrexate)
idoxuridine (IUdR, Allergan 211, Herplex, Stoxil)
Ifex (ifosfamide)
IFN-A (interferon alfa)
ifosfamide (Ifex, IFF, IFM, IFOS)
IgG monoclonal antibody
IgG 2A monoclonal antibody (Immurait)
imidazole carboxamide
Imitrex (sumatriptan)
Immther
immune gamma globulin (leukoglobulin)
immunomodulator class of drugs
immunovar (inosiplex)
ImmuRAID (CEA-^{99m}Tc)
Immurait (IgG 2A monoclonal antibody)
Impact enteral feeding
Imreg-1, Imreg-2
Imudon (PEG-ADA)
Imuthiol (diethyldithiocarbamate)
indecainide (Decabid)
IND (investigational new drug)
indium-111 (^{111}In)
indium-111 labeled human non-specific immunoglobulin imaging agent (^{111}In-IgG)
indium-111 labeled monoclonal antibody (^{111}In)
indium-131 MIBG (^{131}In MIBG)
Infasurg
influenza vaccine
Infumorph solution
Ingram psoriasis regimen
Inhibace (cilazapril)
inosine pranobex (Isoprinosine)

medication *(cont.)*
inosiplex (Isoprinosine)
interferon alfa (IFN-A, Wellferon)
interferon alfa-2a (Roferon-A)
interferon alfa-2b (Intron A)
interferon alfa-n1 (Wellferon)
interferon alfa-n3 (Alferon LDO, Alferon N)
interferon beta (Betaseron)
interleukin-1 (IL-1)
interleukin-1-alpha (IL-1A)
interleukin-1-beta (IL-1B)
interleukin-2 (IL-2)
interleukin-2, recombinant (IL-2, Proleukin, teceleukin)
interleukin-3 (IL-3)
interleukin-4 (IL-4)
interleukin-6 (IL-6)
Intron A (interferon alfa-2b)
investigational new drug (IND)
iodinated contrast medium
iodine-131 labeled monoclonal antibody (^{131}I)
iodine-131 MIBG (^{131}I MIBG)
iododeoxyuridine (IUdR, idoxuridine)
iodophor
iopentol
iophendylate (Ethodian)
Iopidine (apraclonidine)
ioversol
iphosphamide (ifosfamide)
ipomeanol
iproplatin (CHIP)
iridium (IR-192, ^{192}IR, Iriditope)
Iriditope (iridium, IR-192, ^{192}IR)
iscador
Ismo (isosorbide mononitrate)
isobutyl 2-cyanocrylate
Isoprinosine (immunovar, inosine pranobex, inosiplex methisoprinol)
Isoptin (verapamil)
isosorbide mononitrate (Ismo)

medication *(cont.)*
isosulfan blue (Lymphazurin)
isotretinoin (Accutane, 13-CRA, 13-cis-retinoic acid)
IsoVue, IsoVue M
isoxicam (Maxicam)
isradipine (DynaCirc)
itraconazole (Sporanox)
IUdR (idoxuridine, iododeoxy-uridine)
Jevity isotonic liquid nutrition
Karaya powder
Kay Ciel (potassium chloride, KCl)
ketorolac tromethamine (Toradol)
ketotifen (Zaditen)
Kold Kap
Kontrast U
LAAM (L-alpha-acetyl-methadol)
lactated Ringer's solution
lactic acid
ladakamycin
LAF (lymphocyte activating factor) (interleukin-1)
Lamprene (clofazimine)
Lariam (mefloquine)
L-asparaginase (L-ASP, asparagi-nase)
LATS hormone (long-acting thyroid stimulating)
L-buthionine sulfoximine
L-CF (leucovorin-citrovorum factor)
Lente insulin
lentinan
leukoglobulin (immune gamma globulin)
Leucomax (molgramostim)
leucovorin calcium (Wellcovorin)
Leukeran (chlorambucil)
Leukine (sargramostim)
leukopoietin (sargramostim)
leuprolide (Lupron)
leurocristine
levamisole (Ergamisol)
levonorgestrel (Norplant)

medication *(cont.)*
L-5-hydroxytryptophan (L-5HTP)
L-5HTP (L-5-hydroxytryptophan)
LHRH (luteinizing hormone-releasing hormone)
Lipiodol
liposomal daunorubicin
Liquifilm ophthalmic solution
lithium carbonate
L-leucovorin
LM-427 (ansamycin)
Lodine (etodolac)
lomustine (CCNU, CeeNu)
long-acting thyroid stimulating hormone (LATS)
lonidamine (AF 1890)
Lopressor (metoprolol tartrate)
Lorabid (loracarbef)
loracarbef (Lorabid)
loratadine (Claritin)
Losec (omeprazole)
Lotensin (benazepril)
lovastatin (Mevacor)
loxoribine (RWJ 21757)
L-PAM (L-phenylalanine mustard, melphalan)
L-phenylalanine mustard (L-PAM)
LSA_2L_2 chemotherapy protocol
L-17M
Lupron (leuprolide)
luteinizing hormone-releasing hormone (LHRH)
Lutrepulse (gonadorelin acetate)
lym-1 monoclonal antibody
Lymphazurin (isosulfan blue)
lymphocyte activating factor (LAF, interleukin-1)
lymphokines (interleukin-2)
LY186641
Lysodren (mitotane)
Maalox HRF
MAC chemotherapy protocol
MACHO chemotherapy protocol

medication *(cont.)*
MACOP-B chemotherapy protocol
macrolide class of drugs
Macrotec (^{99m}Tc medronate)
MADDOC chemotherapy protocol
mafosfamide
Magnevist (gadopentetate dimeglumine)
MAK-6 cocktail
m-AMSA (amsacrine)
Marinol (dronarinol)
Marogen (erythropoietin)
Matulane (procarbazine)
Maxicam (isoxicam)
MAZE chemotherapy protocol
Mazicon (flumazenil)
mazindol (Sanorex)
M-BACOD chemotherapy protocol
M-BACOS chemotherapy protocol
McCarey-Kaufman medium
MCT oil
MCV chemotherapy protocol
MDAC (multiple dose activated charcoal)
MDLO chemotherapy protocol
Mebadin (dehydroemetine)
MEC chemotherapy protocol
MeCCNU (methyl-CCNU, semustine)
mechlorethamine (Mustargen)
mefenamic acid (Ponstel)
mefloquine (Lariam)
Megace (megestrol acetate)
MeGAG (mitoguazone)
megestrol acetate (Megace)
meglumine diatrizoate
Melacine
Mel-14 F(ab')2 monoclonal antibody
MeliBu (busulfan)
melphalan (Alkeran)
Memorial Sloan-Kettering protocol
menogaril
meralluride (Mercuhydrin)
merbarone
mercaptopurine (Purinethol)

medication *(cont.)*
Mercuhydrin (meralluride)
mesalamine (5-ASA, Asacol, Rowasa)
Mesalt
mesna (Mesnex)
Mesnex (mesna)
metaiodobenzylguanidine (MIBG)
methazolamide (Neptazane)
methiodal sodium (Abrodil, Skiodan)
methionine-enkephalin
methisoprinol (isosiplex)
methotrexate (MTX, Mexate, Folex)
methoxsalen (Oxsoralen)
methyl-CCNU (semustine)
methylmercaptopurine (MMPR)
methyl metolazone (Diulo, Zaroxolyn)
methylprednisolone (MePRDL)
methyl tertiary butyl ether (MTBE)
metipranolol (OptiPranolol)
metoclopramide (Reglan)
metoprolol succinate (Toprol XL)
metoprolol tartrate (Lopressor)
metrizamide
metronidazole (MetroGel)
metyrosine (Demser)
Mevacor (lovastatin)
Mevinolin
Mexate (methotrexate)
mexiletine (Mexitil)
Mexitil (mexiletine)
Mezlin (mezlocillin sodium)
mezlocillin sodium (Mezlin)
MGBG
MG-22 monoclonal antibody
MIBG (metaiodobenzylguanidine)
miconazole nitrate (Monistat)
Micronase (glyburide)
Micturin (terodiline)
Midamor (amiloride)
midodrine
Midrin
mifepristone (RU 486)
Millon's reagent

medication *(cont.)*
milrinone (Primacor)
miltefosine
MINE chemotherapy protocol
Minitran
Miochol solution
misonidazole
Mithracin (mithramycin, plicamycin)
mithramycin (Mithracin, plicamycin)
mitolactol (dibromodulcitrol)
mitomycin (mitomycin-C, MTC, Mutamycin)
mitomycin-C (Mutamycin)
mitotane (Lysodren)
mitoxantrone HCl (Novantrone)
Mivacron (mivacurium)
mivacurium (Mivacron)
MK-906 (finasteride)
MK-217
MMOPP chemotherapy protocol
MMPR (methylmercaptopurine)
MOAB (monoclonal antibody)
MOF chemotherapy protocol
Mogadon (nitrazepam)
molgramostim (Leucomax)
M195 monoclonal antibody
Monistat (miconazole nitrate)
monobactam class of drugs
Monodox (doxycycline, Vibramycin)
Monopril (fosinopril)
Monsel's solution
MOP chemotherapy protocol
MOPP chemotherapy protocol
Moranyl (suramin)
moricizine (Ethmozine)
Motilium (domperidone)
MSL-109 monoclonal antibody
MTBE (methyl tertiary butyl ether)
MTP-PE (muramyl-tripeptide)
muramyl-tripeptide (MTP-PE)
murine monoclonal antibody
Muromonab-CD3 monoclonal antibody

medication *(cont.)*
Mustargen (mechlorethamine)
Mutamycin (mitomycin)
MVAC chemotherapy protocol
M.V.C.9+4
MVF chemotherapy protocol
M.V.I.-12
MVT chemotherapy protocol
Myambutol (ethambutol)
Mycobutin (ansamycin, rifabutin)
Myleran (busulfan)
Myodil
Myoscint
nabumetone (Relafen)
N-acetylated procainamide (NAPA)
nadolol (Corgard)
nafarelin (Synarel)
Naftin
Naganol (suramin)
Napa (acecainide)
NAPA (n-acetylated procainamide)
naphthyalkalone class of drugs
Naphuride (suramin)
native L-asparaginase
N-butyl-deoxynojirmycin (DNJ)
NebuPent (aerosolized pentamidine)
nedocromil (Tilade)
Neosar (cyclophosphamide)
NephrAmine solution
Neptazane (methazolamide)
nerve growth factor (NGF)
Neupogen (filgrastim)
Neurotrast
nevirapine (BI-RG-587)
Nicoderm (nicotine patch)
nimodipine (Nimotop)
nimustine (ACNU)
Nimotop (nimodipine)
N901-blocked ricin conjugate monoclonal antibody
Nipent (pentostatin)
nitrazepam (Mogadon)
nitrendipine (Baypress)
nitrogen mustard (Mustargen)

medication *(cont.)*
nitrogen-13 ammonia
nitroglycerin
Nitrol ointment or paste
Nolvadex (tamoxifen citrate)
nonoxynol 9
nonsteroidal anti-inflammatory drugs (NSAIDs)
norfloxacin (Chibroxin, Noroxin)
Noroxin (norfloxacin)
Norplant (levonorgestrel)
Norvasc (amiodipine)
Novantrone (mitoxantrone HCl)
Novapren
novobiocin
Novolin L synthetic insulin
Novolin N synthetic insulin
Novolin R synthetic insulin
NPH insulin
NR-LU-10 monoclonal antibody
NuLytely solution
Nuromax (doxacurium chloride)
nutrient solution
Nystatin^{LF} (liposomal formulation)
Obecalp (placebo)
OCT medium
octreotide (Sandostatin)
Ocufen (flurbiprofen sodium)
Oculinum (botulinum toxin type A)
ofloxacin (Floxin)
OKB7 monoclonal antibody
OKT3 monoclonal antibody (Orthoclone OKT3)
OKT4 monoclonal antibody
OKT8 monoclonal antibody
olsalazine (Dipentum)
omeprazole (Prilosec)
Omniflox (temafloxacin)
Omnipaque
OMS (oral morphine sulfate) Concentrate
OncoScint CR103
OncoScint OV103
Oncovin (vincristine sulfate)

medication *(cont.)*
ondansetron (Zofran)
One-Alpha (alfacalcidol)
14G2A or 14.G2A monoclonal antibody
14.18 monoclonal antibody
17-1A monoclonal antibody
OPPA chemotherapy protocol
OptiPranolol (metipranolol)
Optiray (ioversol)
Oraflex
Oramorph SR
Ornidyl (DFMO, eflornithine)
orphan drug
Orthoclone OKT3 monoclonal antibody
Ortholinum (botulinum toxin type A)
Osmolite enteral feeding
OTC (over-the-counter) drugs
OTFC (oral transmucosal fentanyl citrate)
over-the-counter drugs
OvuStick
Oxandrin (oxandrolone)
oxandrolone (Oxandrin)
oxiconazole (Oxistat)
Oxistat (oxiconazole)
oxothiazolidine carboxylate (Procysteine)
oxymetholone (Adroyd, Anadrol-50)
PAB-Esc-C chemotherapy protocol
PACE chemotherapy protocol
PALA (N-phosphonoacetyl-L-aspartate)
palladium-103 (Pd103, ^{103}Pd)
pamidronate disodium (Aredia)
Pantopaque
Paraplatin (carboplatin)
parathormone (PTH)
Parnisyl (4-aminosalicylic acid)
paroxetine (Paxil)
PAVe chemotherapy protocol
Paxil (paroxetine)
PCE chemotherapy protocol

medication *(cont.)*
PCP (phencyclidine)
PCV chemotherapy protocol
PEB chemotherapy protocol
PEG-ADA (pegademase bovine, Adagen, Imudon)
pegademase bovine (PEG-ADA, Adagen)
PEG-IL-2
PEG interleukin-2
PEG-L-ASP
Penetrax (enoxacin)
penicilloylpolylysine (PPL, Pre-Pan)
Pentam 300 (pentamidine)
pentamidine, aerosolized (Aeropent, NebuPent)
pentamidine isethionate (Pentam 300)
pentosan polysulfate (PPS)
pentostatin (Nipent)
pentoxifylline
Peptamen isotonic elemental
peptide T
perfluorophenanthrene (Vitreon)
Pergamid (4-HC)
Peridex
Persantine (dipyridamole)
pertechnetate sodium (technetium)
P-glycoprotein
phencyclidine (PCP)
phenformin
PHNO (4-propyl-9-hydroxy-naphthoxazine)
PhosLo (calcium acetate)
phosphonoformate trisodium (foscarnet, Foscavir)
PHRT chemotherapy protocol
physostigmine salicylate
PIA chemotherapy protocol
Pilagan (pilocarpine nitrate)
pilocarpine nitrate (Pilagan)
pinacidil (Pindac)
Pindac (pinacidil)
pipecuronium (Arduan)
PIPIDA (N-para-isopropyl-aceta-nilide-iminodiacetic acid)

medication *(cont.)*
pipobroman (Vercyte)
pirarubicin
pirenzepine (Gastrozepine)
piritrexim isethionate (BW 301U)
piroxantrone (PXT)
placebo (Obecalp)
Plasmalyte, Plasmalyte 148
Plasti-Pore
Platinol (cisplatin)
Plegisol
Plendil (felodipine)
plicamycin (Mithracin, mithramycin)
PM-81 monoclonal antibody
PMFAC chemotherapy protocol
P-MVAC chemotherapy protocol
Pneumopent (aerosolized pentamidine)
POCC chemotherapy protocol
polyribonucleotide (Ampligen)
Polytrim ophthalmic solution
POMP chemotherapy protocol
Ponstel (mefenamic acid)
porfiromycin
Portagen dietary powder
potassium hydroxide (KOH)
potassium sparing diuretic
potassium supplement
potassium wasting diuretic
PPL (penicilloylpolylysine, Pre-Pen)
prednimustine (Sterecyt)
prednisolone (PRDL)
prednisone (PRED)
Premarin
Prepodyne solution
Prilosec (omeprazole)
Primacor (milrinone)
primaquine phosphate
Prinzide
Probenecid (colchicine)
procarbazine (PCB, Matulane)
Procrit (epoetin alfa)
Procysteine (oxothiazolidine carboxylate)
ProHance contrast medium
Prokine (sargramostim)

medication *(cont.)*
Proleukin (interleukin-2, recombinant)
ProMACE-CYTABOM chemotherapy protocol
propafenone (Rythmol)
Propine ophthalmic solution
Proplast
proprietary medicine
ProSom (estazolam)
ProStep (nicotine patch)
protease inhibitor
Prothiaden (dothiepin)
Protocult
Protropin
Prozac (fluoxetine)
pseudomonic acid (mupirocin)
psoralen class of drugs
PTFE (polytetrafluoroethylene)
PTH (parathormone, parathyroid hormone)
P–30 protein
P–32 (chromic phosphate, phosphorus-32)
Pulmo-Aide nebulizer
Purinethol (mercaptopurine)
PVA chemotherapy protocol
PVA (polyvinyl alcohol) particles
PVB chemotherapy protocol
PVDA chemotherapy protocol
PVDR chemotherapy protocol
PVP chemotherapy protocol
pyranocarboxylic acid class of drugs
pyrazine diazohydroxide (PZDH)
pyrazoloacridine
pyridoxilated stroma-free hemoglobin (SFHb)
pyrimethamine (Daraprim)
quaternary ammonium chloride
quazepam (Doral)
quinacrine
quinapril (Accupril)
rabies vaccine, Rhesus diploid cell strain (RDRV)
radioiodine-labeled monoclonal antibody

medication *(cont.)*
radiolabeled monoclonal antibody
ramipril (Altace)
RDRV (Rhesus diploid cell strain rabies vaccine)
Reactine (cetirizine)
Receptin (CD4, recombinant soluble human)
recombinant tissue plasminogen activator (rt-PA)
Reglan (metoclopramide)
Relafen (nabumetone)
Renacidin solution
Renotec (^{99m}Tc iron-ascorbate-DTPA)
Replens gel
Respirgard II nebulizer
Retin-A (tretinoin)
Retrovir (azidothymidine, zidovudine)
Rev-Eyes (dapiprazole)
Rezipas (4-aminosalicylic acid)
RG-83894 AIDS vaccine
RG 12915
r-gp160 vaccine
rHb1.1 (recombinant hemoglobin)
rhenium-186 labeled monoclonal antibody
rHuEPO or EPO (recombinant human erythropoietin)
ribavirin (Virazole)
Rice-Lyte
RIDD chemotherapy protocol
rifabutin (Mycobutin, ansamycin)
rIFN (recombinant interferon)
Rimadyl (carprofen)
rimantadine (Flumadine)
Ringer's lactate
Roferon-A (interferon alfa-2a)
rogletimide
roquinimex
Rovamycin (spiramycin)
Rowasa (mesalamine)
Roxanol CII (morphine sulfate)
rsCD4 (Receptin)
R-75251

medication *(cont.)*
rt-PA (recombinant tissue plasminogen activator)
R24 monoclonal antibody
rubidium-82 (^{82}Rb)
Rubrex (doxorubicin)
RU 486 (mifepristone)
R-verapamil
RWJ 21757 (loxoribine)
RWJ 25213
Sandostatin (octreotide)
Sanorex (mazindol)
sargramostim (leukopoietin, Leukine, Prokine)
sCD4 (soluble CD4, recombinant human CD4)
sCD4-PE40
Schlesinger's solution
Sectral (acebutolol)
Selacryn
Seldane-D
Selecor (celiprolol)
selenium-75 (^{75}Se)
semustine (MeCCNU, methyl-CCNU)
Septacin
Septra (sulfamethoxazole, trimethoprim)
sermorelin acetate (Geref)
serotonin type-3 receptor antagonist drugs
sertraline (Zoloft)
sestamibi (Cardiolite)
SFHb (pyridoxilated stroma-free hemoglobin)
Shohl's solution
simvastatin (Zocor)
6-AN protocol
6-mercaptopurine riboside (mercaptopurine, 6-MP)
Skiodan (methiodol sodium)
Slo-Phyllin Gyrocaps
SMF chemotherapy protocol
SMZ/TMP (sulfamethoxazole and trimethoprim, Bactrim, Septra)

medication *(cont.)*
Sn-protoporphyrin
sodium hyaluronate (Amvisc, Healon)
sodium thiosulfate
somatuline
S 10036 (fotemustine)
sotalol (Betapace)
Sotradecol (sodium tetradecyl sulfate)
sparfloxacin
spiramycin
Sporanox (itraconazole)
Sporicidin
SR-2508 (etanidazole)
SSKI (saturated solution of potassium iodide)
Stadol NS (butorphanol tartrate)
stavudine (d4T, didehydrodideoxythymidine)
STEPA (thiotepa)
Sterecyt (prednimustine)
Stilphostrol (diethylstilbestrol)
Stoxil (idoxuridine)
streptozocin (Zanosar)
stroma-free hemoglobin
Suby's solution G (Suby G)
succimer (Chemet)
sucralfate (Carafate)
Sulamyd (sulfacetamide sodium)
sulfacetamide sodium (Sulamyd)
sulfadoxine-pyrimethamine (Fansidar)
sulindac (Clinoril)
sumatriptan (Imitrex)
Supprelin (histrelin acetate)
suramin (Belganyl, Fourneau 309, Germanin, Moranyl, Naganol, Naphuride)
Surgicel
Surgidine
Surgi-Prep
Survanta (beractant)
Susadrin (nitroglycerin)
Synarel (nafarelin)

medication *(cont.)*
TAC (triamcinolone cream)
TACE (chlorotrianisene)
tacrine (Cognex)
Tagamet (cimetidine)
tamoxifen citrate (Nolvadex, TAM, TMX)
Tao (troleandomycin)
Targocid (teicoplanin)
TAT inhibitor
taxol
Tazidime (ceftazidime)
TcHIDA
TCN-P (triciribine phosphate)
TDR (thymidine deoxyriboside)
TEC chemotherapy protocol
teceleukin (interleukin-2, recombinant)
Techneplex (^{99m}Tc penetate)
Technescan MAG3
technetium 99m albumin
technetium 99m albumin aggregated
technetium 99m albumin colloid
technetium 99m bicisate
technetium 99m colloid
technetium 99m disofenin
technetium 99m etidronate
technetium 99m ferpentetate
technetium 99m glucepate
technetium 99m HIDA
technetium 99m iron-ascorbate-DTPA (Renotec)
technetium 99m lidofenin
technetium 99m macroaggregated albumin (^{99m}TcMAA)
technetium 99m medronate (Macrotec)
technetium 99m mertiatide
technetium 99m oxidronate
technetium 99m penetate (Techneplex)
technetium 99m pertechnetate sodium
technetium 99m PIPIDA
technetium 99m pyrophosphate

medication *(cont.)*
technetium 99m sestamibi (Cardiolite)
technetium 99m siboroxime
technetium 99m sodium
technetium 99m succimer
technetium 99m sulfur colloid (Tesuloid)
technetium 99m teboroxime (CardioTek)
technetium stannous pyrophosphate (TSPP)
teicoplanin (Targocid)
temafloxacin (Omniflox)
TEMP chemotherapy protocol
10-EDAM (EDAM)
teniposide (VM-26)
terazosin (Hytrin)
terlipressin (Glypressin)
teroxirone (alpha-TGI)
TESPA (thiotepa)
Tes-Tape reagent
TestPackChlamydia
Tesuloid
tetracycline
tetrahydrocannabinol (THC)
tetraplatin
thalidomide
thallium-201 (Tl-201)
THC (tetrahydrocannabinol)
Theocon (theophylline)
TheraCys
TheraSeed
Thermophore
thianamycin
thioguanine (6-thioguanine, 6-TG, TSPA)
thiosulfate
thiotepa (STEPA, TESPA, TSPA, TTPA, TTPA)
13-cis-retinoic acid (13-CRA, isotretinoin)
Thorotrast
3F8 monoclonal antibody
thymic humoral factor

medication *(cont.)*
thymidine deoxyriboside (TDR)
thymopentin (Timunox, TP-5)
thymostimuline (TP-1)
tiagabine
tiazofurin
ticarcillin-clavulanate potassium (Timentin)
Tice (intravesical BCG)
Ticlid (ticlopidine)
ticlopidine (Ticlid)
TIL (tumor-infiltrating lymphocytes)
Tilade (nedocromil)
Timentin (ticarcillin-clavulanate potassium)
Timoptic
Timunox (thymopentin)
Tis-U-Sol
tissue plasminogen activator (t-PA)
TI-23 (CMV monoclonal antibody)
TLC G-65 (gentamicin liposome)
TMP-SMZ (trimethoprim-sulfamethoxazole, Bactrim, Septra)
TNF (tumor necrosis factor)
tobramycin sulfate (Nebcin)
tocainide (Tonocard)
tolerogen
tolmetin
tolrestat (Alredase)
T-101 monoclonal antibody
Tonocard (tocainide)
topotecan
Toprol XL (metoprolol succinate)
Toradol (ketorolac tromethamine)
toremifene
Tornalate (bitolterol)
t-PA (tissue plasminogen activator)
TPDCV chemotherapy protocol
TP-1 (thymostimuline)
TP-5 (thymopentin)
TP-40
TRA (all-trans-retinoic acid, tretinoin)
transferrin
Travasorb MCT

medication *(cont.)*
tretinoin (Retin-A)
triazinate (TZT)
triazolam (Halcion)
trichosanthin (compound Q, GLQ223)
triciribine phosphate (TCN-P)
tricyclic antidepressant
trifluoperazine
trimethoprim-sulfamethoxazole (TMP-SMZ, Bactrim, Septra)
trimetrexate gluconate (TMQ, TMTX)
Triphasil
triple antibiotics
trisodium phosphonoformate (foscarnet, Foscavir)
troleandomycin (Tao)
TSPP (technetium stannous pyrophosphate)
T-2 protocol
tumor necrosis factor (TNF)
tumor-infiltrating lymphocytes (TIL)
2A11 monoclonal antibody
2-CdA (2-chlorodeoxyadenosine)
U-87201E
Uendex (dextran sulfate)
Ultradol (etodolac)
Ultravate (halobetasol propionate)
Unicard (dilevalol)
uracil mustard
Uricult
uridine
ursodeoxycholic acid (ursodiol)
ursodiol (Actigall)
urushiol
VAAP chemotherapy protocol
VAB-6 chemotherapy protocol
VAC chemotherapy protocol
VACA chemotherapy protocol
VACAD chemotherapy protocol
VACP chemotherapy protocol
VAD chemotherapy protocol
VAD/V chemotherapy protocol
VAI chemotherapy protocol

medication *(cont.)*
VAM chemotherapy protocol
VAMP chemotherapy protocol
Vascor (bepridil)
VAT chemotherapy protocol
VaxSyn HIV-1
VBC chemotherapy protocol
VBMCP chemotherapy protocol
VBMF chemotherapy protocol
VBP chemotherapy protocol
VeIP chemotherapy protocol
Velban (vinblastine)
Velsar (vinblastine)
VePesid (etoposide, VP-16)
verapamil (Calan, Isoptin, Verelan)
Vercyte (pipobroman)
Verelan (verapamil)
Vibramycin (doxycycline)
VIC chemotherapy protocol
vidarabine (adenine arabinoside, Ara-A, Vira-A)
Videx (didanosine, dideoxyinosine, ddI)
VIE chemotherapy protocol
viloxazine (Vivalan)
VIMRxyn (hypericin)
vinblastine (Velban, VBL, Velsar)
vincaleukoblastine (vinblastine)
Vincasar (vincristine)
vincristine sulfate (Oncovin, Vincasar)
vindesine (Eldisine)
vinorelbine (VOB)
VIP chemotherapy protocol
VIP-B chemotherapy protocol
Vira-A (vidarabine)
Virazole (ribavirin)
Viroptic ophthalmic solution
Viscoat
Visidex, Visidex II
Vitreon (perfluorophenanthrene)
Vivalan (viloxazine)
Vivonex HN

medication *(cont.)*
Vivonex TEN (T.E.N.)
Vleminckx's solution
VM-26 (teniposide)
Voltaren ophthalmic solution
VMCP chemotherapy protocol
VMP chemotherapy protocol
VM–26
VPCA chemotherapy protocol
VPP chemotherapy protocol
VP-16 (etoposide, VePesid)
VP-16-213 or VP-16213 (VP-16)
Wellcovorin (leucovorin calcium)
Wellferon (interferon alfa-n1)
WR-2721 (ethiofos)
Xenon-133 (^{133}Xe)
XomaZyme-H65
yttrium-90 labeled monoclonal antibody
Zaditen (ketotifen)
Zanosar (streptozocin)
Zaroxolyn (methyl metolazone)
ZDV (zidovudine)
Zefazone (cefmetazole)
Zenker's fixative
Zestoretic
zidovudine (AZT, Retrovir)
ZIG vaccine
Zithromax (azithromycin)
Zixoryn (flumecinol)
Zocor (simvastatin)
Zofran (ondansetron)
Zoladex (ZDX, goserelin acetate)
Zoloft (sertraline)
Zomax (zomepirac sodium)
zomepirac sodium (Zomax)
Zovirax (acyclovir)
Zyloprim (allopurinol)

Medicon instruments—for vascular and cardiac surgery.

Medigraphics 2000 analyzer—used in testing exhaled gases in cardiopulmonary exercise study.

Medina ileostomy catheter (Urol).

Medipore Dress-it—a precut surgical dressing of a porous material with a cloth backing.

MediPort—a totally implanted vascular access device for continuous or intermittent outpatient delivery of fluids and medications; can be used on an outpatient basis. May be used with externalized catheters.

Medi-quet surgical tourniquet.

Medi-Vac suction collection container.

Medline—medical bibliographical computer data base, through which a search of the current literature on almost any medical subject can be conducted.

meds—brief form for *medications.*

Medstone STS shock-wave generator (Urol, GI)—used to produce shock waves for dissolving kidney stones and gallstones.

Medtronic Hall heart valve (Cardio).

Medtronic temporary pacemaker (Cardio).

Medtronic Pulsor Intrasound—pain reliever using sound vibrations.

Medtronic SynchroMed pump (Oncol) —an implantable subcutaneous infusion pump used to deliver chemotherapy drugs.

medullaris—conus medullaris.

Mees' lines—transverse lines on the fingernails, strongly suggestive of arsenic poisoning.

mefenamic acid (Ponstel)—used in therapy for arthritis and menstrual cramps.

mefloquine (Lariam)—similar in structure to quinine, this antimalarial drug is effective against some resistant strains of malaria. It is considered the drug of choice for persons traveling in areas where resistant strains of malaria are endemic. Given orally.

Megace—see *megestrol acetate.*

Megadyne/Fann E-Z clean laparoscopic electrodes—Teflon-coated electrodes which do not have to be removed from the operating port for cleaning after coagulation.

megahertz (mHz)—thousand cycles per second, used as measurement in audiograms. See *hertz.*

megestrol acetate (Megace)—used to increase the appetite of HIV-positive patients. Also used in palliation of advanced adenocarcinoma of the breast or endometrium.

meglumine diatrizoate (Radiol)—contrast medium.

meibomian cyst—see *chalazion.*

meibomian froth (Path).

meibomian gland—one of the sebaceous glands of the eyelid.

Melacine (melanoma cell lysate vaccine) (Oncol)—vaccine for advanced melanoma.

melanin—the dark brown to black pigment normally present, predominantly in the hair, skin, the choroid coat of the eye, and substantia nigra of the brain. Also in some tumors, e.g., melanoma. Cf. *melena.*

melanoma cell lysate vaccine—see Melaccine.

melanotic—referring to the presence of melanin. Often confused with "melenic." "Melenic stools," *not* "melanotic stools." Cf. *melenic.*

melenic—referring to or marked by melena, as in "melenic stools." Cf. *melanotic.*

melena—passage of dark, tarry stools, indicating bleeding in the lower gastrointestinal tract. Cf. *melanin.*

melolabial flap—a flap from the medial cheek, used as a transposition flap, to repair a defect on the side of the nose. It is used for deep nasal

melolabial flap *(cont.)* defects, providing thick sebaceous skin and subcutaneous fat for rebuilding tissue lost in surgery and, folded on itself, can recreate an alar rim. Erroneously referred to as nasolabial flap.

meloplasty—face lift; plastic surgery of the cheek (Plas Surg).

melphalan (L-PAM, L-phenylalanine mustard, Alkeran)—used to treat multiple myeloma and unresectable epithelial ovarian carcinoma.

membrane
Bruch's
choroidal neovascular
Descemet's
Gore-Tex surgical
Liliequist

Memorial Sloan-Kettering Cancer Center, New York. Also, MSK Cancer Center. I give this because I remember trying to find it written out, to know whether or not there is a hyphen, and, if so, where. It took a while. So frustrating.

Memorial Sloan-Kettering protocol—a chemotherapy protocol.

MemoryTrace AT (Cardio)—ambulatory cardiac monitor which automatically records an EKG when it senses an arrhythmia in the patient's heart. The EKG is stored electronically and can be transmitted over the telephone to a cardiologist.

MEN I syndrome (multiple endocrine neoplasia, type I).

Mengert's index—in pelvimetry.

meninx—the singular form of the membrane covering the brain and spinal cord; meninges (plural) consist of the dura, pia, and arachnoid.

meniscal *(not* menisceal) (adj.)—usually refers to one of the crescent-shaped structures of the knee joint.

"menisceal"—mispronunciation of *meniscal.* See *meniscal.*

mental status examination—see *test.*

mentis—see *non compos mentis.*

Mentor BVAT (Oph)—computer screen chart used in testing visual acuity.

Mentor two-piece penile implant (Urol).

MEP (motor evoked potential)—used to monitor descending pathways during neurosurgery.

MEP (multimodality evoked potential)—a combination of visual, somatosensory, and brain stem auditory evoked potential.

meralgia paresthetica—a neuropathy, usually due to compression of the lateral femoral cutaneous nerve, producing pain, paresthesias, and sensory disturbances. See *Roth-Bernhardt's disease,* which is synonymous.

M/E ratio (myeloid/erythroid).

mercaptopurine (6-mercaptopurine riboside, 6-MPR, 6-MP, Purinethol) (Oncol)—a chemotherapy drug used to treat acute lymphatic leukemia.

Mercedes tip cannula (Plas Surg)—used for liposuction.

Mercuhydrin (meralluride)—diuretic.

mercury-in-Silastic strain gauge (Vasc Surg)—used for determination of the blood flow.

Merindino procedure (GI)—including distal esophagectomy, 50% gastrectomy, jejunal interposition, with esophagojejunostomy, pyloroplasty and vagotomy, and jejunojejunostomy.

Merocel sponge (ENT)—a compressed, lintfree, nonfiber sponge that expands when in contact with nasal secretions, used in postoperative nasal packing. It may be used in other settings.

Mersilene (*not* Mersiline)—a braided suture; it is nonabsorbable and becomes encapsulated in the body tissues. It is used in general, cardiovascular, and plastic surgery as retention sutures. Colors: green and white.

mesalamine (5-ASA, Asacol, Rowasa) (GI)—anti-inflammatory drug to treat ulcerative colitis. Rowasa is prescribed as a rectal suspension; Oral Asacol is a time-release tablet which dissolves in the terminal ileum.

Mesalt—sterile sodium chloride impregnated dressing.

mesh
- Dexon
- Tanner
- tantalum
- TiMesh

mesna (Mesnex)—used only for patients receiving ifosfamide. It prevents the side effect of hemorrhagic cystitis.

messenger, RNA (mRNA).

Messerklinger sinus endoscopy set (ENT).

met, mets—unit of measurement for treadmill scoring; 1 met = 3.5 ml O_2/kg/min. Cf. *mets, "Metz."*

metacarpal—refers to the bones of the metacarpus, that part of the hand between the wrist and the fingers. Cf. *metatarsal.* The above words are often confused, even by the dictators, so be aware of the anatomic area referred to.

metaiodobenzylguanidine (MIBG).

metaphysis—the wide part at the end of the shaft of a long bone, adjacent to the cartilaginous disk of the epiphysis. In childhood, this is composed of spongy bone and contains the growth zone. In the adult, it is continuous with the epiphysis. Cf. *metastasis.*

metastasis—spread of disease from one organ or part of the body to another not necessarily contiguous with it; it may spread through the lymphatic system or venous system, etc. See *metaphysis. Cf. met, mets.*

metatarsal—refers to the bones of the metatarsus, that part of the foot between the ankle articulation and the toes. See *metacarpal.*

meter
- Accu-Chek II
- Chemstrip MatchMaker blood glucose
- ExacTech blood glucose
- One Touch blood glucose
- Tracer Blood Glucose Micro-monitor

methazolamide tablets (Neptazane).

methemoglobin (metHb). A small amount of methemoglobin is normally present in the blood, but it does not carry oxygen through the blood. If, through injury or exposure to toxic agents, hemoglobin is converted to excess methemoglobin, cyanosis can result.

methiodal sodium (Abrodil).

methionine-enkephalin—a drug used to treat immunodeficiency and AIDS.

methisoprinol (inosiplex).

method (See also *operation; procedure.*)
- bench
- Cherry-Crandall
- CSQI
- Credé's
- flow cytometry
- flush
- intentional transoperative hemodilution
- Ionescu
- Lown and Woolf
- Mauriceau
- Mauriceau-Smellie-Veit
- Oliver-Rosalki

method *(cont.)*
Pfeiffer-Comberg
piggybacking
Pulver-Taft weave
Sigma m. in testing serum CPK
Smellie
Sub-Q-Set
Turner-Warwick
Wheeless
Wroblewski m. of testing serum LDH

methotrexate (MTX, Mexate) (Oncol)—antineoplastic agent, usually used in combination with other chemotherapeutic agents in treatment of various types of cancer. Also used as an immunosuppressive agent.

methoxsalen (Oxsoralen) (Derm)—for treatment of psoriasis; taken orally and then followed by blacklight lamp or sunlamp treatment.

methyl methacrylate—a cement used in orthopedics and neurosurgery.

methyl methacrylate, beads of(Ortho)—a method of providing an antibiotic to prevent postfracture osteomyelitis. Impregnated with an antibiotic, the beads of methyl methacrylate are strung on a surgical wire, implanted in the area of an open fracture (following surgical debridement and irrigation with an antibiotic solution). The beads dissolve, releasing the antibiotic in situ at therapeutic levels over several weeks.

methyl metolazone (Diulo, Zaroxolyn)—a diuretic used in the treatment of peripheral neuropathy, and hypertension.

methyl tertiary butyl ether (MTBE).

metipranolol (OptiPranolol) (Oph)—a topical drug which belongs to the class of beta-blocking agents used to treat chronic open-angle glaucoma. The drug acts to decrease intraocular pressure by decreasing the production of aqueous humor.

metoclopramide (Reglan)—a drug that increases gastric motility and is used to treat gastroesophageal reflux and gastric stasis.

metoprolol succinate (Toprol XL) (Cardio)—a once-a-day treatment for hypertension and angina pectoris in a sustained release tablet. Cf. *metoprolol tartrate.*

metoprolol tartrate (Lopressor) (Cardio)—cardioselective beta blocker drug used for hypertension and angina; also for migraine headaches. Cf. *metoprolol succinate.*

metrizamide (Radiol)—a water soluble contrast medium in myelograms and other studies.

"mets"—slang for *metastases.* Cf. *meds, met, "Metz."*

mets (plural of *met*)—unit of measurement in treadmills. See *met.*

metyrosine (Demser).

"Metz"—slang for *Metzenbaum scissors.* Cf. *mets.*

Mevacor (lovastatin).

Mevinolin—medication to treat hyperlipidemia.

MEWD syndrome (multiple evanescent white dot) (Oph)—a self-limiting problem, occurring more often in women than in men, most common in an age range of 17 to 42. Characterized by blurred vision, decreased visual acuity, with various-sized discrete and confluent white dots appearing as soft, elevated lesions at the level of the retinal pigment epithelium (RPE) and deep retina, and with various degrees of disk edema. The acute phase seems to last for about 18 to 30 days, with a residual of distinct alteration in the appearance of the macula.

Mexate (methotrexate).

Mexitil (mexiletine)—an antiarrhythmic agent (Cardio).

Mezlin (mezlocillin sodium)—a broad-spectrum antibiotic.

mezlocillin—a fourth-generation penicillin. Cf. *Mezlin.*

MGBG—a polyamine synthesis inhibitor; used in the treatment of brain tumors (Neuro).

MHA-TP (microhemagglutination test for *Treponema pallidum,* the organism that causes syphilis).

MHz (megahertz) (1 million hertz). A hertz equals 1 cycle per second. This is a term often used in radiology and audiology.

Miami Acute Care collar (MAC collar)—for cervical support.

Miami J collar—cervical immobilization for ICU patients restricted to the supine position.

MIBG (metaiodobenzylguanidine) (Oncol)—a synthetic antineoplastic drug, used in combination with others, in beginning therapy of nonlymphatic leukemia. It has a cytocidal effect on both proliferating and nonproliferating human cells.

mice, Balb/c—a strain of mice used in laboratories.

MIC gastroenteric tube—a dual-lumen catheter which allows access to the stomach and the jejunum, for use in patients who need both gastric decompression and jejunal feeding (GI, Surg). MIC (Medical Innovations Corp.).

Michel clips (Surg).

Michel deformity—complete failure of development of the inner ear.

Michelis intraocular implant lens.

Micral chemstrip (Lab)—urine test for microalbuminuria.

micro-—prefix meaning small or abnormally small. Cf. *macro-.*

Micro-Aire pulse lavage system (Ortho)—for debriding bone surfaces in hip and knee implantation procedures.

microbipolar forceps (Neuro)—electronic forceps in straight and curved versions; used in microsurgery.

microcalcification (Radiol)—very small deposit of calcium in breast tissue, as seen in a mammogram. Clustered microcalcifications are highly suggestive of malignancy.

Micrococcus sedentarius—a coagulase-negative organism. Can be confused with *Staphylococcus epidermidis,* but *S. epidermidis* ferments glucose and micrococci do not.

Microfoam surgical tape (*not* Microform) (Surg).

micrognathia-glossoptosis syndrome. See *Pierre Robin syndrome.*

Microknit vascular graft prosthesis.

Microlase transpupillary diode laser (Oph).

Micro Minix pacemaker (Cardio)—a new smaller version of the Minix pacemaker. The term *Micro* is part of the trade name.

Micron bobbin ventilation tubes (ENT)—made of titanium; used in surgery.

Micronase (glyburide)—for type II diabetics (NIDDM) who do not respond to diet alone.

Micropuncture introducer
Check-Flo
Desilets-Hoffman
Tuohy-Borst

Micropuncture Peel-Away introducer—used to introduce balloon, electrode, and other catheters. Knobs allow the sheath to be peeled away and removed.

microscope, microscopy
biomicroscope (slit lamp)
dark-field
DIC (differential interference contrast)
Omni operating
OPMI operating
scanning acoustic m. (SAM)
Wild operating

MicroSmooth probe (Oph)—a vitreoretinal probe for attachment to an ocutome.

microsurgical DREZ-otomy (Neuro)—a procedure to treat spasticity and pain in lower limbs. (DREZ, dorsal root entry zone.)

microsurgery—see *transanal endoscopic microsurgery.*

MicroTeq portable belt—a device worn for home treatment as augmentation for TENS.

microtome—see *Stadie-Riggs microtome.*

Microvasive Glidewire—see *Glidewire.*

Microvasive Rigiflex TTS balloon—see *Rigiflex TTS balloon.*

Microvit (Oph)—used in vitreoretinal surgery in cutting the vitreous, in posterior segment surgery.

microwave nonsurgical treatment—for benign prostatic hypertrophy (Urol). Performed under local anesthesia. Ultrasound defines the size and shape of the prostate gland, and the physician uses a computer to guide the procedure. A catheter is inserted through the urethra to the prostate. Microwave energy from an antenna inside the catheter heats and destroys enlarged cells in the gland. The equipment has a cooling and flushing provision. Heated cells dissolve and are absorbed by the body, with resultant shrinkage of the prostate and return of normal urinary function.

Micturin (terodiline).

MID (multi-infarct dementia).

Midas Rex pneumatic instruments (Ortho, Neuro)—used in working on bone and articular cartilage; in cement removal and in polyethylene and metal cutting.

middle cerebral artery (MCA).

midline shift—displacement of a structure that is normally seen at or near the midline of the body, such as the pineal gland or the trachea.

midparental height—a term used in discussion of patients with possible growth hormone deficiency. One of the factors which must be taken into consideration is the height of the patient's parents, as short stature might simply be a familial characteristic. Therefore, the heights of both parents are added together and divided by 2 (the midparental height), and if this is low, it indicates that the patient's short stature is normal for that family and not necessarily a growth hormone failure. Conversely, if the midparental height is relatively high, consideration might be given to institution of supplemental growth hormone therapy.

midodrine—drug used to treat orthostatic hypotension.

Midrin—used for relief of tension headaches and for migraine.

Miege's syndrome—blepharospasm and oromandibular dystonia. First described by Dr. Henry Miege in 1910. Primarily affects middle-aged and elderly adults, women more often than men.

mifepristone (RU 486) (Ob-Gyn)—a progesterone receptor blocker used to induce abortions in early pregnancy.

Mijnhard electrical cycloergometer—a device for measuring the heart rate

Mijnhard *(cont.)* under stress; a type of exercise tolerance test.

mil—unit of measurement equals 0.001 inch. Often used to express diameter of wire sutures.

milestones—see *developmental milestones.*

miliaria—heat rash. Cf. *malaria.*

militate—to affect, to carry weight, used with the word "against": "His long smoking history would militate against a very good prognosis." Cf. *mitigate.*

milk leg disease—the edematous, uniformly swollen, white extremity seen in femoroiliac thrombophlebitis.

Millen technique—retropubic prostatectomy—transverse row of sutures, with the "smile" removed from upper margin of bladder neck (Urol).

Miller-Abbott tube—a double-lumen long gastrointestinal tube.

mill-house murmur—a loud, continuous churning sound heard over the precordium (sometimes even without the use of a stethoscope). May be diagnostic of a venous air embolism.

millicurie (mc, mCi) (1/1000th of a curie)—the unit of measurement of radioactivity.

milliequivalent (mEq)—the unit of measurement used in writing electrolyte values.

Milligan-Morgan technique (Surg)—for treatment of hemorrhoids.

millijoule (mJ) ("mil-e-jul") (1/1000th of a joule)—measurement used in YAG laser and argon laser applications.

Milliknit vascular graft prosthesis.

milliliter (mL).

millimoles per liter (mmol/L).

milliner's needle—a straight needle with an eye; used primarily for suturing skin or readily accessible tissue.

milliosmole (mOsm).

Millon's reagent—a nitric acid/mercuric nitrate solution that reacts with tyrosine and other phenols, turning red or orange in the presence of proteins. Since tyrosine is present in most proteins, Millon's reagent is a good indicator of the presence of protein in urine.

milrinone (Primacor)—a drug used to treat congestive heart failure.

Milroy's disease—manifestated by congenital lymphedema; the patient has an inborn error of development of the lymphatic channels.

Mima polymorpha—see *Acinetobacter lwoffi.*

MINE (mesna, ifosfamide, Novantrone, etoposide)—a chemotherapy protocol used to treat advanced lymphomas.

mini-arousals *(not* many arousals)—a term used in sleep studies.

Mini-Hohmann retractor (Pod).

Minitran (Cardio)—clear plastic patch for transdermal delivery of nitroglycerin.

Minnesota Multiphasic Personality Inventory (MMPI) (Psych)—mental status examination.

Minnesota tube.

miotic—(1) an agent that causes the pupil to contract; (2) pertaining to, or causing, contraction of the pupil.

Mira cautery; reamer (Ortho).

Miragel (Oph)—a hydrophilic sponge material used in the IMEX scleral implant.

mirror image breast biopsy (Path)—a biopsy of the same spot in the oppo-

mirror image breast biopsy *(cont.)* site breast as the location of an earlier lesion (the same, but opposite, as in a mirror).

mirroring (Neuro). One extremity cannot move without the other moving in an identical manner.

Mitchell distal osteotomy (Pod)—to correct hallux valgus.

Mitek anchor system (Ortho)—to provide direct anchoring in the bone with no exposed metal.

MITH—see *plicamycin.*

Mithracin—see *plicamycin.*

mithramycin—see *plicamycin.* Cf. *mitomycin.*

mitigate—to make milder, less severe, as "We might attempt to mitigate his symptoms with phototherapy." Cf. *militate.*

mitolactol (dibromodulcitol)—chemotherapy drug.

mitomycin (mitomycin-C, MTC, Mutamycin) (Oncol)—a chemotherapy drug used to treat gastric, pancreatic, and bladder carcinoma. Cf. *mithramycin.*

mitomycin-C—see *mitomycin.*

mitotic chromosomes.

mitoxantrone (Novantrone).

Mitraflex wound dressing (Surg)—sterile multilayer wound dressing which is very thin and can be used over the entire face or around the shoulder, for example.

mitral valve prolapse (MVP).

mittelschmerz—pain midway between the menstrual periods.

Mittlemeir broach (Ortho).

Mittendorf's dot—also known as hyaloid corpuscle. Represents the attachment of a hyaloid vessel to the posterior capsule.

Mivacron (mivacurium).

mivacurium (Mivacron)—short-acting neuromuscular blocker used in conjunction with general anesthesia to provide muscle relaxation.

mixed connective tissue disease (MCTD).

mixed leukocyte culture (MLC).

MixEvac (made by Stryker)—a closed bone-cement mixer (for mixing polymethyl methacrylate). It keeps the noxious fumes from escaping into the operating room.

Mixtner catheter.

M-K medium (McCarey-Kaufman).

MK-906 (finasteride).

mL (milliliter)—equivalent to a cubic centimeter (cc).

MLC (mixed leukocyte culture)—a trial in a test tube to determine in advance if donor and recipient tissues are compatible.

MLD (minimum lethal dose)—refers to ingestion of poisons or toxins.

MLNS (mucocutaneous lymph node syndrome). See *Kawasaki's disease.* Affects prepubertal children almost exclusively, mostly males, with a peak incidence during the first 18 months.

MMEF (maximum midexpiratory flow rate).

MMK procedure (Marshall-Marchetti-Krantz).

M-mode echocardiogram (Cardio).

mmol/L (millimoles per liter)—an SI (International System) unit of measurement of serum values.

MMOPP (methotrexate, mechlorethamine, Oncovin, procarbazine, prednisone)—chemotherapy protocol used to treat astrocytoma and neuroectodermal tumor.

MOAB, MoAb, MAb (monoclonal antibody).

mobilize—move. Cf. *immobilize.*

Mobin-Uddin umbrella filter (Cardio) —for transvenous vena cava interruption in prevention of pulmonary emboli. See also *Kim-Ray Greenfield filter,* which is not synonymous.

Mobitz I and II AV heart block.

MOBS (Montefiore Organic Brain Scale).

MOCNI (method of collection not indicated) (pronounced "mock-ney") (Path).

MODY (maturity onset diabetes of the young)—a distinct form of noninsulin-dependent diabetes mellitus (abbreviated NIDDM).

Moebius cataract knife.

Moebius' sign (Oph)—in exophthalmos, one or both eyes fail to converge on attempting to look at an object close to midline.

MOF (MeCCNU, Oncovin, fluorouracil)—chemotherapy protocol used to treat rectal adenocarcinoma.

Mogadon (nitrazepam) (Psych, Neuro) —a sedative used in treating myoclonic epilepsy.

Mohs' chemosurgery (named for Frederick E. Mohs, M.D., surgeon). Mohs' fresh tissue chemosurgery is used primarily in basal cell carcinoma. After fixation in vivo with zinc chloride paste, the tumor is then excised under microscopic control.

Mohs' technique—chemotherapy.

molar pregnancy—refers to a hydatidiform mole, an abnormal pregnancy which results from an ovum which has been converted to a mole. (This has nothing to do with molar teeth.)

molars—see *mulberry molars.*

molding—the shaping of the fetal head by the birth canal. Cf. *moulding.*

molgramostim (Leucomax)—a granulocyte/macrophage colony-stimulating factor derived from *E. coli.*

Molnar disk—plastic disk to anchor a nephrostomy tube in place.

Molteno seton (Oph)—a tube which allows aqueous humor to flow from the anterior chamber to the subconjunctival space to decrease intraocular pressure.

molybdenum—see *SMo—stainless steel with molybdenum.*

MOM (milk of magnesia).

Monaghan 300 ventilator—a pressure-cycled ventilator, which forces air into the lungs until an airway pressure (which has previously been determined) is obtained.

Monday crust (Psych)—the phenomenon of patients being less open to analysis after a weekend.

Mondini's dysplasia.

Monistat *(not* Monostat) (miconazole nitrate)—for local treatment of cutaneous or vulvovaginal candidiasis and other superficial fungal infections.

monitor
- actocardiotocograph fetal
- Biotrack coagulation
- BPM^2
- Dinamap blood pressure
- Dopplette
- Doppler
- Doptone
- Holter
- ICP (intracranial pressure)
- Jako facial nerve
- KinetiX ventilation
- Laserflo blood perfusion
- MemoryTrace AT cardiac
- Nicolet Nerve Integrity Monitor-2
- NIM-2
- PressureSense

monitoring, CCTV/EEG (closed circuit television electroencephalographic).

monobactams—a class of antibiotics for gram-negative bacteria. Example: azetreonam (Azactam).

monoclonal antibody (MAb; MoAb; MOAB)—an antibody derived from a single cell ("clone") in the laboratory. Monoclonal antibodies to T-cells are called OKT antibodies and are used to study the T-cell populations (or T-cell subsets) in patients. See *medication.*

Monodox (doxycycline; Vibramycin)—an antibiotic.

Monoflex lens (Oph)—an intraocular lens made of PMMA.

Monojector—see *fingerstick devices for blood glucose testing.*

Monopril (fosinopril).

monosomy 7 syndrome.

Monospot test—a rapidly performed serum agglutination test for infectious mononucleosis.

Monro, foramen of—in brain anatomy (Neuro).

Monsel's solution—a hemostatic solution. "There was a small amount of oozing from the cervical biopsy site, and Monsel's solution was used to stop this bleeding."

monster rongeur.

Montefiore Organic Brain Scale (MOBS).

Monteggia fracture-dislocation—fracture of the ulna, with a radial head dislocation (Ortho).

Montevideo units (Obs)—measurement of the length and strength of uterine contractions.

Monticelli-Spinelli system—a circular external fixation system for fractures of the leg and for leg lengthenings.

moon boot (Ortho)—used as an external support to brace fracture of the distal tibia and fibula.

moon face (or facies)—a pronounced rounding of the cheeks in Cushing's syndrome or prolonged adrenocortical therapy.

MOP (melphalan, Oncovin, mechlorethamine or methylprednisolone, Oncovin, procarbazine)—a chemotherapy protocol used to treat myeloma and malignant glioma.

MOPP (Oncol)—a standard chemotherapy protocol used to treat adult Hodgkin's disease. Consists of the drugs mechlorethamine, Oncovin, procarbazine, and prednisone.

Moranyl (suramin).

Moraxella lwoffi—see *Acinetobacter lwoffi.*

Morgagni's crypt; appendix ("morgah-nyee").

Morganella morganii—newer name for what was formerly called *Proteus morganii.*

moribund—dying.

moricizine (Ethmozine) (Cardio)—a sodium channel blocker used as an antiarrhythmic, and indicated for the treatment of life-threatening ventricular arrhythmias. Similar in its effect and indication to encainide (Enkaid), flecainide (Tambocor), and propafenone (Rythmol). Developed in the Soviet Union and the first such drug to be marketed by a U.S. pharmaceutical company.

Moro reflex (Peds, Neuro). An infant is placed supine, and a sudden noxious stimulus is made (usually a loud noise by slapping the table alongside). The child will respond with the arms extending and then flexing (in

Moro reflex *(cont.)*
a protective or embracing attitude) and the hips and knees will flex.

morselize (ENT, Ortho)—to take small pieces (morsels) of bone or cartilage during nasal surgery or orthopedic surgery. "The distal fibula was morselized and the bone chips packed tightly into the arthrodesis site laterally after the fibrous tissue had been curetted out."

morsicatio buccarum—the nervous habit of biting or chewing the buccal mucosa.

mortise—a slot, or wedge-shaped cut into bone (or timber) into which will fit a tenon (Ortho). This is also a carpenter's or furniture-maker's word. Cf. Webster's definition of *tenon (not* tendon). The ankle mortise is the normal articulation between the talus and the distal tibia and fibula.

mosaicism—see *Turner's mosaicism.*

Moskowitz procedure—obliteration of the cul-de-sac (Gyn).

Mosley method—for anterior shoulder repair (Ortho).

mOsm (milliosmole).

mosquito clamp (Surg).

Moss Suction Buster tube. See *Suction Buster catheter.*

Motilium (domperidone) (GI, Oncol)—a drug which depresses the chemoreceptor trigger zone in the brain to prevent nausea and vomiting in patients receiving chemotherapy.

motorcyclist's knee—see *O'Donahue's Unhappy Triad* (OUT).

motor evoked potential (MEP) (Neuro).

motor meal barium GI series—shows transit time, stomach to colon (normal transit time, 60 minutes).

moulding—See *molding,* which seems to be the preferred spelling.

mouse
joint
peritoneal

mouse units (MU)—used in endocrinology test to measure levels of circulating pituitary hormones.

mouth gag
Dingman
McIvor
Sluder-Jansen

mouthwash—see *Peridex mouthwash.*

moyamoya ("puff of smoke")—angiographic diagnosis of bilateral stenosis or occlusion of the internal carotid arteries above the clinoids.

MPC scissors—automated intravitreal scissors (Oph).

MPHR (maximum predicted heart rate) —a term used in exercise tolerance tests. See *Bruce protocol, ETT.*

M-protein, M-component—used in reference to chemotherapy response in patients with multiple myeloma (and perhaps other diseases).

MRI (magnetic resonance imaging). See MRI terminology list under *magnetic resonance imaging.* Also called *NMR (nuclear magnetic resonance).*

mRNA (messenger RNA).

MRS (magnetic resonance spectroscopy).

MRSA (methicillin-resistant *Staphylococcus aureus)*—a strain of *S. aureus* which is resistant to methicillin, gentamicin, and ciprofloxacin. Now treated with vancomycin. This resistant gram-positive bacterium often inhabits the nares of healthy individuals. See also *MARSA.*

MRU (molecular recognition unit)—pharmacologic technology based on monoclonal antibodies but physically much smaller. MRUs link with drugs or diagnostic radiology agents and

MRU *(cont.)* allow them to reach more fully into body tissues. See *ThromboScan MRU.*

MSAFP (maternal serum alpha-fetoprotein).

"m-site"—**see** *Emcyt.*

MSL-109 monoclonal antibody—drug used to treat patients with AIDS.

MSLT (multiple sleep latency test)—used to diagnose the sleep apnea syndrome, narcolepsy, and other sleep disorders.

MSOF (multisystem organ failure). The most common cause of death in patients in the ICU, multisystem organ failure, by definition, involves the simultaneous failure of two or more of these body systems: lungs, liver, kidneys, GI tract, circulatory system, or central nervous system.

MSUD disease (maple-sugar urine).

MTBE (methyl tertiary butyl ether)—a drug instilled under local anesthesia in the operating room or endoscopy suite to dissolve large cholesterol stones in the gallbladder. Via transhepatic catheter, the bile is aspirated from the gallbladder, and then 5 to 10 ml of MTBE is instilled into the gallbladder. As the stone dissolves, the MTBE containing dissolved cholesterol is removed, and more MTBE instilled. This process is continued until fluoroscopy reveals complete dissolving of the stones. Cf. *Actigall, Chenix, ursodiol.*

MTC (mitomycin).

MTM (modified Thayer-Martin medium, a culture medium) (Path, Lab). Used in culturing *Neisseria gonorrhoeae.*

MTP-PE—see *muramyl-tripeptide.*

MTX (methotrexate).

MU (mouse units).

Much's ("mooks") **granules**—found in the sputa of patients with tuberculosis. They are visible on Gram's stain but not on stain for acid-fast bacilli or by other methods.

mucosa, mucosae (pl.)—the mucous membrane. See *mucous, honeycomb mucosa.*

mucosa-to-mucosa closure.

mucous (adj.)—pertaining to mucus, or secreting mucus, as "mucous membrane"; the epithelium-covered membrane that lines certain organs, the eyes, nose, mouth, throat, vagina, etc. Cf. *mucus.*

mucus (noun)—viscid secretion produced by mucous membranes. See *mucous.*

Mueller Duo-Lock hip prosthesis (Ortho).

Mueller's muscle (or Müller) (Oph)—in the upper and lower eyelids; involved in correction of eyelid retraction in Graves' ophthalmopathy.

Muercke's lines—seen on the fingernails and toenails in patients with hypoalbuminemia. The lines run across the nail and are parallel to each other.

MUGA scan (multiple gated acquisition)—a blood pool radionuclide study of cardiac shape and dynamics in which a radionuclide is introduced into the circulation. Radioactive emissions from the heart are electronically monitored, stored, and analyzed, resulting in a composite scan consisting of a series of successive images all taken at the same point in the cardiac cycle.

Muhlberger orbital implant (Oph).

mulberry molars—five-pointed molars are a sign of congenital syphilis. Also, Hutchinson's teeth and hutchinsonian molars.

Mulder sign (Pod)—to identify a Morton neuroma in the web space of the toes.

Mule vitreous sphere (Oph).

Multiclip—a disposable surgical ligating clip device.

multi-echo images (Radiol)—a series of spin echo images obtained with various pulse sequences in magnetic resonance imaging.

multi-infarct dementia (MID).

multiforme—see *glioblastoma multiforme.*

Multileaf Collimator (MLC) (Oncol)—a device used in radiation oncology which allows the radiation beam to automatically follow the shape of a tumor, thereby irradiating only cancerous tissue not adjacent healthy tissue.

Multi-Med triple-lumen infusion catheter.

multimer assay.

multiplanar mode; technique—MRI terms.

multiple endocrine adenopathies (or abnormalities) (MEA).

multiple endocrine neoplasia (MEN).

multiple endocrine neoplasia type 2b—a syndrome, often familial, characterized by medullary carcinoma of the thyroid, pheochromocytoma, mucosal neuromas, Marfan's body structure, and ophthalmologic manifestations).

multiple gated acquisition scan. See *MUGA.*

Multipoise headrest (Neuro).

multivitamin formula (M.V.I.-12).

Mumford-Gurd procedure (Ortho)—an arthroplasty used in separation of the acromioclavicular joint (Ortho).

Munchausen's syndrome—named for the fictional Baron Munchausen, who told greatly exaggerated tales. In this syndrome the patient gives exaggerated and dramatic symptoms of a disease he does not have. Because the book about the fictional baron was written in English and his name spelled with a single *h* and no umlaut, *Munchausen* is the spelling used today in a medical context.

muramyl-tripeptide (MTP-PE)—drug used to treat patients with Kaposi's sarcoma.

murmur
- Austin Flint
- crescendo-decrescendo
- Docke's
- Graham Steell
- machinery
- mill-house

murmur grades—may use either Roman or Arabic numerals:
- grade I, barely audible, must strain to hear
- grade II, quiet, but clearly audible
- grade III, moderately loud
- grade IV, loud
- grade V, very loud; may be heard with the stethoscope partly off the chest
- grade VI, so loud that it can be heard with the stethoscope just off the chest wall

Muromonab-CD3. The name of this drug tells what it is: a **mu**rine **mono**clonal **antib**ody to the T3 (**CD3**) antigen of human T cells which acts as an immunosuppressant. This drug reverses graft rejection of renal transplants (and probably other transplants as well) by blocking T-cell functions.

muscimol—one of the poisons from the deadly mushroom *Amanita muscaria.*

muscle
- APL (abductor pollicis longus)
- belly of

muscle *(cont.)*
ECRB (extensor carpi radialis brevis)
ECRL (extensor carpi radialis longus)
EDC (extensor digitorum communis)
FCU (flexor carpi ulnaris)
FPL (flexor pollicis longus)
TRAM (transverse rectus abdominis myocutaneous)

muscle-splitting incision (Surg).

mushroom worker's disease—pulmonary symptoms caused by exposure to *Thermoactinomyces* organisms in the compost in which mushrooms grow. Extrinsic allergic alveolitis caused by exposure to mushroom dust. Also, mushroom worker's lung.

musical rhonchi.

mustard—see *L-phenylalanine mustard.*

Mustard procedure (Surg)—for transposition of the great vessels. Cf. *Mustardé procedure.*

Mustardé procedure (ENT)—flap otoplasty. Cf. *Mustard procedure.*

Mutamycin (injectable mitomycin)—used with other chemotherapeutic agents in combination for treatment of disseminated adenocarcinoma of the pancreas or stomach.

mute toe signs (Neuro)—equivocal Babinski reflexes.

mutton fat KPs (keratitic precipitates)—clusters of inflammatory cells and white cells that adhere to the corneal endothelium. Found in patients with uveitis (Oph).

MVAC (methotrexate, vincristine, Adriamycin, and cisplatin)—chemotherapy protocol used to treat adenocarcinoma of the uterus and cervix, and transitional cell carcinoma of the breast.

M.V.C.9+4—a multivitamin complex given intravenously. Contains 9 water-soluble vitamins and 4 fat-soluble vitamins.

MVF (mitoxantrone, vincristine, fluorouracil)—chemotherapy protocol used to treat breast carcinoma.

M.V.I.-12—intravenous **multivitamin** infusion.

MVP (mitral valve prolapse).

MVR blade (Oph).

MVT (mitoxantrone, VP-16, thiotepa)—chemotherapy protocol used to treat multiple myeloma and lymphomas.

MVV (maximal voluntary ventilation).

myalgic encephalomyelitis (ME)—the British term for what in the U.S. is called chronic fatigue syndrome (CFS). Also called postviral fatigue syndrome and yuppie flu.

Myambutol (ethambutol)—a drug used to treat tuberculosis, and now used to treat MAC infection in AIDS patients.

mycelium—a mat of fungal growth consisting of hyphae.

***Mycobacterium avium* complex**—see *MAC infection.*

***Mycobacterium avium-intracellulare* infection**—see *MAI infection.*

Mycobacterium gordonae—has been cultured from tap water, soil, sputum, and gastric lavage specimens.

Mycobutin (ansamycin, rifabutin)—used to treat MAC infection in AIDS patients.

mycosis fungoides—a lymphoma (white blood cell malignancy) which occurs in the skin.

myelographic contrast medium—see *medication.*

myelomere—spinal cord segment.

myeloid/erythroid ratio (M/E).

Myers-Briggs Personality Inventory (Psych).

Myleran (busulfan)—for treatment of chronic myeloid leukemia.

Myobock artificial hand—the Utah artificial arm, a myoelectric prosthesis for amputations above the elbow. Available with either a hook or an artificial Myobock hand.

myopia—nearsightedness.

Myoscint (Radiol)—the monoclonal antibody Fab to myosin, labeled with indium-111. Used to detect myocarditis and signs of rejection in patients after heart transplant.

myxoma—a tumor of mucoid (mucus) material.

N, n

nabumetone (Relafen) (Ortho)—a nonsteroidal anti-inflammatory drug (NSAID) for rheumatoid arthritis and osteoarthritis. It belongs to a class of NSAIDs known as naphthylalkalones and is thought to have fewer GI side effects than other NSAIDs.

NAD (no appreciable disease).

Nadbath akinesia—a facial nerve block that is given behind the ear. Used in preparation for cataract surgery.

nadir—the lowest point; in hematology oncology, the lowest point reached by the white cell count after chemotherapy has been administered. When the WBC count falls below 1000, the chemotherapeutic agent may be discontinued until the white cell count rises. Pronounced like (Ralph) Nader.

nafarelin (Synarel) (Gyn)—a synthetic version of gonadotropin-releasing hormone used to treat endometriosis. The formation of painful endometrial implants within the pelvic area is facilitated by the hormone estrogen. Rising estrogen during the first half of the menstrual cycle causes proliferation of the endometrium and also causes endometrial implants in the pelvic area to swell. Later these implants bleed, slough off, and produce inflammation and scarring within the pelvis and abdomen. Nafarelin suppresses the release of estrogen from the ovaries and stops the menstrual cycle while the patient is on the drug, thereby treating the endometriosis. Note that the usual dose is 400 micrograms per day (not milligrams as is common with many drugs). It is administered intranasally because it cannot be absorbed in the GI tract following oral administration.

Naganol (suramin).

nail bed (*not* nailbed)—the skin surface just under the nail (Ortho).

nail; pin

Deyerle pin
Ender nail
Hagie pin
half and half nails
Inro surgical nail
Jewett nail
Ken nail

nail *(cont.)*
Knowles pin
Kuntscher nail
Nylok self-locking nail
OrthoSorb pin
Rush pin
Russell-Taylor nail
Seidel humeral locking nail
Smith-Petersen nail
Steinmann pin
Terry nails
Zickel nail

NANB hepatitis *(not* NA&B)—non-A, non-B hepatitis. This is an acute viral hepatitis, but does not have antibodies or antigens of either hepatitis A or B.

nanogram (millimicrogram)—used in plasma testosterone measurement, growth hormone assay results; given in nanograms per cubic centimeter (ng/cc).

Napa (''nap-pa'') (acecainide) (Cardio)—antiarrhythmic drug. The chemical name for this drug, n-acetylated procainamide, is abbreviated NAPA. The trade name is Napa.

naphthylalkalones (Ortho)—a class of nonsteroidal anti-inflammatory drugs (NSAIDs) for treating rheumatoid arthritis and osteoarthritis. Thought to have fewer GI side effects than other kinds of NSAIDS. See *nabumetone.*

Naphuride (suramin).

Nardi test (morphine-prostigmine)—for ampullary stenosis of pancreaticobiliary sphincters.

nasal dressing forceps.

nasal flaring (Peds, Cardio)—involuntary outward movement of nasal alae in newborns with respiratory distress and in patients with some types of heart disease. Also called alar flaring.

Nashold TC electrode (Neuro)—for making dorsal root entry zone (DREZ) lesions in the spinal cord.

nasogastric (NG) **feeding; tube.**

nasojejunal (NJ) **feeding; tube.**

natatory ligament (Ortho)—a term you will hear in surgery of the hand, particularly in the context of Dupuytren's contracture.

natriuresis (Urol)—excretion of abnormal amounts of sodium in the urine.

Naughton cardiac exercise treadmill test—used for patients who cannot stand for prolonged periods as required in traditional treadmill tests.

N-butyl-deoxynojirmycin (DNJ)—a drug used in treating AIDS patients.

NCE (new chemical entity).

Nd:YAG laser—neodymium: yttrium-aluminum-garnet. See *neodymium.*

near-miss—adjective describing near fatal occurrence: ''near-miss SIDS,'' ''near-miss drowning.''

nebulizer
Pulmo-Aide
Respirgard II

NebuPent (aerosolized pentamidine) for prevention of *Pneumocystis carinii* pneumonia in AIDS patients.

NEC (''neck'') (necrotizing enterocolitis) (Peds)—develops in premature infants unable to tolerate formula.

NED (no evidence of disease).

necrotizing enterocolitis (NEC).

nedocromil (Tilade)—inhaled drug used to treat reversible obstructive airway disease.

needle
Accucore II biopsy
Addix
Agnew tattooing
Atraloc surgical
atraumatic
B-D spinal
Biopty cut

needle *(cont.)*
bore
Brockenbrough
butterfly
Charles vacuuming
Chiba
Cibis ski
coaxial sheath cut-biopsy
Cobb-Ragde
Control-Release
cut-biopsy
docking
Dos Santos
D-Tach
Fein antrum trocar
French eye
Geuder corneal; keratoplasty
Hawkins breast localization
Hoen ventricular
Howell biopsy aspiration
Huber
Jamshidi
Klatskin
Koch nucleus hydrolysis
Lewis Pair-Pak
milliner's
PC-7
PercuCut cut-biopsy
Pereyra
plum-blossom
pop-off
Reverdin suturing
Sabreloc spatula
Scheie cataract aspirating
SC-1
Seldinger gastrostomy
self-aspirating cut-biopsy
side-cutting spatulated
Simcoe
skinny
SmallPort
SmartNeedle
Solitaire
Stamey
steel-winged butterfly

needle *(cont.)*
stereotactic biopsy
Stifcore aspiration
Tapercut
Terry-Mayo
THI
Tru-Cut
Tuohy
Veirs
Veress
Visi-Black surgical
Voorhees
Wright

needle holder
Ryder (French eye)
Tilderquist
Twisk
Vital Cooley microvascular
Vital Ryder microvascular
Webster

Neer classification of shoulder fractures as I, II, III.

Neer hemiarthroplasty (Ortho).

Neer shoulder replacement prosthesis.

Negri body (inclusion body found in rabies).

Neisseria—now split between the genus *Branhamella* and the genus *Neisseria.*

Neisseria meningitidis—the cause of meningococcal meningitis.

Neivert
dissector
polyp hook
tonsil snare

Nélaton dislocation of the ankle.

Nélaton rubber tube drain (Surg, Ortho).

NEMD (nonspecific esophageal motility disorder) (Radiol).

neodymium: yttrium-aluminum-garnet laser (Nd:YAG laser) (Oph, Neuro). Utilized in a glaucoma procedure combining a nonpenetrating trabeculectomy with a neodymium:

neodymium:YAG laser *(cont.)* YAG trabeculectomy. It forms through-and-through filtration under a scleral flap without actually entering the anterior chamber. See *laser.*

Neoflex bendable knife—an electrocautery with a flexible pencil-like device that provides the surgeon access to difficult-to-reach areas.

NeoKnife electrosurgical instrument, for cutting, fulguration, and desiccation.

neon particle protocol—focal radiation therapy.

NephrAmine—essential amino acid injection formulated for patients with renal disease.

nephrostomy-type catheter (Urol).

nephrotic syndrome—defined as serum albumin greater than 3.0 gm/dl and proteinuria of 3.5 gm or more in 24 hours.

nerve, Arnold's.

nerve block, dorsal penile (DPNB).

nerve growth factor (NGF).

nerve monitor, Jako facial.

nerve of Latarjet (''Lat'ar-zhay'')—continuation of the vagus nerve along the stomach. In a proximal gastric vagotomy procedure, the tiny branches of this nerve to the stomach are divided, which decreases the acid output of the stomach and protects against ulcer disease.

nerve of Wrisberg. There are **two** nerves with the same name: the medial cutaneous nerve of the arm, and the intermediate nerve. Named for an 18th century German anatomist.

nerve stimulator, Axostim.

Neubauer vitreous microextractor forceps.

Neupogen (filgrastim) (Oncol)—a recombinant G-CSF. See *filgrastim, G-CSF.*

Neurairtome (Ortho)—by Zimmer.

neurapraxia *(not* neuropraxia) (Neuro, Ortho)—a conduction block (either partial or total) of a segment of nerve fiber, causing a temporary paralysis, as in ''The patient has a right ulnar nerve neurapraxia.''

neurilemmoma (schwannoma)—proliferation of cells forming a nerve sheath; a common peripheral nerve tumor.

Neurobehavioral Cognitive Status Examination—neurological test.

neurofibrillary tangles—snarled neurofilaments of cortical neurons, seen on biopsy, are diagnostic of Alzheimer's disease (Neuro).

NeuroSectOR (Neuro)—trade name for an ultrasound system. See *real-time ultrasonography.*

neurotmesis—the complete transection of a nerve, which results in cell death.

Neuro-Trace—an instrument that provides pulsating low current stimulation for location of nerves during operative procedures.

Neurotrast (iophendylate) (Radiol)—a radiopaque medium and diagnostic aid.

Neville tracheal and tracheobronchial prostheses—for tracheal reconstruction in patients with benign tumor, primary or secondary carcinoma, or stenosis caused by intubation or other trauma.

nevirapine (BI-RG-587)—a drug used to treat HIV-positive patients. (BI, Boehringer Ingelheim, the manufacturer.)

Nevyas double sharp cystitome.

Nevyas drape retractor (Surg)—a disposable stick-on arched frame, which is placed over the patient's forehead, and the sterile surgical drape is placed over it, thus permitting the patient to breathe more easily.

New England Baptist acetabular cup (Ortho)—used for total hip arthroplasty.

Newvicon vacuum chamber pickup tube—for video camera used in arthroscopy. Also, Circon video camera; Saticon vacuum chamber pickup tube; Vidicon.

Nextep (Ortho)—functional knee brace with a bipivotal hinge.

Nexus implant (Ortho)—a cemented chrome cobalt femoral implant.

Nezelof's syndrome. See *DiGeorge.*

Nezhat-Dorsey Trumpet Valve hydrodissector (Surg)—a device used for tissue dissection, aspiration of fluid, lavage, and smoke evacuation from a laser. The controls are shaped like the valves on a trumpet.

NGF (nerve growth factor) (Neuro)—a substance produced in the brain. Levels of nerve growth factor may be decreased in patients with Alzheimer's disease. Without NGF, neurons die; future therapy for Alzheimer's disease may involve supplementation with NGF.

NG feeding (nasogastric).

Nichol procedure—a vaginal suspension procedure for urinary stress incontinence (Gyn).

Nicoderm—a transdermal patch containing nicotine, available by prescription only, for use by smokers to avoid nicotine withdrawal symptoms when they try to quit smoking. Also, Habitrol, ProStep.

Nicolet Nerve Integrity Monitor-2 (NIM-2)—used in surgery to locate and identify the facial and other cranial nerves quickly. It also helps to map the course of each nerve and to ascertain whether it is functioning.

Nicoll bone graft (Ortho).

nidus—"nest"; the point of origin or focus of a morbid process.

Niebauer prosthesis—Silastic metacarpophalangeal joint.

Niedner anastomosis clamp (Cardio).

Niemann-Pick disease—a rare form of familial lipidosis, resulting in mental retardation, growth retardation, and progressive blindness.

NightBird nasal CPAP (continuous positive airway pressure, or constant positive airway pressure) for treatment of obstructive sleep apnea. (No space in NightBird.)

nil disease—synonym for lipoid nephrosis (so-called because so little evidence of disease is seen on light microscopy of a renal biopsy in a case of lipoid nephrosis).

NIM-2 (Nicolet Nerve Integrity Monitor-2) (Neurosurg).

nimodipine (Nimotop) (Psych)—a calcium channel blocker also used to treat manic-depressive disorder. Its therapeutic action is based on the fact that calcium ions, which it blocks, must enter a nerve cell before a neurotransmitter can be released.

ninety-ninety (90/90) **intraosseous wiring** (Ortho)—used to obtain rigid fixation for digital replantation or for transverse fractures. The two intraosseous wires are placed perpendicular to each other (hence, 90° angle or 90/90).

Nipent (pentostatin) (Oncol)—a drug used to treat patients with hairy cell

Nipent *(cont.)* leukemia who do not respond to alpha interferon.

Nissen fundoplication—procedure to control gastroesophageal reflux.

Nissl's granules—cytoplasmic bodies in nerve cell bodies. (Franz Nissl, German neuropathologist.)

Nissl's stain (Path).

nitrazepam (Mogadon) (Psych, Neuro) —a sedative also used to treat myoclonic epilepsy.

nitrendipine (Baypress) (Cardio)—a vasodilator and calcium channel blocker similar to nifedipine, used to treat hypertension.

nitrogen-13 ammonia (Radiol)—radioactive tracer used to perform a PET scan to evaluate heart function at rest and during stress. Nitrogen-13 ammonia has a longer half-life than rubidium-82. Therefore, the stress portion of the test may be done with an exercise bike or treadmill.

nitroglycerin (Ob-Gyn)—a vasodilator used to treat angina pectoris and now given I.V. to produce uterine relaxation in patients with a contracted, inverted uterus.

Nitrol ointment (or paste)—a topical coronary vasodilator—contains nitroglycerin in a lanolin-petrolatum base. The ointment is spread on the skin, which absorbs the nitroglycerin continuously in a vasodilator effect; used for relief and prevention of anginal attacks. The dosage is given in inches.

NJ feeding (nasojejunal).

NK cell (natural killer cell)—evaluated in specific and nonspecific immunotherapy and in cytotoxicity assays.

NLP (no light perception) (Oph).

NMES (neuromuscular electrical stimulation) protocol—see *ReAct device.*

NMR scan (nuclear magnetic resonance). Early term for what is now called *MRI (magnetic resonance imaging) scan.* The name is said to have been changed because of patients' resistance to the word *nuclear.*

Nocardia—the fungus causing nocardiasis, more devastating than usual in the AIDS patient.

node
- Aschoff-Tawara
- Bouchard's
- Flack's
- jugulodigastric
- Koch's
- Osler's
- SA or S-A (sinoatrial)
- sentinel
- shotty
- signal
- singer's (of a vocal cord)
- Sister Mary Joseph
- Troisier's
- Virchow's

nodules, siderotic—see *siderotic nodules of the spleen.*

Nolvadex (tamoxifen citrate)—adjuvant hormonal therapy for postmenopausal women in breast cancer treatment.

noncholecystokinin—a substance that is thought to be important in regulating gallbladder contraction and emptying.

noncompliant—said of patients who do not follow their physician's directions and advice regarding diet or medicinal treatment.

non compos mentis (Psych)—a psychiatric and legal term for a patient not of sound mind and in need of guardianship.

nonoxynol 9—an over-the-counter spermatocide, a component in most contraceptive creams, gels, and foams,

nonoxynol 9 *(cont.)*
which has been reliably shown to kill the AIDS virus on contact with it.

nonrapid eye movement (NREM).

nonspecific esophageal motility disorder (NEMD) (GI).

nonspecific urethritis (NSU) (Urol).

NoProfile balloon catheter (Cardio).

norfloxacin (Chibroxin, Noroxin) (Oph, Urol)—a fluoroquinolone antibiotic. Chibroxin is used to treat conjunctivitis. Oral Noroxin is used to treat urinary tract infections.

Norland-Cameron photon densitometry.

normal pressure hydrocephalus (NPH).

normal spontaneous vaginal delivery (NSVD).

Norplant (levonorgestrel) (Ob-Gyn)—a synthetic progestin, now used for contraception. Tiny silicone tubes filled with levonorgestrel are implanted under the skin of a woman's upper arm and, over about a five-year period, the hormone is gradually released. This is a reversible method, as the tubes can be removed if fertility is again desired.

Norrie's disease (Oph). One of its manifestations is retinal detachment.

Norvasc (amiodipine).

Norwood procedure—performed for hypoplastic left-sided heart syndrome. See *Fontan; Gill/Jonas; Sade.*

nosocomial disease—disease originating in a hospital.

notch
antegonial
Kernohan

notochord *(not* notocord)—chorda dorsalis—seen in the embryo; in adults the nuclei pulposi are the vestigial notochord.

Nottingham introducer (ENT)—used to place a tube as a palliative procedure in patients with esophageal cancer.

Novafil polybutester monofilament suture.

Novantrone (mitoxantrone HCl)—a synthetic antineoplastic agent used in combination with other drugs in beginning therapy of nonlymphatic leukemia. It has a cytocidal effect on both proliferating and nonproliferating human cells.

Novapren—a drug used to treat HIV-positive patients.

NovolinPen device—holds cartridges of insulin. A patient can select and inject correct dose without need for syringes or insulin vials.

Noyes iridectomy scissors (Oph).

Noyes nasal dressing forceps (ENT).

N.P. (or NP)—nurse practitioner.

NPH insulin—see *insulin.*

NPH (normal pressure hydrocephalus) (Neuro).

NPSG (nocturnal polysomnography).

NREM sleep—non-rapid eye movement in which the heart rate is slowed and regular, the blood pressure is low, the brain waves are slow and of high voltage, and sleep is dreamless, interspersed with occasional periods of REM sleep. See *REM sleep.*

NSAIDs (nonsteroidal anti-inflammatory drugs)—a category of drugs of which the most commonly used for treatment of rheumatoid arthritis and osteoarthritis are acetylsalicylic acid (aspirin) and ibuprofen (Motrin).

NSGCT (nonseminomatous germ cell tumor).

NSO (non-nutritive sucking opportunities) (Neonat)—used to stimulate premature babies suffering from lack of

NSO *(cont.)* stimulation. They were given pacifiers four times a day and did better than other high-risk infants.

NSR (normal sinus rhythm) (Cardio).

NSU (nonspecific urethritis) (Urol).

NSVD (normal spontaneous vaginal delivery) (Obs).

nuchal cord (Obs)—the umbilical cord wrapped around neck of the fetus can result in hypoxia or even death.

nuclear magnetic resonance imaging (NMR)—see *magnetic resonance imaging.*

nuclear sclerosis, lenticular (Oph).

nuclear signal; spin; spin quantum number—MRI terms.

nuclear-tagged red blood cell bleeding study (Radiol).

nuclectomy—excision of nucleus pulposus.

nucleolar pattern of ANA (antinuclear antibodies), associated with scleroderma.

nucleolus (pl., nucleoli)—a part of the nucleus which is spherical and more hyperchromatic than the nucleus.

nucleoside analogue—one of a class of synthetic compounds, like AZT, ddI, and ddC, that inhibit replication of the HIV virus.

Nucleotome system (Ortho)—for performing automated percutaneous lumbar diskectomy procedure for herniated lumbar disk.

Nuclepore prep (Path)—a trademark of General Electric.

nucleus (pl., nuclei)—central cellular core containing DNA. See *Westphal-Edinger nucleus.*

nucleus lateralis of Le Gros Clark—dorsal portion of the lateral mamillary nucleus of Rose (Neuro).

nucleus of Darkschewitsch—located in the rostral part of the midbrain. See *Darkschewitsch.*

nucleus of Gudden—dorsal tegmental nucleus (Neuro).

nucleus of Luys—see *body of Luys.*

nucleus of Perlia—central nucleus of the oculomotor nerve.

nucleus of Rose, see *lateral mamillary nucleus of Rose.*

nucleus pulposus *(not* pulposis)—the semifluid inner portion of the intervertebral disk (Neuro).

NUG (necrotizing ulcerative gingivitis).

Nu Gauze dressing (marketed by Johnson & Johnson). *Not* Nu-gauze.

Nu-Gel (Surg)—clear hydrogel wound dressing for wounds with light to medium exudate, burns, and skin reactions to oncological procedures.

Nu-Knit—see *Surgical Nu-Knit.*

NuKO knee orthosis.

null cell lymphoblastic leukemia.

null type non-Hodgkin's lymphoma.

NuLytely bowel prep—for GI endoscopy.

Nuport PEG tube (GI)—a percutaneous endoscopic gastrostomy tube.

Nurolon suture—a braided nylon suture with extremely low tissue reaction (by Ethicon) (Surg, Neuro).

Nuromax (doxacurium chloride).

nutcracker esophagus (Radiol).

nutmeg appearance of liver (Radiol).

Nutricath (Surg)—a silicone elastomer catheter.

nutrient solutions

FreAmine

HepatAmine

NephrAmine

NWB (nonweightbearing) (Ortho).

nyctalopia—night blindness (Oph).

NYHA (New York Heart Association).

NYHA classification of angina.

NYHA classification of congestive heart failure:

I—asymptomatic

II—slightly symptomatic

III—congestive heart failure symptoms

IV—severe congestive heart failure

Nyhus/Nelson tube (Surg)—gastric decompression and jejunal feeding tube which permits gastric decompression and enteral feeding simultaneously.

Nylen-Bárány maneuver (Neuro).

Nylok self-locking nail (Ortho).

Nyquist limit (Cardio).

nystagmus—a rhythmic horizontal or vertical oscillation of (usually both) eyeballs, generally more pronounced when looking in certain directions. Related terms: periodic alternating nystagmus and optokinetic nystagmus (OKN).

Nystatin[LF] (liposomal formulation)—an antifungal drug.

O, o

O_2 debt (oxygen)—when available oxygen is less than oxygen requirements. Used with reference to resuscitation of newborns and in exercise physiology.

O&P test (ova and parasites). "Stools for O&P x 2 [times two] were obtained and were negative."

Obecalp (*placebo* spelled backwards)—given as a medication.

Ober-Barr procedure (Ortho)—brachioradialis transfer, for weakness of the triceps muscle.

OBS (organic brain syndrome).

obsessive-compulsive disorder (OCD) —a psychiatric disorder characterized by persisting or recurring thoughts or impulses (obsessions) and repetitive, ritualized, stereotyped acts (compulsions) such as handwashing, touching all the posts of a fence, or carrying out a series of actions in a certain order. Sometimes these symptoms overlap with the tics (with the absence of intention)—twitching of the face, blinking, throat-clearing, hyperactivity, tearing hair, gnashing teeth, etc.—of Tourette's disease (Gilles de la Tourette's syndrome).

obturator sign. The flexed thigh is rotated both internally and externally, and hypogastric pain is elicited when there is an inflammatory process in contact with the obturator externus muscle. This may be positive in appendicitis or when there is fluid or blood in the pelvis.

obtuse marginal (OM) **coronary artery.**

Obwegeser periosteal retractor.

Obwegeser sagittal mandibular osteotomy technique (Oral Surg, Plas Surg). There have been many modifications of this procedure, e.g., Salyer and Bardach.

o-cal f.a.—a prescription oral multivitamin containing calcium and folic acid.

occipitofrontal circumference (OFC).

occult—in medicine, something that is present in such a tiny quantity that it's effectively hidden. Usage: "We still must rule out the possibility of occult neoplasm."

occult blood—blood present (as in the stool) in such small quantity that it is not visible, but its presence is determined by lab tests or through the microscope.

occur, occurred (past tense); frequently misspelled.

OCD (obsessive-compulsive disorder).

OCG (oral cholecystogram).

O'Connor shield finger cup—used in performing cystoscopy.

OCT (optimal cutting temperature)—trademark for a synthetic water-soluble glycol and resin mounting medium; used to embed and mount tissue for cutting frozen sections.

OCT (oxytocin challenge test).

octopus test (Oph)—test for measuring peripheral vision. The patient is seated before a large screen, holding a counter. Each time the patient sees a light reflected at any angle on the screen, he presses the hand counter; this is monitored in another room by a technician.

octreotide (Sandostatin)—used to con trol severe diarrhea in patients with vipomas and AIDS.

Ocufen (flurbiprofen sodium) (Oph)—used for inhibition of intraoperative miosis.

ocular density values (OD).

oculi, fundus—*fundus oculi.*

OcuLight SL (Oph)—diode laser. Note: The L is capitalized.

Oculinum—see *botulinum toxin type A.*

oculogyric crisis (Neuro, Oph)—occurs when the eyeballs become fixed in one position for a considerable period of time, minutes to hours. Seen in encephalitis or postencephalitic parkinsonism. "She is having an acute extrapyramidal reaction. She is drooling, unable to speak coherently; no evidence of oculogyric crisis."

oculoplethysmography/carotid phonoangiography (OPG/CPA)—examination used in evaluating suspected intracranial cerebrovascular disease. A noninvasive test, serial angiography of the internal carotid artery, using the OPG-Gee instrument, to determine the degree of occlusion of the internal carotid. The ophthalmic systolic pressure is correlated with the brachial systolic pressure (as determined by arm cuff and auscultation) which is measured immediately after the OPG study.

ocutome (Oph)—a device to remove vitreous; e.g., *O'Malley ocutome.*

o.d. (omni die)—every day (also q.d.).

O.D. *(oculus dexter,* right eye).

OD values (ocular or optical density) —antibody titer determination on amniotic fluid for erythroblastosis fetalis.

OD (overdose).

"OD'd"(overdosed)—slang.

O'Donahue's Unhappy Triad (OUT) (Ortho)—a triple injury of damage, with joint cartilage and both outside and inside knee ligaments being torn. Also called motorcyclist's knee.

Oertli razor bladebreaker knife.

OFC (occipitofrontal circumference) (Peds)—a term used in measurement of the head.

ofloxacin (Floxin)—a broad-spectrum antibiotic of the quinolone group similar to Cipro. It is given either I.V. or orally and is used to treat respiratory and urinary infections as well as sexually transmitted diseases.

Ogura tissue and cartilage forceps (Plas Surg).

Ohashiatsu—a form of shiatsu massage developed by the Ohashi Institute of New York City, consisting of techniques to alleviate symptoms common to pregnancy (fatigue, aching, general discomfort) and the delivery process through the use of pressure to specific body areas.

oil drop change (Derm)—a localized brown color, a sign of psoriasis in the nail bed.

oil red O stain (Oph)—a dye used in histologic demonstration of neutral fats. "Oil red O stain for intracytoplasmic fat was present."

Okamura—see *Schepens-Okamura-Brockhurst technique for retinal detachment repair.*

Oklahoma ankle joint (Pod)—orthosis for ambulation in children with cerebral palsy and myelomeningocele. Made of polypropylene vacuformed in plastic.

OKN (optokinetic nystagmus) (Neuro).

OKT3—see *Orthoclone OKT3.*

OKT4—the monoclonal antibody to human T-4 cells. Also called anti-human T-4 cell, and anti-human inducer/helper T-cell.

OKT8—the monoclonal antibody to human T-8 cells. Also called anti-human T-8 cell, and anti-human suppressor/cytotoxic T-cell.

Olbert balloon dilatation catheter (Urol).

oligoclonal bands.

oligodendroglioma—derived from cells forming and maintaining the myelin sheaths in the central nervous system.

olive wire; ring (Ortho)—used in Ilizarov limb lengthening procedure.

Oliver-Rosalki—method of testing serum CPK. See also *Sigma.*

olsalazine (Dipentum) (GI)—used to treat ulcerative colitis, particularly in patients who cannot tolerate the standard treatment because they are allergic to sulfa drugs (olsalazine is not a sulfa drug). After being given orally, it is converted in the colon to 5-ASA, a topical anti-inflammatory, which is the active ingredient.

Olympus ENF-P2 scope (ENT)—flexible laryngoscope.

Olympus FBK 13 forceps—endoscopic biopsy forceps.

Olympus OSF scope—flexible sigmoidoscope.

Olympus One-Step Button (GI)—a short gastrostomy tube (the thickness of the stomach wall) with an internal button to hold it in place and an external opening with an attached plastic plug. Inserted endoscopically and used for tube feedings.

O'Malley ocutome (Oph).

OMB (obtuse marginal branch)—one of the coronary arteries.

Omed bulldog vascular clamp (Vasc Surg)—for atraumatic occlusion of vessels.

Omega compression hip screw system.

omeprazole (Prilosec) (GI)—used to treat gastroesophageal reflux. Trade name Losec was changed to Prilosec by the manufacturer to avoid confusing Losec with Lasix.

Ommaya reservoir (Neuro).

omni die (o.d.)—every day.

Omnifit HA hip stem (Ortho)—prosthesis of hydroxyapatite.

Omniflox (temafloxacin).

Omni operating microscope.

Omnipaque, nonionic (iohexol) (Radiol)—an imaging agent used like iopamidol or metrizamide in various radiological special procedures.

OMS Concentrate—oral morphine sulfate in solution.

oncogene—tumor gene in the cells of animals and humans.

OncoScint CR103 (colorectal), **OV103** (ovarian) (Radiol)—monoclonal antibody B72.3 labeled with ^{111}indium, used as a radioactive imaging agent to detect colorectal or ovarian carcinomas.

Oncovin (vincristine sulfate)—used in treatment of acute leukemia and in combination with other oncolytic agents in Hodgkin's disease, neuroblastoma, lymphosarcoma, rhabdomyosarcoma, reticulum cell sarcoma, and Wilms' tumor.

ondansetron (Zofran) (Oncol)—an antiemetic drug which decreases nausea by depressing the vomiting center in the brain. It is used for chemotherapy patients and is given I.V.

Ondine's curse—periodic breathing.

One-Alpha (alfacalcidol).

onlay graft—a bone graft, not to be confused with inlay graft. Both are used in craniofacial surgery. Note: No hyphen is used.

1*2*3 Heart Rate. See *Heart Rate.*

One Touch blood glucose meter—for self-testing by diabetics.

"ONP"—see *O&P* (ova and parasites).

opacification (Radiol)—an increase in the density of a tissue or region, with increased resistance to x-rays.

opacities, snowball (Oph).

opening snap (Cardio)—an important finding on physical examination because an audible opening snap in mitral or tricuspid stenosis implies a flexible valve.

open-mouth odontoid view (Radiol)—a view of the odontoid process of the second cervical vertebra for which the x-ray beam is aimed through the patient's open mouth.

open reduction and internal fixation (ORIF)—an orthopedic procedure to correct a severely fractured bone.

open-sky vitrectomy (Oph)—an operative procedure to remove vitreous from the eye by first removing a button of cornea. The vitreous is then removed through the pupil, after the lens has been extracted.

operation (See also *procedure.*)
- Abbe repair
- adenosine echocardiography
- ALT (argon laser trabeculoplasty)
- antecolic anastomosis
- antecolic gastrojejunostomy
- antiperistaltic technique
- Aries-Pitanguy correction of mammary ptosis
- argon laser trabeculoplasty (ALT)
- Auchincloss modified radical mastectomy
- Aufranc-Turner arthroplasty
- Bacon-Babcock rectovaginal fistula
- Baffe's anastomosis
- Baldy-Webster correction of uterus retrodisplacement
- Ball treatment of pruritus ani
- Bankart shoulder dislocation repair
- Bassini inguinal hernia repair
- Belsey Mark IV fundoplication
- Billroth gastroenterostomy
- Blalock–Hanlon cardiac surgery
- Blalock–Taussig cardiac surgery
- Bricker ureteroileostomy
- Brackin ureterointestinal anastomosis
- Bristow repair of shoulder dislocation
- Brooke ileostomy
- Brostrom ankle repair
- Bruhat laser surgery neosalpingostomy
- Buerhenne stone basket
- bunionectomy, tricorrectional
- Bunnell tendon transfer
- Burch iliopectineal ligament urethrovesical suspension
- butterfly flap technique
- CABG (coronary artery bypass graft)
- Camey ileocystoplasty
- capsulorhexis
- cardiomyoplasty
- CAVH (continuous arteriovenous hemofiltration)
- CBWO (closing base wedge osteotomy)

operation *(cont.)*
CCC (continuous curvilinear capsulorhexis)
CCUP (colpocystourethropexy)
cervicectomy
cheilectomy
chevron osteotomy
chorionic villi biopsy
Chrisman and Snook correction of ankle instability
Clagett-Barrett esophagogastrostomy
Clark perineorrhaphy
closing base wedge osteotomy (CBWO)
coagulum pyelolithotomy
Cody tack
Coffey ureterointestinal anastomosis
Collin-Beard resection of levator muscle
Collis-Nissen fundoplication
colocolponeopoiesis
colpocystourethropexy (CCUP)
continent supravesical bowel urinary diversion
continuous arteriovenous hemofiltration (CAVH)
continuous curvilinear capsulorhexis (CCC)
coronary artery bypass graft (CABG)
coronary atherectomy
corset platysmaplasty
Cotton cartilage graft to cricolaryngeal area
coupled suturing
Crawford-Adams arthroplasty
Crikelair otoplasty
Cröhnlein
Cyclops reconstruction to cover defect
Darrach ulnar resection
Davydov vaginal construction
Dennis-Varco pancreatico-duodenostomy
Depage-Janeway gastrostomy

operation *(cont.)*
De Vega tricuspid annuloplasty
direct vision internal urethrotomy (DVIU)
donor island harvesting
Dotter-Judkins PTA
DREZ-otomy
Duecollement hemicolectomy
Duhamel pull-through
duodenal switch
DuVal pancreaticojejunostomy
DuVries hammer toe repair
DVIU (direct vision internal urethrotomy)
Dwyer correction of scoliosis
Dwyer fusion
Dwyer osteotomy
dynamic graciloplasty
EC-IC bypass (extracranial-intracranial)
Eckhout vertical gastroplasty
embryoscopy
Emmet-Studdiford perineorrhaphy
en bloc resection
endoscopic laser cholecystectomy
endoscopic transpapillary catheterization of the gallbladder (ETCG)
endoscopic variceal sclerotherapy (EVS)
enteroenterostomy
enucleation
ETCG (endoscopic transpapillary catheterization of gallbladder)
Evans tenodesis
evisceration
EVS (endoscopic variceal sclerotherapy)
extracorporeal shock-wave lithotripsy
extracranial-intracranial (EC-IC) bypass
Faden retropexy
Fick sacculotomy
Fontan anastomosis

operation *(cont.)*
Fontan-Kreutzer repair
four-flap Z-plasty
Frank vaginal construction
free toe transfer
Furniss ureterointestinal anastomosis
gamete intrafallopian transfer (GIFT)
Giannestras step-down modified osteotomy
GIFT (gamete intrafallopian transfer)
Gillies elevation
Girdlestone–Taylor
Gittes urethral suspension
Goulian mammoplasty
Gustilo-Kyle arthroplasty
Halsted inguinal herniorrhaphy
hammer toe repair
harvesting
Hauser transplantation of patellar tendon insertion
Heineke-Mikulicz pyloroplasty
Heller-Belsey correction of achalasia of esophagus
Heller-Nissen correction of achalasia of esophagus
hemicolectomy
Higgins ureterointestinal anastomosis
Hill cluster harvest micrograft
Hoffa's tendon shortening
Hoffman-Clayton podiatric treatment of rheumatoid arthritis
Hofmeister gastroenterostomy
Hofmeister-Shoemaker gastro-jejunostomy
Hunter open cord tendon implant for hand
Hunter tendon rod insertion
hysterosalpingosonography
Ilizarov limb lengthening
invasive
in vitro fertilization (IVF)
iridectomy
iridencleisis

operation *(cont.)*
IVF (in vitro fertilization)
Jenckel cholecystoduodenostomy
Jones first-toe repair
Judd ventral hernia repair
Kasai peritoneal venous shunt
Keck and Kelly osteotomy
Keller arthroplasty
Keller bunionectomy
Kestenbach-Anderson eye surgery
Kestenbaum repair of nystagmic torticollis
Kiricuta reconstructive breast
Klagsbrun harvest of chondrocytes
Koch lens insertion
Kock modified pouch
Koenig arthroplasty
Kono patch enlargement of aorta
Kreuscher bunionectomy
krypton (red) laser photocoagulation
Kun colocolpopoiesis
LABA (laser-assisted balloon angioplasty)
Ladd correction of malrotation of bowel
Lange tendon lengthening
laparoscopic cholecystectomy
laparoscopic laser cholecystectomy
laparoscopic video-laseroscopy
laser nucleotomy
large loop excision of the trans-formation zone (LLETZ)
laser-assisted balloon angioplasty (LABA)
laser image custom arthroplasty (LICA)
laser uterosacral nerve ablation (LUNA)
Lash hysterectomy
Latzko vesicovaginal fistula
Leadbetter-Politano uretero-vesicoplasty
LeDuc-Camey ileocystoplasty
LEEP (loop electrosurgical excision procedure)

operation *(cont.)*
LeFort I apertognathia
LeFort II and III
LeFort uterine prolapse repair
Lester Martin modification of Duhamel procedure
Lewis-Tanner esophagectomy
LICA (laser image custom arthroplasty)
Lich-Gregoire repair
Lichtenstein hernia repair
LLETZ (large loop excision of the transformation zone)
loop electrosurgical excision procedure (LEEP)
LUNA (laser uterosacral nerve ablation)
Ma and Griffith anastomosis
Madden incisional hernia repair
Madigan prostatectomy
Magnuson-Stack shoulder arthrotomy
MAGPI (meatal advancement, glanduloplasty, penoscrotal junction meatotomy)
mammoplasty
Maquet elevation of tibial crest
Marshall-Marchetti-Krantz vesico-urethral suspension
Masket lens insertion
Mason abdominotranssphincteric resection
Mason vertical-banded gastroplasty
matricectomy
Matsner median episiotomy
McDonald cervical cerclage
McIndoe vaginal construction
McKee-Farrar total hip arthroplasty
McVay hernia repair
meatal advancement, glanduloplasty, penoscrotal junction meatotomy (MAGPI)
median sternotomy
mediastinotomy

operation *(cont.)*
meloplasty
Merindino GI procedure
Millen retropubic prostatectomy
Milligan-Morgan hemorrhoidectomy
Mitchell distal osteotomy
Mohs' chemosurgery
Moskowitz obliteration of cul-de-sac
Mosley anterior shoulder repair
Mumford-Gurd arthroplasty
Mustard transposition of great vessels
Mustardé flap otoplasty
Neer hemiarthroplasty
New England Baptist arthroplasty
Nichol vaginal suspension
ninety-ninety intraosseous wiring
Nissen fundoplication
Norwood (Fontan modification)
Norwood (Gill/Jonas modification)
Norwood (Jonas modification)
Norwood (Sade modification)
nuclectomy
Ober-Barr brachioradialis transfer
Obwegeser's mandibular osteotomy (Salyer modification)
Obwegeser's sagittal mandibular osteotomy
open reduction and internal fixation (ORIF)
Orr-Loygue transabdominal proctopexy
Orr rectal prolapse repair
panretinal photocoagulation and focal laser therapy
pants-over-vest repair
Parker-Kerr closed end-to-end enteroenterostomy
Partipilo gastrostomy
PCCL (percutaneous cholecysto-lithotomy)
PCTCL (percutaneous transhepatic cholecystolithotomy)
Pearce trabeculectomy

operation *(cont.)*
PEG (percutaneous endoscopic gastrostomy)
percutaneous automated diskectomy
percutaneous balloon valvuloplasty
percutaneous cholecystolithotomy (PCCL)
percutaneous endoscopic gastrostomy (PEG)
percutaneous gastroenterostomy (PEG)
percutaneous gastrostomy (PG)
percutaneous mitral balloon valvotomy (PMBV)
percutaneous nephrostolithotomy (PCNL)
percutaneous transhepatic cholecystolithotomy (PCTCL)
percutaneous transluminal angioplasty (PTA)
percutaneous transluminal renal angioplasty (PTRA)
percutaneous transperineal seed implantation
peripheral laser angioplasty (PLA)
peritomy
PG (percutaneous gastrostomy)
PGE (percutaneous gastroenterostomy)
photocoagulation
PLA (peripheral laser angioplasty)
plicectomy
PLIF (posterior lumbar interbody fusion)
PMBV (percutaneous mitral balloon valvotomy)
PMR (posteromedial release) of clubfoot
pneumatic retinopexy
Ponka herniorrhaphy
posteromedial release of clubfoot (PMR)
profundaplasty
proliferative retinopathy photocoagulation

operation *(cont.)*
PTA (percutaneous transluminal angioplasty)
PTRA (percutaneous transluminal renal angioplasty)
Puestow pancreaticojejunostomy
Putti-Platt arthroplasty
radial keratotomy
radiofrequency ablation
Rashkind balloon atrial septotomy
Rastelli cardiac procedure
Raz sling for urinary incontinence
retropubic prostatectomy
Reverdin-Green osteotomy
Ripstein rectal prolapse repair
Rosomoff cordotomy
SAL (suction-assisted lipectomy)
Salter osteotomy
SASMA facelift
Schepens-Okamura-Brockhurst retinal detachment repair
Schlein elbow arthroplasty
Schuknecht cochleosacculotomy
scleral buckling procedure
sclerouvectomy, partial lamellar
second-look laparotomy
Sever-L'Episcopo shoulder repair
SFA (subclavian flap aortoplasty)
Sharrard kyphectomy
Shepherd lens insertion
Shirodkar cervical cerclage
Shouldice hernia repair
Silastic bead embolization
Skoog release of Dupuytren's contracture
Smead-Jones closure
Soave abdominal pull-through
Southwick osteotomy
STA-MCA bypass (superficial temporary-middle cerebral artery)
Stamey bladder suspension
Stamm gastrostomy
Stanmore shoulder arthroplasty
subclavian flap aortoplasty (SFA)
suction-assisted lipectomy (SAL)

operation *(cont.)*
Sugiura paraesophagogastric devascularization
Swanson PIP joint arthroplasty
Swenson's abdominal pull-through
Syme's amputation of foot
Syme's external urethrotomy
TBT (transcervical balloon tuboplasty)
Teflon paste injection for incontinence
TEM (transanal endoscopic microsurgery)
Tennison-Randall cleft lip repair
Thal esophageal stricture repair
Thiersch-Duplay urethroplasty
Thom flap laryngeal reconstruction
THR (total hip replacement)
Torkildsen shunt ventriculo-cisternostomy
total hip replacement (THR)
trachelotomy
tracheotomy
transanal endoscopic microsurgery (TEM)
transcervical balloon tuboplasty (TBT)
Turner-Warwick urethroplasty
ultrasound transcervical tuboplasty
UPPP (uvulopalatopharyngoplasty)
uvulopalatopharyngoplasty (UPPP)
vaginal interruption of pregnancy, with dilatation and curettage (VIP-DAC)
valvuloplasty
VBG (vertical-banded gastroplasty)
vesicourethral suspension
Vineberg cardiac revascularization
VIP-DAC (vaginal interruption of pregnancy, with dilatation and curettage)
vitrectomy
Waldhausen subclavian flap repair
Wardill palatoplasty

operation *(cont.)*
Warthin-Starry
Watson-Jones ankle fracture repair
Watson-Jones tenodesis
Weir nasal alar excision
Wheeless construction of J rectal pouch
Whipple pancreaticoduodenectomy
Witzel duodenostomy
Wyse reduction mammoplasty
Zancolli clawhand deformity repair
ZIFT (zygote intrafallopian transfer)
Z-plasty, four-flap
zygote intrafallopian transfer (ZIFT)

OPG/CPA—see *oculoplethysmography/ carotid phonoangiography.*

ophthalmodynamometry (Oph)—measures the relative central retinal artery pressures and indirectly assesses carotid artery flow on each side. See *Bailliart's ophthalmodynamometer.*

ophthalmoscope
American Optical (AO)
Keeler indirect
Mascot indirect
Primbs-Circon indirect video
Propper

ophthalmoscopy—allows examination of the interior of the eye after dilation.

OPMI operating microscope (Zeiss).

OPPA (Oncovin, procarbazine, prednisone, Adriamycin)—chemotherapy protocol used to treat Hodgkin's lymphoma.

opportunist—normal body flora usually regarded as harmless in a specific location, that may produce disease in another part of the body or if predisposing factors such as neoplasm, trauma, or a compromised immune system is present.

opportunistic infection; organism—a microorganism that does not ordinar-

opportunistic infection *(cont.)* ily cause disease but becomes pathogenic under certain circumstances (e.g., impaired immune response). Patients with AIDS or who are immunocompromised are giving a new meaning to this term and to our understanding of the immune system. Opportunistic infections are responsible for approximately 90% of AIDS-related deaths.

opposition—act of being opposite, or the state of being set in opposite manner, as "The thumb and index finger could be placed in opposition." Cf. *apposition.*

Opraflex incise drape (Ortho).

OpSite (Surg)—a watertight polyurethane dressing. It adheres to the skin around the wound, but not to the wound itself.

opsonizing antibodies—antibodies that make bacteria susceptible to phagocytes.

Optacon—an electronic device that converts the visual image to vibrations that can be felt with the fingertips, providing reading access to the blind and visually impaired. *Not* Opticon. *Optacon* comes from *op*tical *ta*ctile *con*verter.

Op-Temp cautery.

optic neuritis—inflammation of that portion of the optic nerve that is not ophthalmoscopically visible.

Optiflex intraocular lens.

optimal cutting temperature (OCT).

OptiPranolol (metipranolol).

Optiray (ioversol)—a nonionic contrast medium (Radiol).

Optiscope—a flexible fiberoptic angioscope.

optokinetic nystagmus (OKN).

Optotype—an eye testing device.

OR, O.R. (operating room).

oral—pertaining to the mouth, as in oral intake, oral surgery. Cf. *aural.*

Oramorph SR—sustained release tablets of oral morphine sulfate.

orbital implant—see *Muhlberger.*

orbital rim stepoff—an indication of fracture (and slight displacement). "Examination for fracture revealed no orbital rim stepoff."

Oreopoulos-Zellerman catheter—used for peritoneal dialysis.

organic brain syndrome (OBS).

organism—see *opportunistic organism.*

organizer—see *Suture/VesiBand.*

organ—see *Jacobson's organ.*

organ of Corti (in the cochlea)—contains hair cells, transmitting stimuli to the cochlear branch of cranial nerve VIII (the acoustic, or vestibulocochlear, nerve).

orientation (MRI term)
coronal
sagittal
transverse

oriented times four (oriented x 4). We hear "oriented times three" in every neurological examination, but "times four"? A physician who dictates this on every report says the "fourth dimension" is intention—in response to the question "What are your plans?" or "What are you going to do next?"

oriented times three (oriented x 3) (Neuro). This means that the patient is oriented to person, time, and place.

ORIF (open reduction and internal fixation) (Ortho).

origin of a vessel (Radiol)—the commencement of a vessel as it branches off from a larger vessel.

Orion balloon dilatation catheter (Cardio)—used during cardiac catheterization.

ORLAU swivel walker (Ortho)—orthosis for ambulation in children with cerebral palsy and myelomeningocele. (ORLAU, Orthotic Research and Locomotor Assessment Unit.)

Ormond disease—idiopathic retroperitoneal fibrosis.

Ornidyl (eflornithine).

orphan drug—a drug used to treat a rare disease for which the manufacturer could not expect to recoup drug development and production costs due to the small number of patients who would use the drug. The Orphan Drug Act supports the development of orphan drugs by allowing tax credits to the pharmaceutical company and shortened FDA approval time. Recent orphan drugs include GHB, Imuthiol, LAAM, Vivalan, and Wellferon.

Orr-Loygue transabdominal proctopexy—for complete rectal prolapse.

Orr operation (Surg)—to repair rectal prolapse.

"ortho"—when an ophthalmologist uses *ortho,* it usually refers to *orthophoric* or *orthophoria.*

Orthoclone OKT3 (Oncol)—anti-CD3 monoclonal antibody used to treat acute graft rejection in kidney transplant patients.

Ortho-evac (Ortho)—a postoperative autotransfusion system designed especially for orthopedic use, including knee, hip, and spinal surgery.

Orthofix—external fixator.

OrthoGen/OsteoGen—an implantable stimulator for nonunion of fractures.

Ortholav (Ortho)—lavage and suction equipment for pulsed irrigation and suction. Used with any of these tips:
Ritter double-orifice tip
Ritter single-orifice tip
Yankauer multi-orifice tip
Yankauer single-orifice tip

Ortho-mune—the brand name used by Ortho Diagnostic Systems, Inc., for its line of monoclonal antibodies, which includes OKT4 and OKT8, and many others.

OrthoPak II (Ortho)—a bone growth stimulator with electrodes. The battery-powered OrthoPak II weighs only 4 ounces and can be mounted directly on a cast or carried from a belt clip or in a pocket.

orthopedic hardware (Ortho)—wires, pins, screws, plates, and other devices of metal or other material implanted in or attached to bone in the course of a surgical procedure.

orthophoria—parallelism of the visual axes; the normal muscle balance.

orthoplast jacket—a specially molded jacket used for correction of scoliosis. It is worn for 23 hours a day until skeletal maturity has taken place, or the spine has straightened and the correction can be maintained out of the jacket.

orthopnea, three-pillow; two-pillow—difficulty breathing unless positioned in a semi-sitting position. Often measured roughly by how many pillows the patient needs in order to breathe comfortably while sleeping upright in a semi-sitting position.

orthosis—an orthopedic appliance or apparatus used to correct deformities, to support or improve the function of a joint. See also *prosthesis.*
Types of orthosis:
AFO (ankle-foot)
foot (FO)
Gillette joint
GunSlinger shoulder
HKAFO (hip-knee-ankle-foot)
KAFO (knee-ankle-foot)
LSU reciprocating gait
NuKO knee
Oklahoma ankle joint

orthosis *(cont.)*
ORLAU swivel walker
Rochester HKAFO (hip-knee-ankle-foot)
Select joint
SMO (supramalleolar)
TLSO (thoracolumbosacral)
Toronto parapodium
Viscoheel K
Viscoheel N
Viscoheel SofSpot

OrthoSorb absorbable fixation pins (Pod)—especially for use in hallux valgus and hammer toe surgery.

orthotopic transplantation—transplantation of an organ and placing it in the recipient in its normal anatomic position.

Ortolani's sign (Ortho)—a click at the hip joint, in congenital dislocated hip.

O.S. *(oculus sinister,* left eye).

OSA (obstructive sleep apnea).

oscillating saw (Neuro).

Osher intraocular implant lens (Oph).

OS-5/Plus, OS-5/Plus 2 brace (Ortho)—noncustom multifunctional knee brace for postoperative and rehabilitation applications. Made by Omni Scientific (OS).

Osler's nodes—small tender nodules (2 to 5 mm in diameter) seen about the tips of the fingers or toes; may be found in patients with bacterial endocarditis, acute and subacute.

osmolality—a test of concentration of a solution. It is used to determine the concentration of urine or serum, and results are expressed in milliosmoles per kilogram (mOsm/kg). Cf. *osmolarity.*

osmolarity—concentration of an osmotic solution, e.g., urine or blood serum; expressed in osmoles per liter (Osm/l). Cf. *osmolality.*

Osmolite enteral feedings.

osseous—bony.

Ossoff-Karlen laryngoscope (ENT).

osteal—bone (osseous). Cf. *ostial.*

osteoarthritis radiographic grading
grade I—small osteophytes.
grade II—osteophytes without joint space impairment.
grade III—osteophytes with moderate loss of normal joint space.
grade IV—osteophytes with significant loss of joint space and sclerosis of subchondral bone.
grade V—grade IV with subluxation.

osteochondritis dissecans *(not* dessicans). See *König disease.*

Osteonics hip prosthesis.

osteophytes—see *bridging osteophytes.*

Osteo-Stim—implantable bone growth stimulator.

osteotomy
chevron
closing base wedge (CBWO)
Dwyer
Giennestras step-down modified
Keck and Kelly
Mitchell distal
Obwegeser's sagittal mandibular
Reverdin-Green
Salter
Southwick

ostial—pertaining to an ostium (an opening). Cf. *osteal.*

ostium—an opening; an opening into a tubular organ.

OTC drug (over-the-counter).

OTFC (oral transmucosal fentanyl citrate)—fentanyl now available in a candy-like oral tablet (to be sucked); to relieve severe pain in pediatric patients.

otoplasty—see *Crikelair.*

otospongiosis/otosclerosis syndrome (ENT)—a type of genetic deafness.

otospongiosis *(cont.)*
Treatment with sodium fluoride in very low doses is a promising therapy where there is early detection of this syndrome.

Ototemp 3000 (ENT)—measures core body temperature by reading the temperature of the tympanic membrane, without actually touching the membrane, giving an accurate reading in five seconds.

ototoxic—anything harmful to the structures or process of hearing, such as some drugs causing tinnitus, extremely loud noises (or music), etc. "She denied the use of ototoxic drugs and has no history of ear trauma or recurrent infections." Aminoglycoside antibiotics are well known for their ototoxic side effects.

outlet view (Radiol)—an x-ray showing a tangential view of the coracoacromial arch in the sagittal plane of the scapula.

output, insensible fluid—see *insensible fluid output.*

O.U. (*oculus uterque,* each eye).

Ouchterlony double diffusion technique. Usage: "Circulating immune complexes, C3, hemolytic complement, and precipitating antibodies by Ouchterlony are pending."

Outerbridge's ridge (named for R. E. Outerbridge, M.D., British Columbia, Canada)—a ridge of varying height, crossing the medial femoral condyle at its osteochondral junction, described by Outerbridge in 1961. He suggested that at least one cause of patellar chondromalacia might be friction against the medial patellar facet cartilage as the patella rides this ridge in normal movement of the knee. See *Outerbridge scale.*

Outerbridge scale for assessing joint damage or articular surface damage in chondromalacia patellae:
grade 1—softening and swelling of the cartilage
grade 2—fragmentation and fissuring in an area half an inch or less in diameter
grade 3—same as grade 2, but an area more than half an inch is involved
grade 4—erosion of cartilage down to bone

oval window (ENT). See *vestibular window.*

overshooting—failure to stop a voluntary movement when its goal or purpose has been achieved.

over-the-counter drug (OTC) —generally considered safe for consumers to use (as determined by the FDA) if the label directions and warnings are properly followed. Available without a prescription.

OV-1 surgical keratometer (Oph) (mfr. by OV, Ophthalmic Ventures).

OvuStick—a urinary dipstick used to detect luteinizing hormone (LH) surge in infertility patients.

Owen's view.

ox cell hemolysin test.

oxandrolone (Oxandrin)—an anabolic steroid used to treat growth disorders in boys; also used for muscle wasting and weakness in AIDS patients.

oxiconazole (Oxistat)—a topical antifungal agent for athlete's foot and ringworm.

oximeter—a photoelectric device that measures the oxygen saturation of the blood. "Oxygen saturation was monitored by ear or finger oximeter." Used in assessing sleep disorders by polysomnogram.

oxothiazolidine carboxylate (Procysteine).

Oxsoralen (methoxsalen).

oxygen
blow-by
hyperbaric
T-piece

oxygen cisternography—technique of choice by some neurosurgeons and otolaryngologists for the diagnosis of acoustic tumors. In some cases where air will not enter the internal auditory canal, Pantopaque introduced into the posterior fossa for cisternography would be the technique used.

oxymetholone (Adroyd, Anadrol-50, HMD)—used to treat anemias resulting from treatment with chemotherapy drugs.

Oxymizer (Pulm)—oxygen-conserving device used to provide adequate oxygen saturation at lower flow rates. Permits a portable oxygen source to last longer, thus permitting patients to be away from their primary oxygen source for longer periods.

oxyphil cell.

oxytocin challenge test (OCT).

Oxytrak pulse oximeter and Dinamap blood pressure monitor—to measure oxygen saturation.

P, p

p—If you can't find a word anywhere, try looking in the *p*'s in a dictionary; so often the *p* is silent, as in *psoas, psoriasis, psyllium, pterygium, pterygoid, ptosis.*

Pa (pascal). See *pascal.*

PAB-Esc-C (Platinol, Adriamycin, bleomycin, escalating doses of Cytoxan)—chemotherapy protocol.

PAC (papular acrodermatitis of childhood). Cf. *Gianotti-Crosti syndrome.*

PACE (Platinol, Adriamycin, Cytoxan, etoposide)—chemotherapy protocol.

Pacesetter Synchrony pacemaker—a permanent rate-responsive dual-chamber pacemaker.

pacemaker
- Activitrax
- Arco
- Autima II dual-chamber cardiac
- Chardack-Greatbatch implantable cardiac pulse generator
- Command PS
- Cordis Gemini cardiac
- Cordis Sequicor cardiac
- Chorus DDD
- Cyberlith
- Elite dual-chamber

pacemaker *(cont.)*
- Elite dual-chamber rate responsive
- Ergos O_2
- escape
- Medtronic temporary
- Micro Minix
- Pacesetter Synchrony
- Pasar tachycardia reversion
- Spectrax programmable Medtronic
- Triumph VR
- Versatrax cardiac

pacemaker code system (Cardio). A three-letter code is often used to describe various types of pacemakers. The first letter represents the chamber of the heart which is stimulated to contract (i.e., paced) by an attached electrode. The second letter represents the chamber(s) in which the pacemaker can sense ongoing normal electrical activity. The third letter indicates the type of response (i.e., mode) of which the pacemaker is capable (inhibited from competing with normal heart contractions, triggered by abnormal heart activity). Example: A DDD pacemaker serves the electrical activity of both the

pacemaker *(cont.)*
atrium and ventricle, paces (stimulates) both the atrium and ventricle to beat, and may cause (trigger) the atrium to contract while sending no signal (inhibited) to the ventricle depending on what natural electrical activity is occurring in the heart at that time.

Pacing	Sensing	Mode of Response
A Atrium	A Atrium	I Inhibited
V Ventricle	V Ventricle	T Triggered
D Both	D Both	D Atrial triggered but ventricular inhibited
0 None	0 None	0 None

pachometer—an instrument that measures the thickness of the cornea.

pacing system, PASYS.

Packo pars plana cannula (Oph).

pack-year smoking history, as "The patient has a 50-pack-year smoking history." This means the patient has smoked a pack a day for 50 years, or two packs a day for 25 years, or five packs a day for ten years (or ten packs a day for five years!). It is the packs per day multiplied by the number of years of smoking; the cumulative result is the important factor.

PACU (postanesthesia care unit)—a newer name for the recovery room.

Padgett Concorde suction cannula.

Padgett dermatome (Plas Surg)—a drum-type dermatome.

Padgett shark-mouth cannula.

Paecilomyces variotii—a fungus which is an infrequent human pathogen. It has caused complications associated with prosthetic cardiac valves, synthetic lens implants, and cerebrospinal fluid shunts.

PAFD (percutaneous abscess and fluid drainage).

PAG matter (Neuro)—stimulation of the periaqueductal gray (PAG) matter with deep brain electrodes inhibits pain. Cf. *PVG matter.*

PAH acid (para-aminohippuric)—used in kidney function test. See *Stamey test.*

PAIgG (platelet-associated IgG).

painter's encephalopathy (Neuro)—a chronic organic brain syndrome secondary to exposure to fumes from some types of paints.

Palacos cement (Ortho).

palatoplasty—see *Wardill palatoplasty.*

palisading (Path)—a lining up of cells such that their long axis is perpendicular to some other structure. E.g., *peripheral palisading.*

palladium-103 (^{103}Pd) (Rad Oncol)—an isotope used in brachytherapy.

palmar erythema (erythema palmare) —redness of the palms that persists; it may be seen in patients with liver disease, rheumatoid arthritis, and a number of other diverse medical problems.

Palmaz vascular stent (Cardio)—a cylinder of stainless steel mesh. This stent is placed over a balloon catheter and inserted into an occluded artery after angioplasty is performed. The balloon is inflated once the catheter is positioned at the site of the occlusion. The balloon is then deflated, but the stent retains its expanded shape and remains permanently at the site of the occlusion, holding the vessel walls apart and facilitating blood flow. Also, Palmaz-Schatz stent.

palmomental—refers to the palm of the hand and the mentalis muscle. See *palmomental reflex.*

palmomental reflex—contraction of the ipsilateral mentalis and orbicularis oris muscles, with slight elevation and retraction of the angle of the mouth in response to scratching the thenar area of the hand; seen occasionally in an exaggerated form in patients with corticospinal tract lesions. Also called palmomental reflex of Marinesco-Radovici.

palpation—the act of feeling with the fingers in examination of the body. Inspection, palpation, and auscultation are the three methods of examination used most. Cf. *palpitation, papillation.*

palpitation—the subjective feeling of an irregular or abnormally rapid heart beat. Cf. *palpation, papillation.*

palsy—see *tardy palsy.*

Palumbo knee brace (Ortho)—custom-fitted knee brace used with chondromalacia patellae.

PAM (potential acuity meter)—used in testing vision (Oph).

pamidronate disodium (Aredia) (Oncol)—this drug is used to decrease the hypercalcemia associated with malignancy. Also known as disodium pamidronate.

PAN (periodic alternating nystagmus).

pancreatic polypeptide (PP). See *PP.*

pan-cultured, as in "The urine was pan-cultured." The specimen is cultured to determine which, of many, organisms is present; and to determine which, of many, antibiotics is a specific for that organism. The prefix *pan* means *all, every.*

P&K (Polaroids and Kodachromes) (Path)—photographs of specimens. "P&K were taken," or "Polaroids and Kodachromes were taken."

pan-sensitive—sensitive to everything.

Panje voice button ("pan-gee") (ENT)—a laryngeal prosthesis used to improve esophageal speech in patients who have had laryngectomies. See *Blom-Singer valve,* a similar prosthetic device.

panniculus, hanging. See *apron.*

pantaloon embolus. See *saddle embolus.*

pants-over-vest repair.

papilla, optic—point at which the optic nerve fibers leave the eyeball. Also called optic disk.

PAP (peroxidase-antiperoxidase)—see *immunoperoxidase stain.*

papillation—the presence of small projections or elevations (as the papillae on the tongue). Cf. *palpation, palpitation.*

papilledema—swelling of the nerve head from increased intracranial pressure or interference with the venous return from the eye.

papillotome—see *Swenson papillotome.*

papova—an acronym for a group of DNA viruses thought to cause warts in humans. (See *HPV.*) Comes from the first two letters of the names of the viruses:

pa papilloma virus
po polyoma virus
va vacuolative virus

papular acrodermatitis of childhood (PAC).

PAPVR (partial anomalous pulmonary venous return).

para—the number of times a woman has given birth. This word is frequently followed by four numbers (for example, para 3-1-0-3). The first numeral refers to the number of full-term deliveries, in this case three; the second indicates the number of premature births (one); the third numeral is the

para *(cont.)*
number of abortions or miscarriages (none); the fourth numeral indicates the number of living children (three).

para-aminohippuric (PAH).

paradoxus—see *pulsus paradoxus.*

parafascicular thalamotomy (PFT).

paraffin block; section (Path)—tissue embedded in paraffin for sectioning and subsequent staining for microscopy. See *permanent section.*

Paragon immunofixation electrophoresis (Lab).

parallel plate dialyzer. See *hemodialyzer.*

paralysis
Benedikt's ipsilateral oculomotor
rucksack

parameter—one of a number of ways to test, describe, or evaluate a person or an object. Cf. *perimeter.*

parameters—see *pharmacokinetic parameters.*

Paraplatin (carboplatin)—chemotherapy drug.

parathormone (parathyroid hormone, PTH).

parenteral—a route of drug administration not involving the gastrointestinal tract, i.e., intravenous, intramuscular, etc. Cf. *enteral.*

paresthetica—see *meralgia.*

Parham bands (Ortho)—used to hold the fracture fragments of long bones securely in place.

Parinaud's syndrome (Neuro)—paralysis of convergence and vertical gaze (usually upward gaze), and with unequal pupillary reaction to light. There may also be lesions of the third and fourth cranial nerves.

parity—a woman's reproductive history.

Park blade septostomy (Cardio).

Parker-Kerr closed method—of end-to-end enteroenterostomy.

Parker-Kerr intestinal clamps (GI).

Park-Maumenee lid speculum.

Parona's space—the tissue plane over the pronator quadratus in the distal forearm that is deep to the ulnar and radial bursae.

paroxetine (Paxil) (Psych)—a 5HT (serotonin) receptor blocker which inhibits the reuptake of serotonin and increases levels of it. Used to treat depression which is caused by low levels of serotonin.

paroxysmal atrial tachycardia (PAT) (Cardio).

paroxysmal nocturnal hemoglobinuria (PNH).

paroxysmal supraventricular tachycardia (PSVT) (Cardio).

Parrot's sign—dilation of the pupils when the skin of the neck is pinched, as in meningitis (Neuro).

partial agonist—a compound that possesses both agonist and antagonist properties.

partial anomalous pulmonary venous return (PAPVR) (Cardio).

partial saturation technique (Radiol)—a magnetic resonance technique in which single excitation pulses are delivered to tissue at intervals equal to or shorter than T1.

particle, polyvinyl alcohol (PVA).

Partipilo gastrostomy.

party wall—a wall between two contiguous structures.

PASA (proximal articular set angle) (Ortho).

Pasar tachycardia reversion pacemaker (Cardio).

pascal (Pa)—unit of measurement in the SI system; it measures pressure. You will be hearing about this in relation

pascal *(cont.)*
to blood gases. Blood pressures will most probably continue to be given in the form which we are now accustomed to. See *SI, International System.*

P.A.S. port—a peripheral access system port implanted in the antecubital fossa for administration of chemotherapy drugs, for long-term TPN, or for administration of intravenous antibiotics. Also made with double lumens.

P.A.S. Port Fluoro-Free—implantable peripheral access system that incorporates the Cath-Finder catheter tracking system that tracks the catheter tip during placement without the use of fluoroscopy.

Passage catheter (GI)—a balloon catheter used to dilate biliary strictures. Passage is a trade name.

PAS stain—periodic acid-Schiff test for collagen disease. This stain is also a test for the presence of Whipple's disease. See *Whipple's disease.*

Passy-Muir tracheostomy speaking valve (Pulm)—an attachment that allows ventilator-dependent patients to speak more easily.

past-pointing (Neuro) (*not* passed pointing)—a test used to determine the presence of incoordination in voluntary movements. When the patient is asked to touch the examiner's finger or nose, or his own nose, he goes *past* it. A variant of this test is used in otolaryngology to test for vestibular problems.

PASYS ("paces")—a single chamber cardiac **pa**cing **sys**tem (Cardio).

PAT (paroxysmal atrial tachycardia) (Cardio).

patches, Peyer's—see *Peyer's patches.*

patella alta—a "high-riding" patella, associated with some knee problems (Ortho).

Patella disease—pyloric stenosis occurring in tuberculous patients after fibrous stenosis. Named for an Italian physician, V. Patella.

patellar apprehension test (Ortho).

patellaplasty (*not* patelloplasty) (Ortho).

Pathfinder DFA test (Ob-Gyn)—used to detect genital *Chlamydia trachomatis.* (DFA, direct fluorescent antigen.)

pathognomonic—characteristic or diagnostic of a particular disease.

patient-controlled analgesic (PAS) **system.**

Patil stereotaxic system—for biopsy, hematoma evacuation, angiographic targeting, epilepsy implants, stereotaxic craniotomy.

pattern
Christmas tree
crosshatch
echo
fishbone
signet-ring
sine-wave
starry-sky
Wolfe mammographic parenchymal

patty, cottonoid. Also *paddy,* but *patty* seems to be the preferred spelling.

paucity—deficiency, shortage. "There is a paucity of objective findings, so we will have to undertake further laboratory tests before we can make a diagnosis in this patient."

Paufique knife (Oph).

PAVe (Oncol)—a standard chemotherapy protocol used to treat adult Hodgkin's disease. Consists of the drugs procarbazine, melphalan, and vinblastine.

paving stone degeneration—an atrophic condition in which sharply outlined, rounded lesions appear in the peripheral retina. Also, cobblestone degeneration.

Pavlik harness—used to correct congenital hip dysplasia in infants under six months of age.

PAWP (pulmonary artery wedge pressure).

Paxil (paroxetine).

PBLs (peripheral blood lymphocytes).

PBPI (penile brachial pressure index)—Doppler study of blood flow in the penile arteries to assess cardiovascular disease. A value of 0.65 or less indicates possibility of impending myocardial infarction or stroke.

PBV—see *percutaneous balloon valvuloplasty.*

PCA knee prosthesis (porous-coated anatomic) (Ortho)—a cementless implant that permits biologic union between the implant and the bone which infiltrates into the textured surface of the prosthesis.

PCA system (patient-controlled analgesic)—to administer analgesics as needed. Several manufacturers are marketing a portable computerized pump with a chamber that holds a prefilled syringe. The physician programs the pump and determines the total amount of the drug that the patient can receive over a given period of time and the amount of each dose. When the patient is in pain, he can push a button on a cord attached to the pump; the pump then dispenses (like a coffee vending machine) a small dose of the medication into the patient's I.V. line. The patient is quite likely to need less medication this way because he feels in control and therefore less anxious and less tense than when waiting for someone to dispense the medication.

PCBS (percutaneous cardiopulmonary bypass support).

PCCL (percutaneous cholecystolithotomy).

PCE (Platinol, Cytoxan, etoposide)—chemotherapy protocol used to treat small-cell carcinoma of the lung.

PC-IOL (Oph)—posterior chamber intraocular lens.

PCNL (percutaneous nephrostolithotomy)—uses ultrasound waves to disintegrate kidney stones.

PCO (polycystic ovary).

PCP (phencyclidine)—a street drug.

PCP (*Pneumocystis carinii* pneumonia).

PCR technique (polymerase chain reaction)—to detect DNA provirus in HIV and other diseases. Also used in the diagnosis of Lyme disease, for it picks up the Lyme antigen

PC-7 needle (Oph)—a curved needle used during intraocular lens procedures.

PCTCL (percutaneous transhepatic cholecystolithotomy).

PCV (procarbazine, CCNU, vincristine)—chemotherapy protocol used to treat anaplastic astrocytoma.

PCW (pulmonary capillary wedge).

PD (peritoneal dialysis).

PDS (pancreatic duct sphincter).

PDS (polydioxanone suture).

PDT (photodynamic therapy)—a colloquial term for laser surgery.

peak-and-trough levels—maximum and minimum blood levels of a therapeutic agent, determined by drawing blood at strategic intervals after administration. This method provides

peak-and-trough *(cont.)* more precise information than doing random blood levels and is particularly useful with drugs having a narrow margin between effective and toxic levels. "The following studies were considered: blood urea nitrogen (BUN), creatinine clearance, two urinalyses, and three drug assays—one peak-and-trough level each, initially, and a repeat trough level at the end of seven days."

peak flow—see *Wright peak flow.*

peakometer—used in testing the peak flow of the urinary bladder.

peanut—operating room slang for a small sponge.

Pearce nucleus hydrodissector (Oph)—used during cataract surgery.

Pearce trabeculectomy (Oph)—a type of glaucoma surgery in which trabecular meshwork is excised.

Pearce Tripod implant cataract lens.

peau d'orange ("po-do-rahnj"') (Fr., orange peel)—a dimpled appearance of the skin due to interstitial edema and particularly seen in breast cancer.

PEB (Platinol, etoposide, bleomycin)—chemotherapy protocol used to treat malignant germ cell tumor.

pectus excavatum—depression of the sternum. *(Not* pectus excur**v**atum.)

Pedi PEG tube (GI)—a percutaneous endoscopic gastrostomy tube.

peel-away sheath. See *Littleford/Spector introducer.*

PEEP ("peep")—positive end-expiratory pressure.

PEFR (peak expiratory flow rate)—a pulmonary function test.

PEG-ADA—see *pegademase bovine.*

pegademase bovine (PEG-ADA, Adagen, Imudon)—used to treat a rare congenital genetic disorder known as severe combined immunodeficiency disease (SCID) or bubble boy disease, in which the patient is missing the enzyme adenosine deaminase (ADA). Bone marrow transplantation is an alternative treatment that is not always successful. Pegademase replaces the missing ADA enzyme and allows the immune system to produce antibodies in patients who are not candidates for a bone marrow transplant. The term *bovine* refers to the source of the drug—cows. The drug is specially treated to reduce the risk of allergic reactions to this heterologous product.

PEG interleukin-2 (PEG IL-2)—drug used to treat AIDS patients.

PEG tube (percutaneous endoscopic gastrostomy) (GI)—the preferred method for patients who need long-term enteral feedings.

Pelger-Huët cells—seen in acute myelogenous leukemia.

pelgeroid—refers to Pelger-Huët nuclear anomaly of neutrophils and eosinophils.

peliosis hepatis—a rare liver disease which is found in HIV-positive individuals more often now, as more physicians look for it.

Pelizaeus-Merzbacher disease—familial disease of the myelin sheath.

PEMF therapy (pulsed electromagnetic field) (Ortho)—used in treatment of nonunion of bone secondary to trauma.

pencil

Handtrol electrosurgical
Wallach

Penderluft syndrome—a disturbance in air exchange in which the diaphragm is out of synchronization with inhalation and expiration.

Penetrax—see *enoxacin.*

Penicillium—one of the molds most prevalent in damp interior areas. See also *Aspergillus.*

penicilloylpolylysine (PPL, Pre-Pan)—used in skin testing. See *PPL.*

penile brachial pressure index (PBPI).

Pennig dynamic wrist fixator (Ortho)—used to treat distal radius fractures while allowing for use of the hand.

Pennington clamp.

pentagastrin stimulated analysis.

pentalogy, Fallot's—tetralogy of Fallot plus atrial septal defect.

Pentam 300—trade name for *pentamidine.*

pentamidine isethionate (Pentam 300)—an antiprotozoal agent used against *Pneumocystis carinii* pneumonia.

pentamidine isethionate, aerosolized (Aeropent, NebuPent, Pneumopent)—inhaled to prevent *Pneumocystis carinii* pneumonia in AIDS patients.

Peptamen (GI)—a liquid, complete isotonic elemental diet that can be used full strength from the initial feeding.

Pentax flexible sigmoidoscope.

peptide T (Neuro)—a drug used to treat the neurological symptoms of patients with AIDS.

PercuCut cut-biopsy needles (Radiol)—used in soft tissue biopsies.

Percuflex stent (GI)—a flexible biliary stent.

PercuGuide (Radiol)—used in diagnostic radiology for precise localization of nonpalpable lesions.

percussion (Resp Ther)—a rhythmic clapping with cupped hands on the patient's chest and back to loosen pulmonary secretions so they can be coughed up or suctioned out.

percutaneous abscess and fluid drainage (PAFD).

percutaneous automated diskectomy—a procedure which uses a 2 mm suction cutting probe into the disk under fluoroscopy; performed under local anesthesia (Ortho, Neuro).

percutaneous balloon valvuloplasty (PBV)—a balloon is used to dilate a calcified or stenotic heart valve.

percutaneous cardiopulmonary bypass support (PCBS) (Cardio)—used to support patients following cardiac arrest, or used prophylactically for high-risk patients having cardiac catheterization or PTCA.

percutaneous endoscopic gastrostomy (PEG).

percutaneous interosseous nerve (PIN).

percutaneous mitral balloon valvotomy (PMBV).

percutaneous nephrostolithotomy (PCNL)—uses ultrasound waves to disintegrate kidney stones.

percutaneous transluminal angioplasty (PTA).

percutaneous transluminal renal angioplasty (PTRA).

percutaneous transperineal seed implantation (Urol)—a procedure to radiate prostatic cancer locally. Small seeds of ^{15}iodine or ^{103}palladium radioactive material are inserted into prostatic tissue. The procedure is cost-effective and avoids systemic radiation effects.

Pereyra needle (Urol)—a single-prong ligature carrier for use in bladder neck suspension.

perfluoropropane (C_3F_8 gas).

perforator—see *Acra-Cut cranial.*

perfusion—pouring a fluid over an organ or tissue, or through vessels of an organ; used in kidney and heart

perfusion *(cont.)* surgery, and organ transplantation. Cf. *profusion.*

Pergamid (4-HC).

periaqueductal gray electrode—not a proper name; refers to the gray matter (Neuro).

peribronchial cuffing (Radiol)—thickening of bronchial walls by fibrosis, as seen in asthma, emphysema, and other chronic respiratory disorders.

pericardial baffle (Cardio).

pericardium—the fibrous sac surrounding the heart and roots of the great vessels. Cf. *precordium.*

Peridex mouthwash (Oncol)—used to reduce oral mucositis in patients receiving chemotherapy.

perilymphatic fistula (PLF).

perimeter—circumference, edge. Cf. *parameter.*

perineal—refers to the perineum (the area between the scrotum and the anus in the male, and between the vulva and the anus in the female). Cf. *peritoneal, peroneal.*

perineurium—area surrounding nerves; fibrous connective tissue.

periodic acid-Schiff test (PAS stain)—a test for collagen or for presence of Whipple's disease.

periodic lateralized epileptiform discharges (PLEDS)—found in electroencephalograms.

peripheral access system port (P.A.S.)—this implantable port is positioned subcutaneously in the antecubital area of the arm.

peripheral blood lymphocytes (PBLs).

peripheral laser angioplasty (PLA).

peripherally inserted central catheter (PICC).

peripheral vascular disease, arteriosclerotic (Cardio).

peristaltic wave (Radiol)—a wave of muscular contractions passing along a tubular organ (such as the intestine), by which its contents are advanced.

peritomy—an incision of the conjunctiva and the subconjunctival tissues, going around the entire corneal circumference; used in cataract extractions, retinal detachment procedures and in the performance of an enucleation. *Not* peridomy or peridimy.

peritoneal—refers to the peritoneum, the serous membrane lining the abdominal and pelvic cavities. Cf. *perineal, peroneal.*

peritoneal dialysis (PD).

peritoneal mouse—a free body sometimes seen on x-ray in the peritoneal cavity.

peritonealize—to cover with peritoneum. Also, see *peritonize.*

peritoneum—serous membrane lining the abdomen.

peritonize—to cover with peritoneum. See *peritonealize.*

PERK protocol (prospective evaluation of radial keratotomy)—for correction of myopia.

Perkins Brailler—a braille embosser.

Perkins tonometer (Oph)—a hand-held instrument to measure intraocular pressure.

perlèche—another term for cheilitis, or dryness and cracking around the mouth, from repeated licking or from a *Candida* infection.

Perlia, nucleus of.

Perlon suture (size 10-0)—a very fine suture used in eye surgery.

Perma-Hand braided silk suture (Ethicon). See *suture.*

permanent lead introducer. See *Littleford/Spector introducer.*

permanent section (also, paraffin section; paraffin block)—technique in which tissue removed during an operation is embedded in paraffin for microscopic examination of the pathology present. This takes more time than frozen section but has certain advantages in that the specimen is permanent and not deteriorating, as in frozen section. See *frozen section.*

peroneal—refers to the fibula or to the outer side of the leg and the muscles thereof—the peroneus longus and the peroneus brevis. Cf. *perineal, peritoneal.*

peroxidase-antiperoxidase (PAP).

per primam *(not* primum)—first intention; primary union; healing directly, without granulation; the incision closes in minimal time, with no complications and with little resulting scar tissue.

persistent hyperplastic primary vitreous (PHPV).

persistent vegetative state (PVS).

person with AIDS (PWA)—term preferred over "AIDS victim" in AIDS self-help and awareness groups.

pertechnetate sodium (technetium solution) used as a diagnostic aid. See *technetium.*

PET scanning (positron emission tomography). There is some evidence that deoxyglucose on PET scanning can distinguish tumor from necrosis.

petechia (pl., petechiae)—tiny, pinpoint round red spot caused by intradermal or submucous hemorrhage.

petit pas ("petty-pah") (Fr., small step) gait, as in "His gait was petit pas, but was otherwise normal" (Neuro).

Peutz-Jeghers syndrome—familial gastrointestinal polyposis, particularly in the small bowel, with mucocutaneous pigmentation.

Peyer's patches (rhymes with *flyers*)—elevated areas of closely packed lymphoid nodules on the mucosa of the small intestine.

Peyman-Green vitreous forceps.

Peyman vitrector (Oph)—used in cataract extraction.

Pfeiffer-Comberg method (Oph)—radiographically locating a foreign body in the eye.

PF nucleus (parafascicular) (Neuro).

Pfister stone basket (Urol).

PFT (parafascicular thalamotomy) (Neuro).

PFTE shunt (polyfluorotetraethylene) (Urol).

PG (percutaneous gastrostomy) (GI)—a radiologic alternative to surgical and endoscopic gastrostomy. See *PGE.*

PGE (percutaneous gastroenterostomy) (GI)—insertion of a tube into the small bowel, rather than just into the stomach. PG and PGE are used to permit feeding into the stomach, duodenum, or jejunum, and for decompression of a gastric outlet obstruction, or for chronic obstruction of the small bowel. PG and PGE are also used in feeding patients with strokes, with malignancies of the esophagus, and in management of patients with burns or severe trauma.

P-glycoprotein—also known as P-170 glycoprotein (Oncol), this substance is present in some types of cancer cells. When present, it enables those cells to expel chemotherapy drugs and resist their cytotoxic effects. Patients with cancers with P-glycoprotein positive cells (leukemia, multiple myeloma, non-Hodgkin's lymphoma, and renal cell carcinoma) respond poorly to chemotherapy regimens. The P-glycoprotein efflux mechanism has been found to be inactivated by certain calcium channel

P-glycoprotein *(cont.)* blocking drugs which allow the chemotherapy agent to enter the cancer cell and be more effectively cytotoxic. See *calcium channel blockers.*

PgR (progesterone receptor).

pH—the measure of the relative balance between the acids and bases in a system. It has to do with the hydrogen ions in solutions, such as urine or serum. The normal pH of arterial blood is between 7.35 and 7.45. A pH below 7.0 or greater than 7.8 is not compatible with life. See *intracellular pH (pHi).*

PHA (phytohemagglutinin antigen)—a skin test for cellular-based immunity (not antibodies).

phacoemulsification, Kelman.

Phaco-Emulsifier—aspirator used in cataract extractions

PhacoFlex lens (Oph)—see *SingleStitch PhacoFlex lens.*

phage typing of organisms.

phagocyte—"eating cell"; a cell which consumes other cells or foreign material.

phakofragmatome, Girard.

Phalen's maneuver—to determine presence of carpal tunnel syndrome. See *Phalen's sign.*

Phalen's sign; test (*not* Phelan)—in carpal tunnel syndrome. Phalen's sign is present when paresthesias are produced or are exaggerated when the wrist is held in complete flexion for 30 seconds, which presses the median nerve against the upper edge of the transverse carpal ligament.

phantom limb pain—pain felt by the patient in an already-amputated limb, as though the limb were still there.

pharmacokinetic parameters.

phase image—MRI term. See *phased array study.*

phased array study—an inaccurate term for a phase image, which is a form of gated blood pool study, especially processed so that a little more information is obtained from it. See *gated blood (pool) cardiac.*

phase sensitive detector—MRI term.

phenomenon
Arias-Stella
Bell's
dawn
extinction
fern
Gallavardin
Koebner (koebnerization)
Monday crust
R on T
Uhtoff's

phenotype
Cellano
McLeod

pheromones—sexual odors which play an important part in insect, mammalian, and perhaps human reproductive behavior.

pHi (intracellular pH).

Philadelphia chromosome (Ph^1) is a translocation from chromosome number 22 to chromosome number 9. The Philadelphia chromosome is found in the adult form of chronic myeloid leukemia. "A bone biopsy will be done, with Philadelphia chromosome cytogenic analysis."

Philips ultrasound machines—endovaginal and endorectal transducers (Gyn).

phlyctenule ("flick-ten'-yule") (Oph)—a small nodular lesion found at the edge of the cornea; thought to be a cause of neovascularization.

PHNO (4-propyl-9-hydroxynaphthoxazine) (Neuro)—a drug, similar in action to Sinemet, which is used to treat Parkinson's disease.

phonocardiography—noninvasive cardiac diagnostic procedure which tests the occurrence, timing, and duration of the various sounds in the cardiac cycle, determines the frequency (cycles per second) and intensity (amplitude), and can demonstrate murmurs in low frequencies that can be missed by the ear.

Phoropter *(not* Foreopter)—American Optical Company's refractor.

phosphatidylglycerol levels (Neonat)—present with pulmonary maturity in a premature infant; levels decrease with lung maturity.

phosphonoformate, trisodium (PFA, foscarnet, Foscavir)— a drug used to treat AIDS.

photic stimulation—flashing light stimulation, used in electroencephalographic testing.

photocoagulation
Ialo
proliferative retinopathy (PRP)
xenon arc

photodynamic therapy (PDT)—colloquial term for laser surgery.

photometer—see *HemoCue photometer.*

photomotogram—timed Achilles tendon reflex (Neuro).

photon densitometry. See *Norland-Cameron photon densitometry.*

photopenic area—a coined word for the light area on a film or scan.

photophobia—unusual intolerance of light.

photophoresis—treatment used for cutaneous T-cell lymphoma, a rare immune system cancer (Derm). The patient is given doses of psoralen (a light-activated drug) orally. The patient is attached to a device that takes blood from one arm, separates the white cells from the red, and then exposes the white cells to a kind of ultraviolet light. The light-activated psoralen damages the cancerous white cells, which are then reinfused into the patient's other arm. After a few days, the cancerous white cells die. The treatment is repeated at intervals, and over a period of time the patient's immune system will be able to overcome the remaining infected white blood cells. See *psoralen.*

photopsia (Oph)—subjective sensation of sparks or flashes of light in retinal or optic diseases.

PHPV (persistent hyperplastic primary vitreous) (Oph).

PHRT (procarbazine, hydroxyurea, radiotherapy) protocol.

phthisis bulbi (''ty-sis'')—shrinkage and wasting of the eyeball.

Phynox cobalt alloy clip (Neuro).

physostigmine—used in treatment of Alzheimer's disease.

phthisis (''tie-sis'')—a wasting of part of the body. Cf. *ptosis.*

phytohemagglutinin antigen (PHA)—a plant product used for testing human T-cell response. An absent PHA response indicates an abnormally functioning T-cell system.

PIA (Platinol, ifosfamide, Adriamycin)—a chemotherapy protocol.

PIC (peripherally inserted catheter)—intravenous catheter for long-term venous access in patients cared for at home or in nursing homes.

PICA (posterior inferior communicating artery). Cf. *pica.*

pica—eating of materials not usually considered edible or nourishing (e.g., starch, dirt, clay, paint), usually by pregnant women or malnourished children. Cf. *PICA.*

PICC (peripherally inserted central catheter) (Cardio)—inserted into the

PICC *(cont.)* cephalic or basilic vein in the arm and threaded into the superior vena cava. Made of silicone rubber (which is soft, flexible, durable, and reduces the risk of thrombosis).

Pick inclusion body—in Pick's disease.

Picket Fence leg positioner (Ortho).

picornavirus—extremely small, ether-resistant RNA virus, one of the group comprising the enteroviruses and the rhinoviruses.

picture element (pixel)—MRI term.

Pierre Robin syndrome ("pe-air ro-ban")—consisting of brachygnathia and cleft palate, giving a rather bird-like appearance; may also include displacement of the larynx backward and upward, and may produce feeding problems because sucking and swallowing are difficult. Often associated with glossoptosis. Cf. *Robin's syndrome; micrognathia-glossoptosis syndrome.*

Pierse corneal forceps (Oph).

Piezolith EPL—see *EPL.*

piggyback, piggybacking—a method by which more than one solution, and medication, can be infused simultaneously by introducing additional intravenous lines to the main solution line.

piggyback probe.

pigskin (Surg, Plas Surg), as in pigskin graft. See *porcine xenografts.*

pigtail catheter.

PIH (pregnancy-induced hypertension).

Pilagan (pilocarpine nitrate) (Oph)—used for control of intraocular pressure in glaucoma.

Pillet hand prosthesis (Hand Surg).

pillion fracture (Ortho). Caused by a severe blow to the knee, it is a T-shaped fracture involving the distal femur, and posterior displacement of the condyles. "The patient is now status post grade II open fracture of the left tibia, with an ipsilateral minimally displaced left pillion fracture which was treated immediately following his injury."

pill-rolling tremor—involuntary rhythmic opposing movements, or circular rolling motion, of the thumb and index finger, characteristic of Parkinson's disease.

pilocarpine iontophoresis method—to measure sweat chloride levels. An elevated level of chloride in perspiration is a sign of cystic fibrosis.

pilosebaceous unit—the combination of a hair follicle with its oil gland, considered as an anatomic unit.

PIMS (programmable implantable medication system).

pin—see *nail.*

PIN (percutaneous interosseous nerve) (Hand Surg).

pinacidil (Pindac) (Cardio)—a vasodilator used to treat hypertension.

Pinard's sign (Ob-Gyn)—in pregnancy, pain on pressure over the uterine fundus, after the sixth month. An indication of possible breech presentation.

pinchcock mechanism—at the esophagogastric junction.

Pindac—see *pinacidil.*

ping-pong fracture—an actual fracture or simply a concavity and depression in the skull, resembling the indentation that results from pressure by the fingers on a ping-pong ball.

pinguecula—a degenerative lesion of the conjunctiva appearing as a yellowish nodule near the limbus.

pin headrest (Neuro). See *headrest.*

pinked up (verb) (Cardio).

pinkeye—any condition causing hyperemia of one or both eyes; usually, bacterial or viral conjunctivitis.

pink puffer—a patient with early respiratory failure, showing dyspnea but no cyanosis. Cf. *blue bloater.*

pink tetralogy of Fallot—tetralogy of Fallot with only mild cyanosis, mild pulmonary stenosis, and left-to-right shunt, and with the pulmonary pressure higher than normal. See *tetralogy of Fallot.* Cf. *Fallot's trilogy, Fallot's pentalogy.*

Pinky—see *Super Pinky.*

Pins' sign—disappearance of pleuritic pain when the patient assumes a knee-chest position.

pinwheel, Taylor.

pipecuronium (Arduan)—a neuromuscular blocking agent similar to Pavulon. Used during anesthesia to relax skeletal muscles. Does not induce tachycardia, thus offering increased safety for cardiac patients undergoing surgery.

Pipelle endometrial suction catheter (Gyn)—for endometrial dating, cancer screening, and monitoring the effects of hormone treatment.

pipestem sheathing (Oph)—appearance created by lipid deposition along retinal arterioles.

PIPIDA scan—^{99m}Tc-PIPIDA hepatobiliary scan in acute cholecystitis. (PIPIDA, N-para-isopropyl-acetanilide-iminodiacetic acid.)

pipobroman (Vercyte).

pirenzepine (Gastrozepine) (GI)—a drug for treating peptic ulcer disease.

piritrexim isethionate—used to treat *Pneumocystis carinii, Toxoplasma,* and *Mycobacterium avium-intracellulare* in AIDS patients.

Pisces spinal cord stimulation system (Neuro) (electrical stimulation of nerve structures, delivered by percutaneously implanted epidural electrodes).

pisotriquetral joint (Hand Surg)—in the area of the flexor carpi ulnaris.

Pitt talking tracheostomy tube—used in patients with ventilator-dependent quadriplegia with severe phrenic nerve damage.

pitting edema—on firm finger pressure, a depression lasts for several minutes; due to fluid retention.

pivot-shift sign; test (Ortho).

PLA (peripheral laser angioplasty).

placebo (''plah-see'bo'') (Obecalp—*placebo* spelled backwards). Placebo is Latin for ''I will please.''

plafond, as in tibial plafond (Ortho)—the undersurface of a plateau.

PLA-I—a platelet antigen. This protein is sometimes lacking on the surface of platelets in patients who have received red cell transfusions from donors who are PLA-I positive, causing severe bleeding, and may also cause post-transfusion purpura.

plain—simple, open, clear; used often in *plain film,* a radiographic study performed without contrast medium, as differentiated from contrast studies and tomograms. Cf. *plane.*

planar spin imaging—MRI term.

plane—(1) a specified level, as the plane of anesthesia; (2) an anatomical area between two tissue layers where an incision may be placed. Cf. *plain.*

PLAP (placental alkaline phosphatase) (Oncol). It has been noted that serum levels of placental alkaline phosphatase are elevated in patients with seminomas and nonseminomatous malignant germ cell tumors, so it would appear that PLAP may be useful as a serum marker in patients undergoing treatment for one of these tumors to determine progression or regression of the tumor. It should be noted, however, that

PLAP *(cont.)*
PLAP is elevated in patients who are smokers, so that must be taken into consideration in determining the usefulness of this test in those patients.

plaques —see *Hollenhorst plaques.*

plasma expander, Hespan, or hetastarch.

plasma F—another term for cortisol.

Plasmalyte—used for priming the pump in liver transplant procedures.

Plasmalyte 148—used as an irrigating solution during phacoemulsification.

plasmapheresis—removal of plasma from blood taken from the patient, with retransfusion of the solid elements (red cells, platelets) into the patient. May be used for therapeutic purposes, or for laboratory studies. Spelling note: Different root words in plasmaph**er**esis and electroph**ore**sis. Cf. *electrophoresis.*

plasma thromboplastin component (PTC) in bleeding diseases.

plasmids—pieces of double-stranded circular DNA outside chromosomes, thought to be responsible for bacterial resistance.

plaster—see *Hapset plaster.*

plaster slab splint (Ortho).

plaster splint—see *sugar-tong.*

Plastibell—used in circumcising infants.

Plasti-Pore—porous high density polyethylene material employed for the fabrication of ossicular replacement prostheses in otolaryngology, and for other grafts. It is used in the same way as Proplast. Cf. *Proplast.*

Plastiport TORP (total ossicular replacement prosthesis) (ENT).

Plastizote collar (Ortho).

plate form—see *tantalum.*

platelet antigen—see *PLA-I.*

plates—see *Ishihara.*

Platina Clip implant cataract lens.

Platinol (cisplatin)—used in treatment of advanced carcinoma of the bladder.

platysmaplasty—see *corset platysmaplasty.*

pledgets, usually cotton (Surg). Cotton balls (sponges), rolled so that they have somewhat pointed ends; used to absorb blood or fluids at the operative site. In some parts of the country they are called ''pollywogs.''

PLEDs (periodic lateralized epileptiform discharges)—in electroencephalogram.

Plegisol (Cardio)—a cardioplegic solution.

Plendil (felodipine) (Cardio)—a once-a-day calcium channel blocker for mild to moderate hypertension.

plesiotherapy (Rad Oncol)—the same as brachytherapy. See *brachytherapy.*

plethysmography
impedance (IPG)
thermistor

pleural—refers to the pleura, the serous membrane lining each half of the thorax: pleural cavity, pleural effusion. Cf. *plural.*

pleural effusion (Radiol)—an abnormal accumulation of fluid in the pleural cavity, as seen on chest x-ray.

plexus of Santorini.

PLF (perilymphatic fistula).

plica (pl., plicae)—a ridge, fold, band, or shelf of synovial tissue, as in the transverse suprapatellar, medial suprapatellar, mediopatellar, and infrapatellar plicae. These usually cause few problems, but occasionally are large enough to become symptomatic and may require surgical intervention. See *plicectomy.*

plicamycin (mithramycin, MITH, Mithracin) (Oncol)—chemotherapy drug used to treat testicular carcinoma

plicamycin *(cont.)* when surgery or radiation is not an option.

plicectomy ("ply-kek'-to-me")—excision of a plica (Ortho). See *plica.*

PLIF (posterior lumbar interbody fusion) (Neuro).

plombage, as in "bone or chest plombage" ("plom-bahzh") (Surg)—the surgical filling of an empty space in the body with an inert material such as methyl methacrylate.

plop, tumor—heard with cardiac tumors on auscultation.

plug
- Biomet
- Dohlman
- Eagle Vision-Freeman punctum
- Freeman Punctum
- punctum

plum-blossom needle—used for acupuncture.

Plummer-Vinson syndrome—iron-deficiency anemia and esophageal webs or mucous membrane abnormalities; often associated with carcinoma of the upper third of the esophagus.

plural—more than one. Cf. *pleural.*

PMBV (percutaneous mitral balloon valvotomy).

PMFAC (prednisone, methotrexate, FAC)—chemotherapy protocol.

PM-81 monoclonal antibody (Oncol)—used to treat patients with acute myelogenous leukemia prior to bone marrow transplant.

PML (progressive multifocal leukoencephalopathy)—catastrophic HIV-related encephalopathy for which there is, at present, no treatment.

PMMA lens (Oph)—a hard contact lens or intraocular lens made of polymethylmethacrylate.

PMR (posteromedial release) (Pod)—a one-stage correction for talipes equinovarus (clubfoot).

PMT AccuSpan tissue expander. Cf. *tissue expander, AccuSpan.*

P-MVAC (Platinol, methotrexate, vinblastine, Adriamycin, carboplatin)—chemotherapy protocol.

PND (paroxysmal nocturnal dyspnea).

pneumatic retinopexy (Oph)—the fixation of the retina in its proper position with the injection of a bubble of gas into the interior of the eye in the vitreous cavity. With proper postoperative positioning, the retina can be pushed back into proper position and then the gas will spontaneously disappear in a few weeks. Gases used in this procedure may be either perfluoropropane (C_3F_8) or sulfur hexafluoride (SF_6).

***Pneumocystis carinii* pneumonia** (PCP)—once a rare pneumonia, caused by a protozoan parasite, seen only in immunosuppressed patients, such as transplant patients or patients on chemotherapy; now one of the leading causes of death in AIDS. See *AIDS; HIV; Kaposi's syndrome.*

pneumoniae—see *Klebsiella pneumoniae.*

Pneumopent (aerosolized pentamidine isethionate)—used to prevent *Pneumocystis carinii* infection in AIDS patients.

pneumophila, Legionella—the organism causing legionnaires' disease.

PNH (paroxysmal nocturnal hemoglobinuria).

"PNK"—see *P&K* ("P and K").

POCC (procarbazine, Oncovin, Cytoxan, CCNU)—chemotherapy protocol.

podagra—gout. "She comes to the emergency room complaining of acute podagra to the right big toe for the past two days."

podophyllum—caustic agent used for removal of papillomas.

POEMS syndrome

P polyneuropathy
O organomegaly
E endocrinopathy
M monoclonal (M-) protein
S skin change

This is a combination of sclerotic myeloma, polyneuropathy, and endocrinological disorder. Hepatomegaly may also be seen in these patients.

poikilocyte—an atypical red blood cell.

Poland's syndrome.

Polar-Mate Model 27-400 bipolar micro-coagulator by ASSI (Surg).

Polatest vision tester (Zeiss) (Oph)—tests binocular vision.

pole of kidney (Radiol, Surg)—the upper or lower extremity of a kidney.

Pollock forceps (Oph).

"pollywogs"—see *pledgets.*

Polaroids and Kodachromes (P&K) (Path)—photographs of specimens. "Polaroids and Kodachromes were taken," or "P&K were taken."

polyamines—putrescine, spermidine.

polycystic ovary (PCO).

Polydek—a coated polyester suture used in plastic surgery (Ethicon).

polydioxanone suture (PDS).

polymerase chain reaction (PCR)—test for viral activity at the cell level.

polyp hook, Neivert.

polyribonucleotide—see *Ampligen.*

polysomnogram—performed for evaluation of sleep apnea syndrome and sleep efficiency. Sleep stages are determined by EEG, EMG, and EOG (electro-oculogram) recordings. Oxygen saturation is monitored by ear or finger oximeter, and EKG is used to monitor cardiac rhythm. REM and NREM sleep, slow wave sleep, number of arousals, microarousals, awakenings, respiratory events (hypoxic and apneic) are recorded. Respiratory parameters are monitored by nasal and oral thermistors.

Polystan perfusion cannula and venous return catheter (Cardio).

Polytef (Teflon paste).

polytene chromosomes.

Polytrim solution (trimethoprim sulfate, polymyxin B sulfate) (Oph)—a broad-spectrum ophthalmic anti-infective.

polyurethane foam embolus (Neuro)—used in treatment of fistula of the carotid cavernous sinus. Under local anesthesia, a small compressed piece of polyurethane foam is attached to a suture, and the common carotid artery is entered and the foam embolus placed in the artery. Blood flow carries the embolus to the fistula site, and after a few minutes the foam expands and occludes the fistula site. Then the suture is attached to the arterial wall. Blood flow through the carotid artery continues unimpeded; only the fistula site is occluded.

polyvinylalcohol splinting material—Its advantages are said to be that it is easily molded, hypoallergenic, lighter than plaster of Paris, and transparent to x-rays (Ortho).

POMP (prednisone, Oncovin, methotrexate, mercaptopurine) (Oncol)—a chemotherapy protocol used to treat promyelocytic leukemia.

pomum adami (Adam's apple)—the prominence in the neck that is the thyroid cartilage.

Ponka technique—for local anesthesia in herniorrhaphy.

Pontiac fever—a nonpulmonary flu-like form of legionellosis. See *legionnaires' disease.*

pooling of blood in extremities (Cardio).

POP—plaster of Paris (Ortho). You may hear of POP ("pop") bandages.

pop-off needle (Surg, Ob-Gyn). Pre-attached needle is used to take one stitch, only; the needle is then twisted slightly, and the suture "pops" off, leaving a long suture for later tying. A series of sutures can then be tied sequentially. Used in hard-to-get-at places, as deep in the abdomen. Is faster to use than having needles threaded by a nurse. Trade names: D-Tach (Davis-Geck); Control-Release (Ethicon).

Poppen forceps (Neuro).

porcine xenograft (Surg, Plas Surg). When autograft material is not available in a severely burned patient, split-thickness grafts of pigskin are used to cover the burned areas. This is a temporary graft that reduces the pain, permits the wound to heal more rapidly, and helps prevent the loss of fluids through evaporation. It also helps to protect the wound from infection.

pores of Kohn—communications between alveoli.

Porites coral—see *madreporic coral.*

Porocoat—a porous coating used in the interfacing surfaces of DePuy's interlocking (Tri-Lock Cup) acetabular cups. See *Proplast* and *Plasti-Pore* for other porous prosthetic materials.

porous-coated anatomic (PCA) knee prosthesis.

porous prosthetic materials—Plasti-Pore, Porocoat, Proplast.

PORP (partial ossicular replacement prosthesis) (ENT).

porphyria, acute intermittent (AIP).

porphyrins—biochemical compounds in hemoglobin.

port—a small rubber stopper on the side of intravenous tubing used to administer drugs by I.V. push or to insert a needle to piggyback another smaller I.V. solution. See also *I.V. push; piggyback.*

port (implantable)

A Port
Chemoport
Groshong
Hickman
Implantofix
Infus-a-port
Life port
Medtronic
Norport
Norport SP
P.A.S. Port
Port-a-Cath
Q-Port
SEA (side entry access)
Vasport

portable film (Radiol)—an x-ray picture taken with movable equipment at the bedside or in the emergency department or operating room, when it is not feasible to move the patient to the radiology department.

Port-A-Cath—an implantable port of plastic or stainless steel with a rubber-covered entry site for inserting drugs. The port is connected to a central venous catheter which is positioned in the subclavian vein. Both the port and the catheter are implanted subcutaneously. Drugs are injected by inserting the needle through the skin and subcutaneous tissue and into the rubber-covered entry site on the port.

Portagen diet—medium chain triglyceride diet.

Porta Pulse 3—portable defibrillator.

Portex tracheostomy tube.

Portnoy ventricular cannula (Neuro).

position
- Bertel's
- dorsal lithotomy
- Gaynor-Hart
- jackknife
- Kraske's (in surgery)
- Rose head extension

positioner, Picket Fence leg.

position sense, joint (JPS).

positive end-expiratory pressure (PEEP).

positron emission tomography (PET) —a scanning technique in radiology using computers and radioactive isotopes to aid imaging and diagnosis. PET scanning depicts blood flow and measures metabolism.

posterior blue (Oph).

posterior subcapsular cataract (PSC).

posterior sulcus (Radiol)—the groove formed by the intersection of the diaphragm and the posterior thoracic wall, as seen in a lateral chest film.

posteromedial release (PMR).

post-poliomyelitis muscular atrophy—see *PPMA*.

post-tussive—after coughing. Applied to rales and rhonchi that do not disappear after the patient tries to clear his trachea and bronchi by coughing.

posturing, decorticate and decerebrate (Neuro)—rigid involuntary positioning of unconscious patient giving evidence of brain damage.

postviral fatigue syndrome—see *myalgic encephalomyelitis, chronic fatigue syndrome, yuppie flu.*

potassium—see *SSKI* (saturated solution of potassium iodide); *Kay Ciel.*

potassium hydroxide (KOH). When added to a specimen of skin, other tissue, or vaginal secretions before microscopic examination, potassium hydroxide destroys human cells and thus facilitates identification of funguses or yeasts in the specimen.

potential acuity meter (PAM)—used in testing vision (Oph).

Pott's puffy tumor (named for P. Pott). Post-traumatic osteomyelitis of the skull, with resultant edema, but without laceration of the overlying scalp (Neuro). Also, subperiosteal abscess of frontal sinus origin (ENT).

pouch
- Dennis-Brown
- Florida
- Indiana
- Kock
- Mainz urinary reservoir

poudrage (''poo-drahj'')—application of a powder to a surface, as done to promote fusion of serous membranes (e.g., two layers of pericardium or pleura).

powder—see *Karaya powder.*

PP (pancreatic polypeptide). ''PP is associated with bronchogenic carcinoma, and is also associated with diarrhea, possibly mediated by prostaglandins.''

PPD test (purified protein derivative)—a skin test for tuberculosis.

PPK (palmoplantar keratoderma)—see *Voerner's disease.*

PPL (penicilloylpolylysine, Pre-Pen)—used in skin testing along with penicillin G and penicilloic acid, for detecting IgE antipenicillin antibodies; to identify patients who are at risk for allergic reactions to penicillin.

PPMA (post-poliomyelitis muscular atrophy)—in 15% of people who have had polio in the past. It appears about 30 years later and manifests itself by extreme fatigue, often severe muscle pain, and with a muscular

PPMA *(cont.)* weakness that may be slowly progressive over a long period of time.

PPMD (posterior polymorphous dystrophy) of the cornea—a bilateral autosomal, dominantly determined condition, usually nonprogressive, affecting the deepest layers of the cornea. Associated with this may be secondary alterations in Descemet's membrane.

P pulmonale—an electrocardiographic syndrome of tall, narrow, peaked P-waves seen in leads II, III, and aVF, with a prominent initial positive P-wave component in V_1 and V_2.

Praeger iris hook.

PRA test (plasma renin activity) (Cardio).

Pravachol (pravastatin).

pravastatin (Pravachol) (Cardio)—a drug used to lower the levels of LDL in patients with hypercholesterolemia that has not responded to dietary measures.

preceding *(not* preceeding). Occurring before. Cf. *proceeding.*

precessional frequency—MRI term.

Precise disposable skin stapler (Surg).

Precision Osteolock (Ortho)—femoral component design system using LPPS (low-pressure plasma spray) hydroxyapatite for a stable cementless fixation.

precordial honk—an abnormal heart sound.

precordium—the area over the heart and the lower part of the thorax. See *pericardium.*

prednimustine—a drug used in treatment of non-Hodgkin's lymphoma.

premature rupture of the membranes (amniotic) (PROM) (Obs).

Premium CEEA circular stapler—with a detachable anvil and stem; used in end-to-end anastomosis, as in the rectum.

Prepodyne solution—used as an operating room skin preparation.

prepped—"The patient was prepped and draped in the usual sterile manner." A brief form for *prepared.*

PREs (progressive resistive exercises) (Phys Ther, Ortho).

presbyopia—defect of vision in advancing age, involving loss of accommodation, or recession of near point. Onset usually occurs betwen 40 and 45 years of age. Synonym: farsightedness.

present (verb)—to present oneself to a physician, clinic, or hospital for treatment.

presentation—the initial overt features of an illness; also, the part of a fetus that enters the birth canal first—the presenting part.

Press-Fit Condylar Total Knee.

pressure support ventilation (PSV).

pressured speech—a rapid, tense manner of speaking that betrays the anxiety of the speaker.

PressureSense Monitor—used to check for compartment syndrome (Ortho).

Preston pinch gauge—used to quantify pinch strength of the fingers (Ortho, Hand Surg).

prickle-cell layer of epidermis.

Prilosec (omeprazole) (GI)—trade name replacing Losec by the manufacturer at the request of the FDA because of reports of confusion between Losec and Lasix in drug orders.

Primacor (milrinone) (Cardio)—used to treat patients with congestive heart failure.

primaquine phosphate—antimalarial drug combined with the antibiotic clindamycin to treat *Pneumocystis carinii* pneumonia in AIDS patients.

Primbs-Circon indirect video ophthalmoscope system (Oph)—can be used with either AO (American Optical) or Keeler indirect ophthalmoscope. It utilizes a beamsplitter; a portion of the light goes to the eyepiece used by the surgeon, and the rest of the light goes to a video camera which televises (in color) the image seen through the ophthalmoscope (the televised image of intraocular, retinal, and vitreal pathology) to members of the surgical team.

Prinzide (Cardio)—combination of the diuretic hydrochlorothiazide and the ACE inhibitor lisinopril. Used to treat hypertension.

Prinzmetal's angina—an angina pectoris variant in which the patient has attacks while resting, and exercise tolerance is not significantly decreased.

proarrhythmic effect (Cardio)—the tendency of certain antiarrhythmic drugs to actually worsen a minor cardiac arrhythmia; such drugs are given only for life-threatening arrhythmias. See *propafenone.*

proband—a person, affected with what is probably a familial disease, diagnosed independently of his family in a genetic study. "A proband of this family was a seven-year-old girl with hyperextensible joints. Note: The family has several members with Ehlers-Danlos syndrome."

probe
- ArthroProbe laser
- Becker
- Bruel–Kjaer transvaginal ultrasound
- Buie fistula

probe *(cont.)*
- Circon-ACMI electrohydraulic lithotriptor
- Endo-P-Probe
- Frigitonics
- Gherini-Kauffman endo-otoprobe laser
- Girard Fragmatome
- HeatProbe
- Horn endo-otoprobe laser
- IntraDop Doppler
- Maloney endo-otoprobe
- MicroSmooth
- piggyback
- quartz fiberoptic
- Quickert
- Quickert-Dryden
- Robicsek Vascular
- Sarns temperature
- tulip
- Versadopp 10 ultrasonic
- vitrector

procedure (diagnostic, radiographic, and nonsurgical) (See also *operation; test.*)
- adenosine echocardiography
- air contrast barium enema
- ALT-RCC (autolymphocyte-based treatment for renal cell carcinoma)
- antifibrin antibody imaging
- A-scan ultrasound
- autolymphocyte-based treatment for renal cell carcinoma (ALT-RCC)
- BEAM (brain electrical activity mapping)
- blind esophageal brushing (BEB)
- B-mode ultrasound
- body surface Laplacian mapping
- B-scan ultrasound
- bubble ventriculography
- cardiokymography
- Cardiolite scan
- CardioTek scan
- CAVH (continuous arteriovenous hemofiltration)

procedure *(cont.)*
celiacography
cholescintography radionuclide
chromohydrotubation
chymonucleolysis
cine CT (computed tomography)
cinematography
continuous arteriovenous hemofiltration (CAVH)
contrast material enhanced scan
counterflow centrifugal elutriation
cribogram
CT (computed tomography)
dermabrasion
digital subtraction angiography (DSA)
dipyridamole echocardiography
donor-specific transfusion
double contrast barium enema
DSA (digital subtraction angiography)
dual photon absorptiometry
dual photon densitometry
duplex ultrasound
dynamic computerized tomography
ECMO (extracorporeal membrane oxygenation)
Egan's mammography
electro-oculogram
electroretinogram
embryoscopy
endoscopic retrograde cholangiopancreatography (ERCP)
endoscopic ultrasonography
ERCP (endoscopic retrograde cholangiopancreatography)
ErecAid treatment of erectile impotence
EVAL embolization
fiberoptic bronchoscopy
fluorescein angiography
flush aortogram
full-bladder ultrasound
full-column barium enema

procedure *(cont.)*
gallium scan
heavy ion irradiation
hemodilution
hemofiltration
HIDA scan
HSSG (hysterosalpingosonography)
hyperbaric oxygen therapy
hyperthermia, whole body
hysterosalpingosonography (HSSG)
impedance plethysmography (IPG)
incentive spirometry
indium-111 leukocyte scintigraphy scan
intentional transoperative hemodilution
intravenous fluorescein angiography (IVFA)
intravenous pyelogram (IVP)
invasive
in vitro fertilization (IVF)
iontophoresis
isolated heat perfusion of an extremity
IVF (in vitro fertilization)
IVFA (intravenous fluorescein angiography)
IVOX (intravascular oxygenator) artificial lung
IVP (intravenous pyelogram)
Judkins coronary arteriography
liquid crystal thermography
loopogram (ileostogram)
low-dose screen-film technique
lympharesis
MAA lung scan
magnetic resonance spectroscopy (MRS)
magnetic stimulation of fracture
medronate scan
metrizamide CT cisternogram
microwave treatment for benign prostatic hypertrophy
M-mode echocardiogram

procedure *(cont.)*
MRS (magnetic resonance spectroscopy)
MUGA (multiple gated acquisition)
noninvasive
oculoplethysmography-carotid phonoangiography (OPG/CPA)
oral cholecystogram
oxygen cisternography
percutaneous transhepatic cholangiogram (PTHC)
PET scan (positron emission tomography)
phonocardiography
PIPIDA scan
plasmapheresis
positron emission tomography (PET)
psoralen inactivation technique
PYP scan (pyrophosphate)
quantitative computed tomography (QCT)
radiofrequency ablation
radionuclide cholescintography
radionuclide scan
real-time ultrasonography
rectilinear bone scan
remote afterloading brachytherapy (RAB)
scintigraphy
sector scan echocardiography
serial scans
sestamibi stress test
small-bowel enteroscopy (SBE)
Sones coronary arteriography
SPECT scan (single photon emission computed tomography)
stacked scans
stereotaxy
stress cystogram
TcHIDA scan
teboroxime scan
TechneScan MAG3
technetium scan
Teflon paste injection for incontinence

procedure *(cont.)*
thallium stress test
thermistor-plethysmography
3DFT magnetic resonance angiography
ThromboScan MRU
thyroxine radioisotope assay (T_4 RIA)
total lymphoid irradiation (TLI)
transesophageal echocardiogram
transnasal endoluminal ultrasonography
transrectal ultrasonography (TRUS)
TSPP rectilinear bone scan
two-dimensional echocardiography
unenhanced
urocytogram
VCUG (vesicoureterogram; voiding cystourethrogram)
vectorcardiography
velolaryngeal endoscopy
vesicoureterogram (VCUG)
video-laseroscopy
voiding cystourethrogram (VCUG)
V/Q (ventilation/perfusion)
zonulolysis

proceeding—progressing. Cf. *preceding.*

procrastination (delayed action)—as in "His basic suggestions were that treatment remain conservative, and that procrastination be the procedure of choice for the time being." See also *tincture of time.*

Procysteine (oxothiazolidine carboxylate)—a drug used to treat AIDS.

Prodigy lens inserter (Oph)—an intraocular lens inserter that requires little manipulation of the eye.

profile—see *PULSES profile.*

profundaplasty, profundoplasty (Vasc Surg)—procedure used in treatment of femoropopliteal occlusive disease; surgical reconstruction of the profunda femoris.

profusion—abundance. "There was normal hair distribution and profusion." Cf. *perfusion.*

progesterone receptor (PgR).

progressive systemic sclerosis (PSS).

ProHance—a magnetic resonance imaging contrast agent.

Prokine—see *sargramostim.*

Prokop intraocular lens (implant).

prolapse, mitral valve (MVP).

Prolene (*not* Proline)—suture material.

Proleukin (interleukin-2).

proliferative retinopathy photocoagulation (PRP).

PROM (premature rupture of membranes, amniotic) (Obs).

ProMACE-CYTABOM (Oncol)—chemotherapy protocol, consisting of prednisone, methotrexate, Adriamycin, Cytoxan, etoposide, cytarabine, bleomycin, Oncovin, and mechlorethamine. Used to treat Hodgkin's lymphoma.

propafenone (Rythmol) (Cardio)—an oral antiarrhythmic drug that decreases electrical conduction across the atria and ventricles. It is indicated for life-threatening arrhythmias only, as it may actually make minor arrhythmias more severe.

proper lamina; ligament; membrane (L., *propria).* Anglicized form of *lamina propria,* which is the form usually dictated.

Proplast—trade name of a composite of Teflon polymer and elemental carbon. It resembles a black felt sponge and is 70 to 90% porous. It is used as graft material in fashioning prostheses. The host tissue, in effect, *invades* the pores of this material and transforms it into a similar tissue; it is biocompatible with many tissues, such as bone, soft tissue, dura, etc. Used in repair of dural defects, CSF leaks, etc. See also *Plasti-Pore.*

Propper ophthalmoscope (Oph).

Propper retinoscope (Oph).

proprietary medicine—nonprescription medicine.

proprioception (Neuro)—relates to the sensory system mechanism that has to do with movement of the body, its posture, balance, and coordination.

Propionibacterium—an anaerobic organism, one of a group of normal skin flora.

proptosis—a forward displacement of the eyeball in exophthalmic goiter or in an inflammatory condition of the orbit. Cf. *ptosis.*

ProSom (estazolam)—a benzodiazepine type of sedative drug.

prostate—the prostate gland, which surrounds the beginning of the urethra in the male. Cf. *prostrate.*

prostate-specific antigen (PSA).

prostatectomy
- Madigan
- Millen retropubic

ProStep—see *Nicoderm.*

prosthesis (See also *orthosis.)*
- Angelchik anti-reflux
- aortic valve
- Arthropor cup
- Aufranc-Turner
- Austin Moore hip
- Autophor femoral
- Bankart shoulder
- Bateman UPF
- Bechtol hip
- Björk-Shiley
- Bucholz
- Caffinière
- Calnan-Nicolle synthetic joint
- Carrion penile
- Charnley-Muller hip
- Cintor knee
- Cutter-Smeloff cardiac valve
- De La Caffinière trapeziometacarpal
- Deon hip
- Dilamezinsert penile

prosthesis *(cont.)*
Duracon
Duraphase penile
ELP femoral
Endo-Model rotating knee joint
endoprosthesis
Finney Flexi-Rod penile
Flatt finger/thumb
Flexi-Rod II penile
Freeman-Swanson knee
Galante hip
Geomedic total knee
Geometric knee
Gianturco
Gillette joint
GSB elbow
Guepar hinge knee
Hall-Kaster mitral valve
Harris HD hip
Harris-Galante hip
HD II (or HD2)
Hexcel total condylar knee system
Heyer-Schulte breast implant
Howmedica
Judet hip
Kastec mitral valve
Kinematic rotating hinge knee
Leinbach
Lo-Por vascular graft
Lord total hip
McKee-Farrar total hip
McKeever Vitallium cap
McNaught keel—laryngeal
Microknit vascular graft
Miller-Galante hip
Milliknit vascular graft
Mueller Duo-Lock hip
Muhlberger orbital implant
Neer II shoulder
Neer shoulder replacement
Neville tracheal and tracheobronchial
Niebauer
Omnifit HA hip stem
Osteonics hip
Panje voice button—laryngeal

prosthesis *(cont.)*
partial ossicular replacement
PCA (porous-coated anatomic) knee
Pillet hand
Plastiport TORP
PORP (partial ossicular replacement)
Richards hydroxyapatite PORP
Richards hydroxyapatite TORP
SAF (self-articulating femoral) hip replacement
Sbarbaro tibial plateau
Starr-Edwards Silastic ball valve
St. Jude Medical valve
Sheehy incus replacement
Shier total knee
Sivash
Small-Carrion penile
Starr-Edwards aortic valve
Sutter-Smelloff heart valve
Surgitek mammary
Surgitek penile
TARA (total articular replacement arthroplasty)
TORP (total osssicular replacement)
Townley TARA
UPF (universal proximal femur)
Wada valve
Wall stent biliary endoprosthesis
Wehrs incus
Xenophor femoral
Zirconia orthopedic
Z stent
Zweymuller cementless hip

prostrate—lying prone. Cf. *prostate.*

protean—said of a disease having various symptoms in different patients.

protease inhibitor —a drug used to treat patients with AIDS and ARC.

Prothiaden (dothiepin)—an antidepressant drug.

"pro time"—medical slang for prothrombin time (PT), a test for defects in blood clotting.

protocol
Balke

protocol *(cont.)*
Bruce
chemotherapy
Goeckerman

Protocult—stool sampling device that reduces the chance of contamination.

proton density images—MRI term.

Protouch—synthetic orthopedic padding (Ortho).

Pro-Trac—cruciate reconstruction measurement device (Ortho).

Protropin—human growth hormone, genetically entineered. See *Genentech biosynthetic human growth hormone.*

protrusio shill (Ortho).

proverbs, Benjamin (Psych).

Providencia rettgeri—newer name for the former *Proteus rettgeri;* commonly found in stool.

proximal articular set angle (PASA) (Ortho).

Proximate flexible linear stapler (Surg).

PRP (proliferative retinopathy photocoagulation).

Pruitt-Inahara carotid shunt—a long polyvinyl tube with an inflatable balloon at each end. The inflated balloon keeps the shunt tube within the vessel; thus no clamps are utilized, with resultant less trauma to the blood vessel. This shunt may also be used in some patients undergoing vascular reconstruction of the leg.

Pruitt occlusion and irrigation catheters.

prune-belly syndrome—see *Eagle-Barrett syndrome.*

PSA (prostate-specific antigen).

psammoma ("sah-mo'mah")—a tumor, especially a meningioma, that contains psammoma bodies.

psammoma bodies—microscopic laminated calcified bodies commonly seen in thyroid and ovarian cancer.

PSC (posterior subcapsular cataract) (Oph).

Pseudallescheria boydii—fungus originally identified as one of the agents thought responsible for Madura foot. *P. boydii* is an opportunistic pathogen, and has been recognized with increasing frequency as a cause of pulmonary, central nervous system, prostatic, osteomyelitic, ophthalmological, otitic, and disseminated infections, particularly in patients who are immunocompromised.

Pseudomonas maltophilia *(Alcaligenes bookeri)*—an organism found in soil, plants, water, sewage, animals, raw milk, etc. Seen in meningitis, septicemia, pleuritis, infected wounds. An opportunistic pathogen.

Pseudomonas stutzeri—found in soil, but occasionally in sputum specimens, in wounds, ear drainage, and infected eyes; found also on aerosol equipment.

pseudomonic acid—old name for *mupirocin.*

p.s.i., psi ("sigh") (pounds per square inch)—the unit of measurement used in procedures involving pressure. See *Brown-McHardy pneumatic dilator.*

psomophagia (the initial *p* is silent)—swallowing food without chewing it thoroughly.

psoralen—a light-activated drug, used in treatment of psoriasis, and in T-cell lymphoma. See *photophoresis.*

psoralen inactivation technique—used to inactivate a variety of infectious agents including some that are considered more difficult to inactivate than HIV. Involves exposing an active infectious agent to psoralen or one of its derivatives, and thereafter exposing it to ultraviolet light, by which process the psoralen forms

psoralen *(cont.)* chemical bonds with the nucleic acids (DNA or RNA) in the infectious agents.

PSS (progressive systemic sclerosis). Scleroderma is a form of this disease.

PSV (pressure support ventilation)—a setting for respirators, it allows patients to breathe on their own while still maintaining a positive airway pressure.

PSVT (paroxysmal supraventricular tachycardia).

psychedelic drugs (*not* psychodelic)—refers to certain types of drugs that act on the central nervous system, e.g., LSD, mescaline, etc., producing heightened perception, visual hallucinations, delusions.

PTA (percutaneous transluminal angioplasty). Cf. *Dotter-Judkins technique* and *PTCA.*

PTAH (phosphotungstic acid-hematoxylin)—a histochemical diagnostic stain (Path). See *Mallory's PTAH.*

PTBD (percutaneous transhepatic biliary drainage).

PTC (plasma thromboplastin component) in bleeding diseases.

PTCA (percutaneous transluminal coronary angioplasty). See *Grüntzig* or *Gruentzig.*

PTFE (polytetrafluoroethylene)—an arterial graft material. PTFE is manufactured by Impra and also by Gore-Tex (Vasc Surg). PTFE does not need pre-clotting, as does Dacron. It is also used as vascular access in hemodialysis.

PTH (parathormone, parathyroid hormone).

PTHC (percutaneous transhepatic cholangiogram) (GI).

P-32 (Oncol)—a chromic phosphate suspension given via intraperitoneal administration to patients with ovarian cancer. It is used only after a second-look laparotomy has yielded negative findings and its purpose is to attempt to improve survival time.

P300—a test for dementia.

ptosis, noun ("toe-sis")—a prolapse or drooping of an anatomic structure, such as the upper eyelid. Cf. *proptosis, phthisis.*

ptotic (adj.) ("tot'tic")—see *ptosis.*

PTRA (percutaneous transluminal renal angioplasty) (Radiol).

P24 or p24 antigen level—a virologic marker used to study the effects of AIDS drugs; a sensitivity test for the presence of the AIDS virus.

PUD (peptic ulcer disease).

puddle sign—a quick, if unsophisticated, method of differentiating minimal ascites from edema. The patient lies prone for five minutes and then assumes the knee-chest position; dullness on percussion in the periumbilical region indicates ascites rather than edema.

Puestow pancreaticojejunostomy—an operation performed on patients with obstruction of the pancreatic ductal system resulting in dilated duct, with points of stenosis and distal calculi.

"puff of smoke" (moyamoya)—angiographic diagnosis of bilateral stenosis or occlusion of the internal carotid arteries above the clinoids.

puffer, pink—a patient with early respiratory failure, showing dyspnea but no cyanosis. Cf. *blue bloater.*

Pulmo-Aide nebulizer—used to permit easier breathing in patients with

Pulmo-Aide nebulizer *(cont.)* allergies, asthma, chronic obstructive pulmonary disease, cystic fibrosis.

pulmonary artery wedge pressure (PAWP).

pulmonary toilet—postural drainage, percussion, hydration, and other means of clearing the respiratory tract.

pulmonary vascular markings (Radiol)—as seen on chest x-ray, the normal radiographic appearance of the branches of the pulmonary arteries and veins about the hila of the lungs.

pulmonary vascular redistribution (Radiol)—on chest x-ray, increased prominence of upper pulmonary vessels and reduced prominence of lower pulmonary vessels at the lung hila in left ventricular failure and other disturbances of circulatory dynamics.

pulse deficit—the arithmetical difference between the apical pulse and the radial or other peripheral pulse. Generally it indicates the number of cardiac contractions per minute that are not sufficiently strong to generate a peripheral pulse.

pulse oximetry devices (Pulm). Pulse oximetry devices are used extensively in the intensive care unit and operating room to continuously monitor the patient's arterial blood oxygen saturation. They are composed of a sensor which emits two types of light (red and infrared) and a photodetector. The red and infrared light beams are transmitted through the patient's tissue, including through the arterial blood vessels. When they reach the photodetector on the other side, a computer calculates how much of each type of light was transmitted. Oxygenated hemoglobin within the arteries absorbs more infrared light, while deoxygenated blood absorbs more red light. These devices can be placed around the patient's finger, over the bridge of the nose and, on newborns, around the foot or even around the great toe.

PulseSpray (Radiol)—a pulsed infusion system consisting of a syringe and catheter. PulseSpray is used to inject thrombolytic agents into a vessel. Injection can be done by a radiologist or other physician, or with a pump.

pulsed gradient—MRI term.

pulse (MRI terms)
length
radiofrequency
sequence
width

PULSES profile (Neuro)—a disability profile:
P physical condition
U upper extremity function
L lower extremity function
S sensory and communication abilities
E excretory control
S social support
Scored from 1 (total independence) to 4 (total dependence). A score of 2 represents symptomatology, but no impairment in activities of daily living. A score of 3 means impairment and need for assistance from others.

pulsing current (electrostimulation) (Ortho)—used in nonunion of fractures. When bone is placed in an electromagnetic field, and the field switched on and off, a current in the microampere range is generated in the bone, causing changes in the environment of the cells in the gap region. This leads to bone healing.

Pulsolith laser lithotripter—for nonsurgical removal of gallstones and urinary tract stones.

pulsus bisferiens (biferious pulse)—a pulse with two beats, sometimes palpable in combined aortic stenosis and aortic regurgitation.

pulsus paradoxus (*not* paradoxicus). Also, *paradoxical pulse.*

Pulver-Taft weave—a method used in microsurgical tendon transfer.

pump
  Autosyringe insulin
  Barron
  CADD-PLUS infusion
  Cormed ambulatory infusion
  Entera-Flo feeding
  Felig insulin
  Hakim-Cordis
  Harvard
  Hemopump
  Infusaid programmable insulin
  IVAC infusion
  Master Flow Pumpette
  McGaw volumetric
  Medtronic SynchroMed
  Servo
  Stat 2 Pumpette
  SynchroMed
  SynchroMed infusion

punch
  Citelli-Meltzer atticus
  DyoVac suction
  Gass scleral
  Goosen vascular
  Hajek-Koffler sphenoid
  Hardy-Sella
  Klein
  Rhoton
  Stammberger antrum

punctum plug (Oph). See *Freeman Punctum Plugs.*

Puntenney forceps (Oph).

pupil
  Adie's
  cat's eye

Purkinje's (''per-kin-jees) (Oph)
  cells
  fibers
  images
  shift

purpura
  Henoch-Schönlein
  Schönlein-Henoch
  thrombotic thrombocytopenic

pursestring, or *purse-string suture*—a continuous running suture placed about an opening, and then drawn tight, like a drawstring purse.

pursuit mechanism—the slow, involuntary movement of both eyes as they follow a moving object (Oph).

pursuit—see *saccadic pursuit.*

putrefaciens
  Alteromonas
  Pseudomonas

Putti-Platt arthroplasty—for acromioclavicular separation (Ortho). Subscapularis muscle and capsular repair, for chronic shoulder separation.

PUVA regimen; therapy (''poo-vah'') (Derm) for psoriasis. (PUVA, psoralens, ultraviolet A.) Ultraviolet A is a long-wave ray.

PVA (polyvinyl alcohol) particles—an embolic material used in embolization of the potential blood supply to a cranial nerve in interventional radiology procedures of the extracranial head and neck.

PVA (prednisone, vincristine, asparaginase)—chemotherapy protocol used to treat acute lymphoblastic leukemia.

PVB (Platinol, vinblastine, bleomycin)—chemotherapy protocol used to treat germ cell tumors.

PVDA (prednisone, vincristine, daunorubicin, asparaginase)—chemotherapy protocol used to treat non-Hodgkin's lymphoma and acute lymphoblastic leukemia.

PVG matter (periventricular gray) (Neuro)—stimulation of the PVG matter with deep brain electrodes inhibits pain. Cf. *PAG matter.*

PVP (Platinol, VP-16)—chemotherapy protocol used to treat neuroblastoma.

PVR (postvoiding residual).

PVS (persistent vegetative state).

PWA (person with AIDS)—term preferred over AIDS victim in AIDS self-help and awareness groups.

pyknosis—a phenomenon where the cell becomes opaque and darkly stained under the microscope, as seen in cell death.

Pylori Fiax—an objective quantitative IFA (indirect fluorescent antibody) serology assay for *Helicobacter pylori.*

Pylori Stat—rapid EIA (enzyme-linked immunoassay) serology assay for *Helicobacter pylori.*

pyloric string sign—an elongated, narrowed pyloric canal—a sign of pyloric hypertrophy; this does not change on administration of antispasmodics.

pyogenic granuloma, or **granuloma pyogenicum**—a benign polypoid growth containing proliferating capillaries. It may result from trauma and often becomes infected.

PYP scan (technetium pyrophosphate)—used for myocardial infarct imaging.

pyranocarboxylic acid class (Ortho)—a new class of drugs chemically different from nonsteroidal anti-inflammatory drugs such as ibuprofen, but which exert the same effects in treating inflammation, pain, and fever as NSAIDs. Also see *etodolac.*

pyridoxilated stroma-free hemoglobin (SFHb)—an artificial blood capable of carrying oxygen, can sustain life at a hematocrit of zero, and is nontoxic to the kidneys.

pyrimethamine (Daraprim)—a drug used to prevent toxoplasmosis in AIDS patients.

pyrophosphate scan (PYP).

pyrosis—heartburn.

Pyrost (Ortho)—bone replacement material used as a complement to homologous or heterologous bone grafts.

Q, q

13q-deletion syndrome (46 Dr or 46 Dq) is due to a deletion of the long arms of chromosome 13 (one of the group D chromosomes). The syndrome may include mental retardation and physical retardation, broad nasal bridge, large and prominent low-set ears, facial asymmetry, hypertelorism, ptosis, epicanthus, microcephaly, microphthalmia, imperforate anus, and a number of other anomalies.

QCT (quantitative computed tomography).

Q fever—a disease endemic to sheep in the western part of the U.S. It causes flu-like symptoms in humans who are exposed to diseased sheep. These symptoms can be mild, occasionally severe, and can prove fatal. The organism causing Q fever is *Coxiella burnetii,* a rickettsia.

QHS (quantitative hepatobiliary scintigraphy) (GI, Radiol).

q.n.—every night.

q.o.d., QOD—every other day.

Q-T$_c$ interval—corrected Q-T interval.

Quad-Lumen drain for closed wound drainage (Surg). This is a perforated drain with a radiopaque stripe, which permits postoperative monitoring.

quadrature detector—MRI term.

quadriceps muscle (*not* quadricep), as in "the quadriceps and hamstring muscles." It is, in effect, one muscle with four heads (Ortho).

quadriplegia—*not* quadraplegia.

quality factor—MRI term.

quantitative computed tomography (QCT) (Radiol). Using single photon absorptiometry, this is a noninvasive test for assessment of the skeleton with regard to bone mineral density in osteoporosis, hyperparathyroidism, Cushing's syndrome, and other metabolic diseases known to affect the bones.

quantitative hepatobiliary scintigraphy (QHS).

QUART (quadrantectomy, axillary dissection, and radiotherapy). Used in treatment of carcinoma of the breast.

quartz fiberoptic probe (Oph).

quaternary ammonium chloride *(not* quarternary)—a skin cleansing compound, used in skin preparation prior to surgery.

Quantum pacemaker (Cardio).

quazepam (Doral) (Psych)—benzodiazepine for insomnia, related chemically to Halcion, Restoril, and Dalmane.

Queckenstedt's sign—failure of cerebrospinal fluid pressure to rise and then fall when neck veins are compressed; indicative of a vertebral CSF canal block.

quellung reaction (swelling)—a technique for demonstrating the presence of capsular polysaccharide antigen. It is used to diagnose pneumococcal pneumonia. (Note: *not* quelling.)

quench, quenching—a term used when the magnet of the MRI equipment fails or goes down.

Quervain abdominal retractor (Surg).

Quervain's disease—see *de Quervain's disease.*

Quervain fracture (Ortho).

questionnaire, McGill pain.

Queyrat—see *erythroplasia of Queyrat.*

Quickert probe (Oph).

Quickert-Dryden probe; tube (Oph).

quinapril (Accupril) (Cardio)—a once-a-day ACE inhibitor for hypertension.

quinacrine (Pulm)—drug used in patients at high risk for repeat pneumothorax.

Quinton Mahurkar dual-lumen catheter—for hemodialysis and peritoneal use; comes in femoral and subclavian sizes. Also, Mahurkar dual-lumen catheter.

Quinton-Scribner shunt (Urol)—a vascular shunt used in dialysis patients.

Quinton suction biopsy instrument (Rubin tube)—used in esophageal biopsies.

Quinton tube—used for small bowel biopsy.

Quire mechanical finger forceps (ENT)—for removal of foreign bodies from the ear.

R, r

Raaf Cath—vascular catheter (Quinton).

RAB (remote afterloading brachytherapy)—a remote-controlled method of implanting a radioactive source in a patient for brief treatment without exposing the physician or nurse to radioactivity. The applicator is placed manually by the physician, and the radioisotope is administered under computer control by machine, after the physician or nurse has left the treatment room.

rabbit nose—habitual repeated wrinkling of the nose by a person with itching of the nares due to allergic rhinitis.

rabbit stools—stools expelled as small pellets.

rabies vaccine, Rhesus diploid cell strain (RDRV) (adsorbed).

raccoon eyes (Neuro)—discoloration below or around the eyes due to subcutaneous hemorrhage, sometimes seen in basal skull fracture.

racemic epinephrine (''rah-see'mik'').

rachitic—pertaining to rickets.

rachitic rosary—seen in patients with rickets. So-called because the enlargement of the cartilages at the costochondral junctions has the appearance of a string of beads.

rad (radiation absorbed dose)—see *centigray; gray; joule.*

radial keratotomy (Oph)—a procedure for improving vision in myopic patients. Developed by Dr. Fydorov in the Soviet Union. Radial cuts (8 or 16) are made in the cornea, not quite all the way through. This flattens the shape of the eye, and changes myopia to more normal vision.

radiation dosages—may be given as rads in a tissue dose (usually in histories before 1960), and in roentgens as an air dose. See *centigray; gray; joule.*

radical—(1) going to the root or source of a morbid process; directed to the cause, as in ''radical excision of a tumor''; (2) a fundamental constituent of a molecule; ''free radical.'' Cf. *radicle.*

radicle—one of the smallest branches of a nerve or a vessel, as in ''intrahepatic biliary radicles.'' Cf. *radical.*

radioactive iodinated serum albumin study (RISA).

radioallergosorbent test (RAST).

Radiofocus Glidewire (*not* guide wire) (Radiol)—trade name for an angiographic polymer-coated guide wire. It reduces friction and the risk of thrombus formation. The tip of the wire is flexible, to minimize trauma to the vessel.

radiofrequency ablation (RFA) (Cardio)—Using fluoroscopy, a catheter is positioned in the heart, and radiofrequency current is conducted from a patch placed on the patient to the tip of the ablation catheter positioned in the heart. The current is used to destroy accessory conduction pathways causing arrhythmias unresponsive to medical therapy.

radiofrequency coil; pulse (RF)—MRI term.

radioimmunodetection (RAID).

radiolucent (Radiol)—offering relatively little resistance to x-rays (by analogy with *translucent*).

radioisotope
- Cardiolite (^{99m}Tc sestamibi)
- CardioTek (^{99m}Tc teborixime)
- CEAker
- fluorodeoxyglucose (FDG)
- Hedspa
- ImmuRAID (CEA-Tc99m)
- indium-111 labeled human nonspecific immunoglobulin G (^{111}In-IgG)
- iodine-131 MIBG
- iridium-192 (Iriditope)
- nitrogen-13 ammonia
- OncoScint CR103 MOAB labeled with indium-111 (^{111}In)
- OncoScint OV103 MOAB labeled with indium-111 (^{111}In)
- palladium-103 (Pd103)
- rubidium-82
- selenium-75 (^{75}Se)
- technetium 99m colloid

radioisotope *(cont.)*
- technetium 99m medronate
- technetium 99m mertiatide
- technetium 99m teboroxime
- technetium 99m sestamibi
- technetium 99m macroaggregated albumin (^{99m}TcMAA)
- technetium 99m sulfur colloid (^{99m}Tc SC)
- technetium pertechnetate
- technetium stannous pyrophosphate (TSPP)
- thallium-201 (Tl-201)
- xenon-133 (^{133}Xe)

radionuclide (Radiol)—radioactive isotope; a species of atom that spontaneously emits radioactivity.

radionuclide scan (Radiol)—the introduction into the body of a radioactive substance whose distribution in tissues, vessels, or cavities can be detected and recorded by a device that senses radiation. The choice of radioactive substances (radionuclides, isotopes) is governed by the tendency of certain organs or tissues to take up (absorb, concentrate) certain elements or compounds. Radionuclides may be swallowed, inhaled, or injected into a body cavity or into the circulation. Scanning may be performed immediately after the material is administered (as in studies of blood flow) or after an interval (as when absorption or concentration of a substance in an organ must occur first). The standard lung scan procedure includes two separate scans of the lungs, one after inhalation of a radionuclide and the other after injection of a second radionuclide into the circulation. The scanning is done with a scintillation camera (scintiscanner, gamma camera) which creates a picture on film representing the

radionuclide scan *(cont.)* distribution and intensity of gamma radiation emitted by the patient. Also, *radionuclide spleen scan.*

radiopaque—resisting penetration by x-rays.

Radovan tissue expander (Plas Surg).

RAE endotracheal tubes (ENT); both oral and nasal tubes can be bent to keep them out of the respective surgical fields.

RA factor (rheumatoid arthritis)—a protein in the blood of most patients with rheumatoid arthritis. It is detected by a blood test. Cf. *Rh factor.*

Ragnell hand-held retractor (Pod).

RAID (radioimmunodetection) (Radiol) —used in combination with a monoclonal antibody against carcinoembryonic antigen. See *ImmuRAID.*

Raimondi ventricular catheter (Neuro).

Raji cell assay test—for immune complexes.

rale—a fine crackling, static-like sound heard through the stethoscope, indicating a pathologic condition. Take a lock of hair and roll it between your thumb and index finger near your ear; you've just heard what a crackling rale sounds like. Also, *Velcro rales.*

rale de retour (Fr., rattle of return). See *rale redux.*

rale indux—a crepitant rale that is heard in patients with pneumonia at the stage when consolidation begins. Cf. *rale redux.*

rale redux—an unequal subcrepitant sound caused by the passage of air through the fluid in bronchial tubes. This rale is heard when pneumonia is resolving. See *rale de retour.*

RAM (rapid alternating movements).

ramipril (Altace) (Cardio)—an antihypertensive belonging to the group of drugs known as ACE inhibitors. See also *fosinopril.*

Rand microballoon (Cardio)—used in microballoon embolization of cerebral aneurysms, arteriovenous malformations, and carotid cavernous fistula occlusion.

randomize—This term is used in testing new medications or chemotherapy protocols. Patients are selected at random, rather than in any predetermined manner, to test responses.

Randot test (''ran-dot'') (Oph)—not a physician's name; it is a coined word for the **ran**dom **dot**s that become recognizable as geometric figures when the patient wears a certain kind of eyeglasses. This is a test of binocular depth perception.

Raney clip (Neuro, Plas Surg)—used in repair of facial fractures requiring bicoronal incision, to obtain hemostasis of the galea and skin.

Ranfac cholangiographic catheters:
- LAP-13 for insertion through the lateral port
- ORC-B for open procedure
- XL-11 for percutaneous or three-puncture technique

range of motion (ROM).

Ranke complex—calcified node, or mass, or granuloma in the chest, from old tuberculosis.

RAP (recurrent abdominal pain).

rapid alternating movements (RAM).

rapid eye movement (REM).

rash, butterfly—rash seen over the malar area and bridge of the nose in patients with systemic lupus erythematosus.

Rashkind balloon atrial septotomy—a procedure in which a cardiac catheter with a balloon is inserted; the

Rashkind balloon septotomy *(cont.)* balloon is inflated, thus enlarging the aperture.

RAST (radioallergosorbent test).

Rastelli procedure (Cardio).

ratbite fever—see *Haverhill fever.*

ratio
- C/N (contrast-to-noise)
- CT (cardiothoracic)
- cup-to-disk
- gyromagnetic
- helper/suppressor cell
- I/E (inspiration/expiration)
- L/S (lecithin/sphingomyelin) (in amniocentesis)
- M/E (myeloid/erythroid)
- RV/TLC (residual volume/total lung capacity)
- S/N (signal-to-noise)
- T-lymphocyte subset

Raulerson syringe (Cardio)—used with guide wire insertion during the Seldinger technique.

Rayleigh scattering law (Neuro).

Ray-Tec sponge—x-ray detectable surgical sponge. Cf. *Vistec.*

Raz double-prong ligature carrier (Urol)—for performing bladder and bladder neck suspensions.

Raz sling operation (Urol)—for urinary incontinence. (Shlomo Raz, M.D.)

Razi cannula introducer (Surg)—used to simplify the procedure and diminish postoperative strokes and memory loss following aortic cannulation.

rCBF (regional cerebral blood flow) (Neuro). PET (positron emission tomography) term. See also *rCBV.*

rCBV (regional cerebral blood volume) (Neuro). PET (positron emission tomography) term. See also *rCBF.*

rCD4 (recombinant CD4). See *CD4.*

rCPP (regional cerebral perfusion pressure) (Neuro).

rd., abbreviation for *rutherford,* a unit of radioactivity.

RDRV (adsorbed)—Rhesus diploid cell strain rabies vaccine. See *HDRV.*

RDS (respiratory distress syndrome, formerly hyaline membrane disease) (Pulm, Neonat)—occurs in the lungs of premature infants due to the lack of surfactant (lubricant). It is this lubricant which helps keep the air sacs in the lungs open on exhalation. Without surfactant, the walls of the air sacs collapse and stick together, making it difficult or impossible to inhale. See the surfactants *Exosurf* and *Survanta.*

RDW (**r**ed cell **d**iameter **w**idth) (in the context of hematology).

ReAct NMES device—neuromuscular electrical stimulation used in physical therapy to treat disuse atrophy and other neuromuscular disorders. The system uses Multi-Ply or Soft-EZ reusable electrodes.

reaction
- Arthus
- Kveim
- quellung
- Sgambati's

Reactine (cetirizine).

reagent—substance involved in a chemical reaction; also a substance used to detect the presence of another substance by chemical means. See *Millon's reagent.* Cf. *reagin.*

reagin—a type of antibody. See *RPR* and *reagent.*

real-time Color Flow Doppler—permits two-dimensional color-coded imaging of blood flow (Radiol).

real-time ultrasonography—intraoperative scanning technique (frequency around 30 cycles per second [cps]) which permits physiological move-

real-time ultrasonography *(cont.)* ment to be observed while it is happening, e.g., it is possible to see a cyst collapsing as its wall is entered. It is used for determining the precise location of tumors of the brain, beneath the cerebral cortex, for removal through very small and accurately placed incisions. It also permits the accurate guiding of biopsy needles, localizing of intracranial cysts, aneurysms or abscesses, or foreign bodies, and makes it possible to position catheters in the ventricles for draining fluids or to measure pressure. In a laminectomy, the spinal cord can be visualized without opening the dura. It is also used for noninvasive exploration of the pelvis and abdomen. It is particularly useful in that the examination can be taped on magnetic tape and individual frames can be placed in the patient's record. There is no radiation hazard associated with the use of real-time ultrasonography. Also called real-time examination. See *ultrasound.*

reamer
- chamfer
- Indiana
- Kuntscher
- Mira

rebound tenderness. To test for rebound tenderness, the fingers are pushed into an area far from the area of suspected inflammation and then quickly removed. The rebound of the indented structures causes pain in the area of inflammation.

Rebuck window.

recanalization—see *transcervical balloon tuboplasty.*

Receptin (CD4)—a drug used to treat patients with AIDS and ARC.

receptor
- E-rosette
- estrogen
- H_1
- H_2
- progesterone (PgR)

recession (Oph)—the moving of the end of an eye muscle (usually the medial rectus or lateral rectus, that adducts or abducts, respectively, the eyeball) and reimplanting it in a slightly different position, for correction of strabismus. Cf. *resection.*

reciprocating saw (Ortho, Plas Surg).

recombinant alpha interferon—see *interferon.*

recombinant hemoglobin—see *rHb1.1.*

recombinant tissue plasminogen activator (rt-PA)

reconstitution (Radiol)—a term used in angiography for maintenance of flow in an artery beyond an area of narrowing or obstruction by establishment of collateral circulation.

reconstruction study (Radiol)—generation of an image by computer processing of scan data. Used in computed tomography (CT) scan.

recording, bipolar esophageal.

recovery, saturation—MRI term.

recruitment (Audiol)—when, in testing hearing, a slight increase in decibel level causes a disproportionate increase in loudness perceived.

Rector-Gordon-Healey-Mendoza-Spitzer type IV renal tubular acidosis—a rare type named for five physicians in different cities who first found and identified it.

recurred *(not* reoccurred), as "The symptoms recurred with the advent of cold weather."

recurrent abdominal pain (RAP).

red cell diameter width (RDW).

red reflex (Oph). When the light from the ophthalmoscope is flashed on the patient's pupil at a slight angle lateral to the patient's line of vision and at about a distance of 12 inches, a bright orange glow will be noted.

Reddick cystic duct cholangiogram catheter (Surg)—used during laparoscopic cholecystectomy.

Redifurl TaperSeal IAB catheter (Radiol)—for percutaneous insertion in the femoral artery.

reducing substances (Peds)—positive in stools of premature infants who are not properly digesting formula, consists of various sugars tested by making a mixture of stool and water and Clinitest tablet.

Redy 2000 hemodialysis system.

reefing—folding, or tucking of skin or other tissue: "We then performed arthrotomy, lateral release, medial reefing of the right patella for lateral subluxation."

Reese dermatome—a drum-type dermatome that makes grafts from .008 to .034 inch.

Reese-Ellsworth classification of retinoblastoma. Groups I through V.

Reese stimulator—used in recurrent nerve sectioning, for spastic dysphonia (ENT).

refer, referred—also, referring, referral, *but* referable.

reference, ideas of (Psych)—delusions that strangers such as radio or television broadcasters are referring to the patient.

re-flex (verb)—a hyphen is needed to distinguish *re-flex* (to flex again) from the noun *reflex* (an involuntary action).

reflex—a reflected action or movement. Cf. *reflux.* Types of reflex:
abdominal

reflex *(cont.)*
Achilles
anal
ankle jerk (AJ)
asymmetric tonic neck (ATNR)
Babinski's
biceps jerk (BJ)
brachioradialis
cat's eye
Chaddock's
consensual light
corneal
cremasteric
crossed
deep tendon
direct light
gag
gastrocnemius
Gordon
grasp
H
Hoffmann
knee jerk (KJ)
light
Mayer's
Moro
Oppenheim
palmomental
patellar
pathologic
plantar
pupillary
quadriceps
red
Romberg
rooting
startle
swallowing
tendon
triceps
vestibular
Wartenberg

reflexes (deep tendon reflexes).
0 absent
1+ decreased

reflexes *(cont.)*
2+ normal
3+ hyperactive
4+ clonus

reflex sympathetic dystrophy (RSD)—a response to an injury consisting of vasomotor instability, trophic skin changes, swelling, and pain.

reflux—a backward or return flow. Cf. *reflex.*
gastroesophageal
hepatojugular
intrarenal
vesicoureteral

reflux esophagitis, classification. Written as grades, with Roman numerals:
EI erythema, edema
EII erosions
EIII localized deformity
EIV stricture

refraction—determination of the refractive errors of the eye for distance and near vision.

Regen's flexion exercises (Ortho), pronounced like "region."

regime—government or social system; mode of rule or management. Often misused in medicine for *regimen.* Cf. *regimen.*

regimen *(not* regime)—a systematic course of therapy, diet, or exercise meant to achieve certain ends:
CMF r. for breast cancer
Einhorn r. of chemotherapy
Goeckerman r. for psoriasis
Ingram r. for psoriasis
leucovorin rescue
PUVA r. for psoriasis
uridine rescue

regional cerebral blood flow (rCBF).

regional cerebral blood volume (rCBV).

regional cerebral perfusion pressure (rCPP).

Reglan (metoclopramide).

Reichert SC-5 sigmoidoscope.

Reichling corneal scissors (Oph).

Reil, island of, in the brain.

Reinke crystals—crystals contained in interstitial cells (Leydig cells) of human testes. See *Leydig cell.*

Reitman-Frankel—test for SGOT and SGPT.

Relafen (nabumetone).

relaxation rate; time—MRI terms.

relaxing incision (or relief incision)—an incision made to relieve tension in tissue.

Relia-Vac drain—manufactured by Davol. Used like the Hemovac.

rem—unit of measurement of maximum tolerance dose of radiation (to hospital personnel). A permissible dose is 0.1 rem/week, or 5 rems per year. See *gray.*

REM sleep (rapid eye movement)—that period of sleep when the heart rate and respiration are irregular, brain waves are rapid and of low voltage, and dreaming occurs. Cf. *NREM sleep.*

remote afterloading brachytherapy. See *RAB.*

Renacidin (GU)—genitourinary irrigating solution used to dissolve stones.

renal tubular acidosis, Rector-Gordon-Healey-Mendoza-Spitzer type IV.

renin (Cardio). In addition to cholesterol and triglyceride levels in cardiac patients, you will be hearing about serum renin levels. Studies have shown that elevated cholesterol and triglycerides are not the only factors responsible for an increased risk of heart attacks. It has been found that the risk of heart attack is seven times higher in patients with elevated renin levels. In addition, elevated

renin *(cont.)*
renin levels may provide the key to the question of why more than half of patients experiencing a myocardial infarction have normal cholesterol levels.

repair—see *operation.*

repeated FID (free induction decay)—MRI term.

Repel—a surgical glove resistant to tear and puncture. Made of Kevlar and Lycra.

repetition time (RT)—given in seconds; MRI term.

repetitive strain injury (RSI)—see *carpal tunnel syndrome.*

rephasing gradient—MRI term.

re-place (verb)—a hyphen is needed to distinguish *re-place* (to place again) from *replace* (to take the place of).

Replens gel (Gyn)—for vaginal dryness.

Replogle tube (Neonat).

rescue
citrovorum
folinic acid
leucovorin
stem cell
uridine

resection—excision of a portion of an organ or of a structure. Cf. *recession.*

resectoscope, Iglesias fiberoptic.

reservoir
Camey
double bubble flushing
Florida pouch
Kock pouch
Ommaya
Rickham
Salmon-Rickham
Seroma-Cath wound drainage catheter and suction

residual—lasting effect of disease or injury.

residual volume/total lung capacity (RV/TLC) ratio.

resolution (Radiol)—the ability of an optical, radiographic, or other image-forming device to distinguish or separate two closely adjacent points in the subject. In computed tomography, resolution is measured in lines per millimeter; the higher the resolution, the sharper and more faithful the image.

Respiradyne—an electronic instrument that measures pulmonary function.

respirations
Cheyne-Stokes
Kussmaul

respirator—see *ventilator.*

respiratory syncytial ("sin-sish-ul") **virus** (RSV).

Respirgard II nebulizer—used to deliver aerosolized pentamidine (Pentam 300, NebuPent). See *NebuPent.*

Respironics CPAP machine—continuous positive airway pressure (CPAP) device for treatment of sleep apnea and in all-night polysomnogram.

Res-Q AICD (Cardio)—an automatic implantable cardioverter/defibrillator.

rete ridges ("ree-tee") (Path)—epidermal projections into dermal tissue.

retention sutures (also, stay sutures)—heavy nonabsorbable sutures used to reinforce wound closure where there is likely to be unusual postoperative stress.

Rethi incision—in the nose (Plas Surg).

reticent—reserved, quiet, not inclined to speak out. With some frequency, I hear dictators use it incorrectly thus: "We discussed having an upper GI and barium enema, which she was reticent to get." Of course, what is meant is *reluctant.*

retina—innermost, or third tunic, of the eye, that receives the image formed by the lens, and is the immediate instrument of vision.

retinal commotio (concussion)—usually a result of trauma to the eyeball.

retinal detachment—pathological condition where the retina, or part of it, becomes separated from the choroid. Surgical correction includes cryotherapy (cold therapy), diathermy (heat therapy), photocoagulation (laser therapy), and scleral buckling. These therapies induce a sterile inflammatory reaction that causes retinal re-adherence. See *pneumatic retinopexy; rhegmatogenous retinal detachment;* and *Schepens-Okamura-Brockhurst technique for retinal detachment repair.*

retinal pigment epithelium (RPE).

retinal tear; hole—injuries, disease, or degeneration may cause small holes or tears in the retina, allowing the vitreous humor from the large chamber in the back of the eye to seep in between the retina and the choroid, causing the two layers to separate, reducing the blood supply to the retina, and resulting in retinal detachment.

retinopathy—any disorder of the retina, including:
- arteriosclerotic
- central serous
- chloroquine
- circinate
- diabetic
- hypertensive

retinopathy of prematurity (ROP) (Neonat).

retinopexy—see *pneumatic retinopexy.*

retinoschisis (Oph)—splitting of the sensory layers of the retina, usually due to aging.

retractor
- Agricola lacrimal sac
- Army-Navy
- Aufricht
- Berkeley-Bonney self-retaining 3-blade
- Bookwalter
- Bronson-Turtz iris
- Burford rib
- Deaver
- De Lee
- Desmarres
- Echols
- Favoloro sternal
- Finochietto rib
- Fomon
- Gelpi
- Gilvernet
- Goligher
- Harrington
- Henning knee
- Hohmann
- Jannetta
- Joe's hoe
- Judd-Masson bladder
- Klemme laminectomy
- Leyla
- Lone Star
- Magrina-Bookwalter vaginal
- malleable
- Mark II Chandler
- Mini-Hohmann
- Nevyas drape
- Obwegeser peritoneal
- Quervain abdominal
- Ragnell hand-held
- Richardson-Eastman
- Rizzuti iris
- Sachs vein
- Schindler
- Semb
- Sewell
- Tuffier rib
- Upper Hands
- Weinberg

retrobulbar neuritis—inflammation of the orbital portion of the optic nerve, usually unilateral.

retrolisthesis (Ortho)—the displacement posteriorly of a vertebra on the one below.

retropubic prostatectomy.

retrospectoscope—a physician's coined term for 20/20 hindsight.

Retrovir (zidovudine, AZT)—approved by the FDA to treat patients with AIDS and ARC.

retroviruses—RNA viruses; leukoviruses and lentiviruses are in this group. Retroviruses were not considered to be pathogenic in humans, until the identification of HTLV-I, which causes a leukemia, and HIV. See *HIV.*

Reuter bobbin tube (ENT). The tube looks like a sewing machine bobbin (the round kind).

Reverdin-Green osteotomy (Pod)—osteotomy of the metatarsal head.

Reverdin suturing needles (Plas Surg).

reversible ischemic neurological deficit (RIND).

reversible obstructive airway disease (ROAD)—used synonymously with *asthma.*

Rev-Eyes (dapiprazole).

Rey and Taylor Complex Figure Test—a neurological test.

Rey Auditory Verbal Learning Test.

Reye's syndrome—a rare, but often fatal, disease in children, marked by edema of the brain, fatty infiltration of the liver, unconsciousness, and seizures. Seen after viral illnesses such as chickenpox and influenza. Thought possibly related to the administration of aspirin during these illnesses.

RF coil; pulse (radiofrequency)—MRI terms.

RGB (Roux-en-Y gastric bypass).

RGO (reciprocating gait orthosis).

RG-83894—an AIDS vaccine.

RG 12915 (Oncol)—an antiemetic given to cancer patients who have experienced severe nausea during a prior cycle of chemotherapy.

r-gp160—a potential vaccine for HIV developed by MicroGeneSys, Inc.

rhabdomyolysis (disintegration or dissolution of muscle)—newly recognized as a complication following cocaine use.

rhagades—white linear scars at the corners of the mouth; a sign of congenital syphilis.

rhegmatogenous retinal detachment (Oph)—caused by a retinal tear.

Rhesus diploid cell strain rabies vaccine (RDRV) (adsorbed).

Rh factor (Rhesus)—an antigen, genetically determined, which is found on the surface of erythrocytes. Incompatibility of the antigens in a mother and fetus is the cause of erythroblastosis fetalis. See *RhoGam.*

RH factor (rheumatoid). See *rheumatoid factor.* Not to be confused with Rh (Rhesus) factor.

rHb1.1 (recombinant hemoglobin)—a genetically engineered hemoglobin that is used as a blood substitute in order to prevent transmission of infectious diseases through transfusions.

rheumatic fever diagnosis—see *Jones criteria, revised.*

rheumatoid factor (RH factor, *not* Rh). An abnormal protein in the blood of most patients with rheumatoid arthritis. Testing for RH factor helps to make a diagnosis of this disease.

Rhino Rocket—nasal packing in a disposable plastic applicator, used for control of postoperative bleeding and for epistaxis.

Rhizopus nigricans—an allergen.
Rhoton punch (Neuro).
Rhoton ring tumor forceps.
Rhoton round dissector (Oph).
Rhoton titanium microsurgical forceps.
rHuEPO or **EPO** (recombinant human erythropoietin). See *epoetin alfa.*
ribavirin (Virazole)—a drug used to treat ARC and HIV-positive patients.
ribbon stools—stools of greatly narrowed diameter, often due to partial obstruction of the lower bowel by a tumor.
ribonuclear protein (RNP)—results of ENA testing.
RICE (rest, ice, compression, elevation (Ortho)—an acronym for basic treatment for most sprains, strains, and other closed soft-tissue injuries, particularly of the extremities. Also used in instructions to patients who have undergone orthopedic surgery or arthroscopy.
Rice-Lyte (Peds)—a product by Mead Johnson, manufacturer of infant formulas. Rice-Lyte is an over-the-counter solution containing rice and electrolytes found to be effective in controlling infant diarrhea.
Richards hydroxyapatite PORP and TORP prostheses (ENT)—made of a biocompatible material for ossicular reconstruction.
Richardson-Eastman retractor.
Richards Solcotrans Plus (Ortho). See *Solcotrans Plus.*
Richter's hernia—a strangulated hernia in which the constricting ring has caught only a portion of loop of intestine.
rickettsia—see *Coxiella burnetii.*
Rickham reservoir—used in obtaining serum methotrexate levels.
RIDD (recombinant interleukin-2, dacarbazine, DDP [cisplatin])—chemotherapy protocol.
ridges, rete (''ree-tee'') (Path)—epidermal projections into dermal tissue.
Ridley implant cataract lens.
Riedel's struma—a thyroiditis in which the gland is slowly replaced by hard dense fibrous tissue which is difficult to distinguish from cancer. Surgery may be necessary to relieve tracheal compression.
rifabutin (Mycobutin, ansamycin)—used to treat MAC infection.
rigidity
decerebrate
decorticate
Rigiflex balloon dilator (GI)—used to dilate strictures.
Rigiflex TTS balloon catheter (GI)—a through-the-scope catheter with a balloon at the tip that is inserted through the patient's mouth, into the GI tract. Used to dilate a stenosis in the ileum or colon resulting from Crohn's disease. Also called Microvasive Rigiflex TTS balloon.
rigor—rigidity, stiffness (as in rigor mortis). Cf. *rigors.*
rigors—chills. Cf. *rigor.*
Rimadyl (carprofen) (Ortho)—a nonsteroidal anti-inflammatory drug.
rimantadine (Flumadine)—an antiviral drug used to prevent infections by influenza type A viruses.
RIND (reversible ischemic neurological deficit). Episode may last several hours, longer than a transient ischemic attack.
ring
BAR (biofragmentable anastomotic)
Falope
fixation

ring *(cont.)*
Fleischer
Flieringa scleral
hymenal
Kayser-Fleischer
Klein-Tolentino
Landoldt
olive
Schatzki's
signet-ring pattern
silicone
Soemmering's
tantalum
Tolentino
Valtrac BAR
Woronoff's

ring forceps *(not* Ring forceps); also called sponge forceps.

ring fracture (Neuro)—encircles the foramen magnum; may be considered a basilar or occipital fracture.

Ringer's lactate. See *lactated Ringer's solution.*

Ringer's solution—a physiologic salt solution used for irrigation in surgery. See *lactated Ringer's solution.*

Ring hip prosthesis (Ortho).

Ring-McLean sump tube (Surg). "The tract was dilated to 12 French, and a 12 French Ring-McLean sump tube was placed."

Rinne test ("rin-nay") (ENT). This test uses air and bone conduction. A tuning fork is stroked or tapped and held close to the external auditory meatus until it is no longer heard. Then the base of the tuning fork is placed near the mastoid bone. If the patient cannot hear it on the mastoid bone, the test is considered normal (positive). If the patient can hear it better by bone conduction, the Rinne is negative, and the patient has a conductive hearing loss.

Ripstein procedure—for rectal prolapse (Surg).

RISA (radioactive iodinated serum albumin) study.

Risser localizer cast—used in treatment of scoliosis (Ortho).

Rizzuti expressor; iris retractor.

RM stereotaxic system (Riechert/Mundinger) (Neuro)—used in performing stereotaxic craniotomy. Also for 3-D stereotaxic treatment planning for convergent beam irradiation and radioactive seed implantation.

RNP (ribonuclear protein)—result of ENA testing.

ROAD (reversible obstructive airway disease)—another term for asthma.

Robicsek Vascular Probe (RVP) (Surg) —intravascular flexible surgical probe. Has different sizes of bulbs at the end of the probe and has a flexible one-piece construction without a metal stylet to be removed.

Robin's syndrome ("ro-banz"). See *Pierre Robin syndrome* and *micrognathia-glossoptosis syndrome.*

Robotrac passive retraction system—mounted on the operating room table, this apparatus holds all types of retractors in a fixed position until repositioned, thus allowing surgical assistants to perform other duties.

Rochester HKAFO (Ortho, Pod)—a hip-knee-ankle-foot orthosis which has separate hip and knee joint locks. For ambulation in children with cerebral palsy and myelomeningocele.

rocker, Carolina—see *Carolina rocker.*

rockerbottom foot—congenital vertical talus foot deformity (Ortho).

Rockey-Davis incision *(not* Rocky).

rod
Auer
Biofix system bioabsorbable fixation

rod *(cont.)*
Ender fixation
Harrington
Hunter tendon
Kuntscher
Luque
Maddox
silicone flexor
Wiltse
Wissinger

rod fixation, Luque.

rod test, Maddox.

roentgen knife (Neuro)—not a knife, but a type of stereotaxic radiosurgical device used in surgery to reach deep-seated tumors or arteriovenous malformations in the brain. See *Gamma knife.*

Roferon-A (interferon alfa-2a)—a drug used to treat leukemia, carcinoma, AIDS, and Kaposi's sarcoma.

rogletimide (Oncol)—a chemotherapy drug given to women with metastatic breast cancer with positive estrogen and progesterone receptor status.

Rogozinski spinal fixation system (Ortho, Neuro)—system of rods, hooks, and screws used to provide sacral fixation. Provides two points of spinal fixation combined with cross-linking to create strong, stable fixation. Also called Richards Rogozinski spinal fixation system.

Roho mattress—an air-filled device that helps prevent pressure sores (decubitus ulcers) (Surg).

Rokitansky-Aschoff sinuses—small outpouchings of the gallbladder mucosa extending through the lamina propria and muscular layer (GI).

Rokitansky's disease—see *Budd-Chiari syndrome.*

rolandic epilepsy (also jacksonian). See *jacksonian seizure.* Note: The word *rolandic* is not capitalized, except at the beginning of a sentence.

rolfing—a type of massage therapy.

Rolyan foot drop splint (Ortho).

Rolyan tibial fracture brace (Ortho).

ROM (range of motion).

Romberg test (Neuro). The patient stands with feet together, first with the eyes closed, then with the eyes open. The examiner evaluates the amount of body swaying. Some swaying is normal. If the Romberg is positive or equivocal, the patient may be asked to hop in place on one foot and then the other.

"romi"—used as a verb, as in "The patient was romied." Medical slang; it means a myocardial infarction was ruled out—**r**ule **o**ut **m**yocardial **i**nfarction.

rongeur
Adson
Beyer
Citelli
Decker pituitary
Ivy mastoid
Leksell
monster
Semb
Spurling-Kerrison

R on T phenomenon (Cardio)—premature ventricular contractions coming so closely together that ventricles are stimulated in their resting period, which can lead to fatal ventricular tachycardia or fibrillation; the name reflects the electrocardiogram appearance.

Roos test—a maneuver performed to detect thoracic outlet syndrome (Vasc Surg).

rooting reflex (Peds). An infant will turn its head toward the stimulus when its cheek is gently touched (as if it is searching for food).

root signs—signs of compression or injury of spinal nerve roots, such as absence of deep tendon reflexes in a

root signs *(cont.)* patient with a slipped intervertebral disk.

ROP (retinopathy of prematurity) (Neonat).

ROPA (Regional Organ Procurement Agency)—matches potential donors and recipients for organ transplants.

roquinimex—a chemotherapy drug used to treat advanced renal cell carcinoma as well as AIDS.

Rorschach test (Psych)—ink blot test.

Rösch-Thurmond fallopian tube catheterization set (Gyn).

rose bengal (Oph)—a dye, used as a stain to demonstrate the presence of abrasion of the corneal surface in Sjögren's syndrome—"dry eye."

Rose position—head extension (ENT).

Rosenmueller's fossa.

Rosenthal fibers—seen in pilocytic astrocytoma (Neuro).

rosettes, Homer-Wright—sometimes seen on histologic examination of medulloblastomas.

Rosomoff cordotomy (Neuro)—a percutaneous radiofrequency cervical cordotomy.

Rotablator (Cardio)—a rotating bur with diamond blades only 10 microns each in size. Used to pulverize calcified atheroma causing coronary artery stenosis.

rotating frame of reference—MRI term.

rotating hinge, Kinematic.

rotator, Bechert nucleus.

rotavirus—a group of viruses involved in acute gastroenteritis in infants.

Rotazyme diagnostic procedure—an enzyme immunology kit from Abbott Labs for rotavirus antigen in stool and liver aspirates.

Roth-Bernhardt disease—see *meralgia paresthetica.*

Roth's spots—small hemorrhages, round or oval lesions with small white centers; may be seen in the ocular fundi in cases of subacute bacterial endocarditis.

Rothmund-Thomson syndrome—oculocutaneous disorder seen with linitis plastica (a gastric carcinoma), and characterized by skin changes including atrophy, telangiectasias, alterations in pigmentation, and sparse or absent eyelashes and eyebrows. Some patients are also found to have cataracts, bone defects, dystrophic nails, and small stature.

Roto-Rest bed.

Rous sarcoma virus—oncogenic retrovirus.

Roux-Y chimney ("roo-Y") (Radiol, Surg). "Transjejunal approaches have been used to examine patients following Kasai procedures, to dilate stenotic hepaticojejunostomies in a retrograde manner, to place a U tube percutaneously, to perform percutaneous hepaticojejunostomy, and to accomplish intermittent biliary access in patients with Roux-Y chimneys brought up to the skin." Also, Roux-en-Y anastomosis.

rovamycin—British name for an antibiotic tried against AIDS, called *spiramycin* by the USAN.

Rovsing's sign—pain elicited at McBurney's point (in the lower right abdomen) when the corresponding point in the lower left is pressed. Indicative of acute appendicitis.

Rowasa enema—used for ulcerative colitis, proctosigmoiditis, proctitis.

Rowe disimpaction forceps.

Roxanol CII (morphine sulfate) oral solution—for severe acute and severe chronic pain.

Royal Flush angiographic flush catheter (Rad).

Royalite body jacket (Ortho).

RPE dropout; clumping (retinal pigment epithelium) (Oph).

RPR (rapid plasma reagin)—a test for syphilis, faster than the VDRL, and macroscopic rather than microscopic. See *reagin.*

RPR-CT (rapid plasma reagin circle-card test)—for syphilis. Cf. *RPR.*

RRA (registered record administrator).

rsCD4 (recombinant soluble CD4, Receptin)—a drug used to treat patients with AIDS and ARC.

RSI (repetitive strain injury).

RSLT (reduced size liver transplant) (GI)—in pediatric patients with liver failure, used to fit the donor liver into the smaller intra-abdominal space of the recipient.

RSV (respiratory syncytial virus).

rt-PA (recombinant tissue plasminogen activator).

rub—a sound heard on auscultation of the chest that sounds like . . . a rub. (Also called saddle leather friction rub.) Caused by a serous surface rubbing against another. (To duplicate the sound, rub your thumb and index finger together close to your ear.)

rubeosis iridis—a condition in which new blood vessels form on the anterior surface of the iris, associated with some ischemic vascular or ocular diseases which may lead to painful hemorrhagic glaucoma.

rubidium-82 (^{82}Rb) (Radiol)—a radioactive tracer used to perform a PET scan to evaluate heart function at rest and during stress. It has a half-life of only 75 seconds—too short to be helpful in evaluating the patient if a treadmill test is done. Therefore, it is combined with the vasodilator dipyridamole (Persantine) and injected intravenously. Stress is evaluated as the patient squeezes a dynamometer.

Rubin Brandborg biopsy tube.

"ruby" lens—see *Hruby lens.*

rucksack paralysis—backpack straps can compress the upper trunk of the brachial plexus, compromising the peripheral nerves to the shoulder.

Rudd-Clinic hemorrhoidal ligator and Rudd-Clinic hemorrhoidal forceps.

RU 486—see *mifepristone.*

ruga (pl., rugae)—rugal folds; folding of the gastric mucosa.

Rule of Nines—formula by which the percentage of body surface which has been burned is determined. The head is figured at 9%, as is each arm. Each leg is 18% (2 x 9), as are the anterior trunk and the posterior trunk. This all adds up to 99%. The perineum is figured at 1%. See also *Berkow formula.*

Rumel technique; tourniquet.

rumination—(1) Constant obsession or preoccupation with certain thoughts, with the patient being unable "to let go" of them. "Special symptoms include some ruminations, insomnia, and vacillatory appetite." (2) A condition in which infants regurgitate food after almost every meal, vomiting part of it and swallowing the rest.

runoff (Radiol)—the flow of blood (and contrast medium) through the branches of an artery into which the medium has been injected.

Rush pin—used in hand surgery, and other orthopedic surgery procedures.

Russell dwarf.

Russell traction—used as a temporary measure to stabilize femoral fractures until the patient can be taken to surgery.

Russian forceps (Ob-Gyn, Surg).

RUT (modified rapid urease test) (GI)—the most rapid and accurate test available to detect *Helicobacter pylori* in gastric lesions. The test produces a color change in one minute with a specimen of gastric mucosa obtained via endoscopic biopsy. Other tests for *Helicobacter pylori* take much longer: Gram stain (1 to 3 hours); culture (4 to 7 days). The RUT allows appropriate treatment to be initiated immediately.

rutherford unit—a unit of radioactivity; abbreviated *rd.*

Rutzen ileostomy bag (Surg).

RVH (right ventricular hypertrophy) (Cardio, Radiol).

RV/TLC ratio (residual volume/total lung capacity).

RWJ 25213—used to treat HIV-positive patients. (RWJ, R. W. Johnson Pharmaceutic Research Institute.)

Ryder (French eye) **needle holder.**

Rye histopathologic classification of Hodgkin's disease.

Rythmol—see *propafenone.* Note the spelling of this drug—*Ry,* not *Rhy,* although it affects the rhythm of the heart.

S, s

SA, S-A node (sinoatrial).
Sabouraud's medium—culture medium for growing fungi.
sabre shin deformity—in congenital syphilis, the leading edge of the tibia bows forward.
Sabreloc spatula needle.
saccade—series of involuntary, abrupt, rapid small movements or jerks of both eyes simultaneously in changing the point of fixation.
saccadic pursuit—following movements of the eyes.
saccadic slowing (Oph, Neuro).
sacculotomy—see *Fick sacculotomy.*
SACH heels (solid ankle cushioned heel)—for orthopedic appliances.
Sachs nerve spatula; tissue forceps; vein retractor (Neuro).
Sacks-Vine PEG (percutaneous endoscopic gastrostomy) **tube.** Also called Sacks-Vine feeding gastrostomy tube.
sacralization—abnormal bony fusion between the fifth lumbar vertebra and the sacrum.
saddle coil—MRI term.
saddle embolus—a blood clot that has lodged at the bifurcation of an artery, thus blocking both branches. Also called pantaloon embolus or straddling embolus. ''Her significant past history includes a history of a saddle embolus.''
saddle leather friction rub—on heart examination.
Sade modification of the Norwood procedure for hypoplastic left-sided heart syndrome (Card Surg). See *Fontan; Gill/Jonas.*
Sadowsky hook wire—used in breast surgery.
SAE (subcortical atherosclerotic encephalopathy).
Saethre-Chotzen syndrome (''say-ther-cho-tzen'')—a form of craniofacial anomaly, familial, in which there may be cranial synostoses and other anomalies.
SAF hip replacement (self-articulating femoral).
sagittal orientation (Radiol).
sagittal roll spondylolisthesis (Ortho).
SAH (subarachnoid hemorrhage).
sail sign (Ortho)—anterior and superior elevation of the fat pad in the elbow joint. The sail sign is highly suggestive of intra-articular fracture.

SAL (suction-assisted lipectomy) (Plas Surg).

salaam activity—a form of seizures.

Salmon's law—a method of locating the internal opening of an anal fistula.

salmon-patch hemorrhage (Oph). The hemorrhages (usually found in patients with sickle cell disease) occur in the midperipheral part of the fundus. They are initially red but often turn a salmon color after several days.

Salmon-Rickham reservoir (Neuro).

Salter fracture (Ortho)

Salter I—fracture through the plate only.

Salter II—fracture through the growth plate and through a portion of the metaphysis.

Salter III—fracture through the growth plate and through the epiphysis.

Salter IV—fracture through the growth plate, the metaphysis, and the epiphysis.

Salter V—a crushing fracture injury of the growth plate.

Salter VI—fracture of the perichondrial ring surrounding the epiphysis.

Salter osteotomy (Ortho).

saluresis—excretion of sodium and chloride ions in the urine.

saluting—repeated rubbing of the nose upward to scratch an itchy nose and open the obstructed airway (seen in patients with allergies). Also called allergic salute.

Salyer modification—of Obwegeser's mandibular osteotomy.

SAM (scanning acoustic microscope).

SAM (systolic anterior motion)—on 2-D echocardiogram.

"sammoma"—see *psammoma.*

Sam splint (Ortho)—foam pad with aluminum center which is invisible on x-ray, waterproof, and reusable.

Sandifer syndrome (Surg)—rare manifestation of gastroesophageal reflux in children that is associated with abnormal movements and postures of the head, neck, and trunk; treated with Nissen fundoplication and a Heineke-Mikulicz pyloroplasty.

Sandostatin (octreotide)—a drug used to control severe diarrhea in patients with vipomas and AIDS.

Sandoz suction/feeding tube (GI).

Sanger-Brown syndrome.

sanguineous—bloody.

Sanorex (mazindol).

Santorini plexus—a network of veins in the region of the prostate gland.

SaO_2 (arterial oxygen saturation)—the percentage of hemoglobin in the arterial blood that is saturated with oxygen. Normal values are 95% to 100%.

sargramostim (Leukine, leukopoietin, Prokine) (Oncol)—a granulocyte/macrophage colony-stimulating factor (GM-CSF) used in autologous bone marrow transplantation and to treat Kaposi's sarcoma and CMV retinitis. See *GM-CSF.*

Sarmiento cast (Ortho).

Sarns aortic arch cannula (Cardio).

Sarns saw (Surg).

Sarns temperature probe (Surg).

Sarot bronchus clamp (Thor Surg).

SAS (sleep apnea syndrome).

SASMA system (skin-adipose superficial musculoaponeurotic) (Plas Surg)—a face-lift technique said to achieve more lasting results than other techniques.

satellite lesion—a smaller lesion, near the primary lesion; accompanying,

satellite lesion *(cont.)*
nearby, subordinate lesions. "There was an indurated, excoriated rash which had no satellite lesions or any appearance of tinea." "Examination reveals an erosive vaginal lesion at 6 o'clock, consistent with herpes, and several satellite lesions which are also erosive, ulcerative lesions."

Saticon vacuum chamber pickup tube for video camera used in arthroscopy. Cf. *Circon; Newvicon; Vidicon.*

Sattler veil—see *bedewing of cornea.*

saturation recovery technique—MRI term.

saucerize—to create a saucer-shaped excavation surgically.

Sauflon PW (lidofilcon B)—soft, extended-use hydrophilic contact lens for aphakia in children (Oph).

sausaging of a vein—refers to a narrowing of the vein so that it looks like a string of sausages.

Sauvage graft (Vasc Surg)—filamentous velour Dacron arterial graft material.

saw
Aesculap reciprocating
Charriere bone
Gigli
Hall sternum
oscillating
reciprocating
Sarns
Williams microsurgery

Sbarbaro tibial plateau prosthesis.

SBE (small bowel enteroscopy).

SBE (subacute bacterial endocarditis).

SBP (spontaneous bacterial peritonitis).

SBRN (sensory branch of the radial nerve).

scale (See also *score; test.*)
Abbreviated Injury Scale
Bayley Scales of Infant Development

scale *(cont.)*
Brazelton Neonatal Assessment
Cattell Infant Intelligence
CIWA-A (Clinical Institute Withdrawal Assessment–Alcohol)
Dubowitz
Esterman
French (sizing)
Glasgow Coma Scale
Glasgow Outcome Scale
Injury Severity Score
Karnofsky
MOBS (Montefiore Organic Brain Scale)
Outerbridge
Tanner Developmental
Vineland Social Maturity
visual analogue
WAIS (Wechsler Adult Intelligence Scale)
Wechsler Memory Scale
Zung Depression Scale

scalloping of vertebrae (Radiol)—sometimes seen on x-ray of patient with sickle cell anemia.

scalp—the layers covering the skull: skin, subcutaneous tissue, galea aponeurotica, loose connective tissue, and periosteum.

scalp electrode (Obs)—EKG lead attached to scalp of infant about to be delivered to evaluate intrauterine heart rate.

scalp pH (Obs)—blood sample taken from scalp of infant about to be delivered to evaluate intrauterine oxygenation.

scan (See also *procedure.*)
B-scan
Cardiolite
CardioTek
contrast material enhanced
CT (computed tomography)
gallium
HIDA, or TcHIDA

scan *(cont.)*
indium-111 leucocyte scintigraphy
MAA lung
medronate
MUGA (multiple gated acquisition)
PET (positron emission tomography)
PIPIDA, or TcPIPIDA
PYP (pyrophosphate)
radionuclide
rectilinear bone
sector echocardiography
serial
sestamibi stress
SPECT (single photon emission CT)
stacked
teboroxime
TechneScan MAG3
technetium
ThromboScan
TSPP rectilinear bone
unenhanced
V/Q (ventilation/perfusion)
xenon-133 (^{133}Xe)

scanner
Aloka
ATL real-time NeurosectOR
Bruel–Kjaer ultrasound
cine CT
CT/T 8800
EMI
General Electric CT/T
high field strength
linear
sector

scanning acoustic microscope (SAM).

Scaphoid-Microstaple system (Pod)—a system for osteosynthesis using a simple staple device.

scapholunate arthritic collapse (SLAC). See *SLAC wrist.*

scatoma—stercoroma; a tumorlike mass in the rectum formed by an accumulation of fecal material. Cf. *scotoma.*

SCC (small-cell cancer) of the lung. Also, squamous cell carcinoma.

sCD4 (soluble recombinant human CD4). See *CD4.*

sCD4-PE40—a drug used to treat patients with AIDS.

Schaaf foreign body forceps (Oph).

Schachar implant cataract lens (Oph).

Scharf implant cataract lens.

Schatzki's esophageal ring (ENT).

Scheie
anterior chamber cannula
cataract aspirating needle
goniopuncture knife
ophthalmic cautery

Schepens–Okamura–Brockhurst technique (Oph)—for retinal detachment repair.

Scheuermann juvenile kyphosis (Ortho).

Scheuermann's disease (Ortho)—osteochondrosis of vertebral epiphyses in the young.

Schiff, in *periodic acid-Schiff test.*

Schiller test—when iodine is painted on the cervix, healthy tissue is stained but cancerous tissue is not.

Schindler esophagoscope; retractor (ENT).

Schiötz tonometry (Oph)—measures intraocular pressure. See *applanation tonometry.*

Schirmer's tear strips (Oph)—used in measuring tear secretion.

Schirmer's test—A strip of filter paper or soft tissue paper is placed between the eyelids to determine the quantity of tear production. Used in the diagnosis of Sjögren's syndrome and one of its elements, keratoconjunctivitis sicca ("dry eye").

Schlein elbow arthroplasty (Ortho).

Schlemm's canal (Oph)—in the inner scleral sulcus, against the sclera, a large vessel filled with aqueous humor, closely resembling a large lymphatic channel.

Schlesinger's solution—a morphine solution used for palliative purposes in patients with far-advanced carcinoma.

Schlichting posterior polymorphous dystrophy.

Schober test (Rheum)—a test for evaluation of spondylitis; measures lumbar flexion. Measurements are given in degrees, with normal being 20° or more.

Schönlein-Henoch purpura—a kidney disease with urticaria, erythema, arthritis, arthropathy.

Schüffner's dots—cytoplasmic stippling.

Schuknecht cochleosacculotomy (ENT)—for treatment of progressive endolymphatic hydrops (Ménière's disease). Involves the placement of an endolymphatic shunt to control a chronic state of excessive accumulation of endolymph.

Schuller's view.

Schwachman's syndrome.

schwannoma—see *neurilemmoma.*

Schwartz test—for patency of the deep saphenous veins.

SCID (severe combined immunodeficiency disease).

scintigraphy, quantitative hepatobiliary (QHS).

scintillating scotoma—flashing lights and expanding circles of light—seen in migraine headache and in disorders of the occipital lobe of the brain.

scirrhous ("skir-us")—refers to a hard cancer, e.g., scirrhous carcinoma of the breast. Cf. *serous.*

scissors
- Aebli corneal section
- automated intravitreal
- Belluci stapedectomy
- Bruel-Kjaer ultrasound
- Castroviejo
- Converse nasal tip
- Dandy

scissors *(cont.)*
- DeWecker iris
- Diethrich valve
- Haenig irrigating
- Jabaley-Stille Super Cut
- Katzin corneal transplant
- Knapt
- Littauer
- Littler
- Litwak mitral valve
- Lloyd-Davies
- McPherson-Vannas iris
- MPC automated intravitreal
- Noyes iridectomy
- Reichling corneal
- Stevens tenotomy
- Stille-Mayo
- Sutherland
- Sutherland-Grieshaber
- Toennis anastomosis
- Twisk needleholder/forceps/scissors.
- Vannas capsulotomy
- Westcott tenotomy
- Yasargil bayonet

scissors gait.

sclera (pl., sclerae)—the tough white tissue which covers the so-called white of the eye.

scleral buckling procedure (Oph)—used as treatment for primary retinal detachment. Silicone sponge, solid silicone, or fascia lata are attached to the sclera or buried in it. The sclera indents (or buckles) toward the center of the eye. Subretinal fluid is drained, and the retina is reattached (after the fluid has been drained or resorbed) and is in contact with the pigment epithelium. The buckling element can be applied locally or can encircle the eye, as appropriate. Cf. *pneumatic retinopexy,* a newer procedure.

scleroderma—a form of progressive systemic sclerosis.

sclerotherapy—see *EVS.*

sclerotome—see *Lundsgaard.*
sclerouvectomy, partial lamellar (Oph)—used to remove a uveal tumor and leave intact outer sclera and sensory retina.
SC-1 needle (Oph)—used to reposition a subluxated lens in intraocular surgery.
SCOOP 1—a transtracheal oxygen catheter with an opening at the distal tip for oxygen flow.
SCOOP 2—a transtracheal oxygen catheter with a distal opening and side openings to facilitate oxygen flow.
scorbutic white line—radiologic finding in scurvy.
score (See also *scale; test.*)
Abbreviated Injury Scale (AIS)
APACHE II
Apgar
cardiac morbidity
Cooperman event probability
Detsky modified risk index score
Dripps-Aemrican Surgical Association
Eagle equation
Eastman visual function
Glasgow Coma
Gleason
Goldman cardiac risk index
Hughston knee
Kurtzke disability
LAP (leukocyte alkaline phosphatase)
Lysholm knee
McGill pain
PULSES profile
treadmill duration (TDS)
scoring incision—"This allowed a vertical scoring incision posteriorly, as well as another scoring incision along the bone ridge, permitting swiveling of the cartilage to a more midline position."
Scotchcast 2 casting tape (Ortho).
scotoma—an area of depressed vision in the visual field surrounded by an area of more normal vision. Examples: Bjerrum's; scintillating; Seidel's. Cf. *scatoma.*
"scrim"—ENT slang for speech or auditory discrimination.
scultetus binder; bandage (Ob-Gyn).
scurf—flaky material seen around the eyelashes, usually, but also other parts of the body.
scybalous stool ("sib-uh-lus")—hard, dry fecal matter. I mention this not because it is not in the dictionaries (it is), but simply to save your going through the *ci, cy, si, sy, psi, psy,* etc., routine to find the word. Used thus: "He was taking laxatives and enemas, with production of scant, scybalous stools."
scyphoid ("si'foid")—cup-shaped. Cf. *xiphoid.*
SD antigens (serologically-determined).
SDAT (senile dementia of the Alzheimer type) (Neuro).
sea fan (Oph)—in patients with sickle cell retinopathy, major nutrient arterioles and draining venules grow in neovascular patches. The neovascular channels develop slightly dilated aneurysmal tips resembling the typical fan shape of *Gongonia flabellum* (sea fan).
sea fronds—description of neovascularization seen on eye examination.
seagull bruit.
SEA port (side entry access).
seat belt fracture—see *Chance fracture.*
seat belt sign (Ortho)—abrasion across the abdomen following trauma in an automobile accident in which the lumbar vertebrae are fractured from extreme forward flexion. See *Chance fracture.*

second-look laparotomy—reoperation, for further investigation.

sector scan echocardiography—see *two-dimensional echocardiography.*

Secu clip ("C-Q") (Gyn)—clip used in tubal ligation.

secundum atrial septal defect (ASD) (*not* secundim) (Cardio).

sediment—see *spun urine sediment.*

sed rate (sedimentation rate). This test is a good indicator of the possible presence (or absence) of generalized systemic illness. My own preference is to write it out. I would certainly never type *sed rate* if *sedimentation rate* had been dictated.

"see-pap"—see *CPAP.*

SeeQuence disposable lens (Oph).

segments—middle cerebral artery
M_1 sphenoidal
M_2 insular
M_3 opercular
M_4 cortical

Seguin's sign (Neuro)—involuntary contracture of muscles just prior to an epileptic seizure.

Seidel humeral locking nail (Ortho).

Seidel intramedullary fixation (Ortho).

Seidel test—used with fluorescein dye to locate wound leaks.

SE image (spin-echo) (Radiol)—a magnetic resonance image obtained by the spin-echo technique; with this technique, T2 is determined indirectly, as a function of TE, the echo time.

Selacryn—antihypertensive medication.

Seldane-D (ENT)—the nonsedating antihistamine, Seldane, combined with the decongestant pseudoephedrine.

Seldinger gastrostomy needle (GI).

Selecor (celiprolol).

selective excitation; irradiation—MRI terms.

Select joint (Ortho)—orthosis for ambulation in children with cerebral palsy and myelomeningocele.

selenium-75 (^{75}Se)—radioisotope used in pancreatic scan.

self-articulating femoral (SAF) **hip replacement.**

self-aspirating cut-biopsy needle (Radiol)—see *PercuCut cut-biopsy needle.*

Sellick maneuver—pressure on the cricoid during anesthesia induction/intubation. Used to prevent aspiration of stomach contents. Pressure is maintained until the anesthesiologist inflates the cuff on the endotracheal or nasoendotracheal tube.

Selverstone clamp (Neuro). (*Not* Silverstone.)

Semb
retractor
rib shears
rongeur

semisynthetic human insulin:
Novolin N (equivalent to NPH)
Novolin L (equivalent to lente)
Novolin R (equivalent to regular)

Senning intra-atrial baffle—for repair of transposition of the great vessels).

sensitize (Radiol)—to introduce radioactive material into a fluid, tissue, or space for purposes of performing a radioactive scan; essentially the same as *label.* Cf. *label.*

sensorimotor skills—alertness, responsiveness, interest in surroundings. *Not* sensory-motor.

sensorineural (*not* sensory neural).

sensory branch of the radial nerve (SBRN).

sensory nerve action potential (SNAP).

sentinel loop (Radiol)—an isolated, gas-filled, distended loop of small bowel that represents paralytic ileus.

sentinel node—an enlarged lymph node in the left supraclavicular fossa containing cancer metastatic from the stomach; also called Virchow's or Troisier's node.

sentinel pile—a hemorrhoid or hemorrhoid-like nodule of tissue that forms below an anal fissure.

SEP (somatosensory evoked potential) (Neuro); used to monitor spinal cord function in spinal injury, and in spinal cord monitoring in surgery. See also *SSEP,* which is synonymous.

Septacin (Ortho)—an implant used to treat osteomyelitis. This flexible chain of oval beads, made from the biodegradable polymer Biodel, contains the antibiotic gentamicin. The implant is left in situ following surgery to remove necrotic tissue in the bone of patients with osteomyelitis. The Septacin implant delivers the gentamicin in high concentrations directly to the site of the infection, releasing the drug over a three-week period as the beads are absorbed by the body. See also *Biodel, Gliadel.*

Septra—see *TMP-SMZ.*

sequela (pl., sequelae; usually used in the plural)—a persistent effect of an illness or injury, such as paralysis after a stroke.

sequence (MRI terms)
Carr-Purcell
Carr-Purcell-Meiboom-Gill

sequential multiple analyzer (SMA).

SER (somatosensory evoked response) (Neurol).

SER-IV (supination, external rotation-type IV fracture) (Ortho).

serial scans (Radiol)—a series of scans made at regular intervals along one dimension of a body region.

sermorelin acetate (Geref)—given I.V. to assess the ability of the pituitary gland to secrete growth hormone.

Seroma-Cath (Ob-Gyn)—wound drainage catheter and suction reservoir used to drain seromas that develop after mastectomy.

serotonin type-3 receptor antagonists (Oncol)—a new class of drugs used to treat chemotherapy-induced nausea and vomiting. See *ondansetron.*

serous (''se'rus'')—pertaining to serum, resembling serum, or containing serum (as in serous cystadenoma). Cf. *scirrhous.*

serpiginous—snake-like.

Serratia liquefaciens—formerly classified as *Enterobacter liquefaciens*; it has been isolated from the intestinal tract, respiratory tract, blood, and urine.

Sertoli-cell-only syndrome (Urol)—characterized clinically by aspermia and histologically by complete loss of the epithelium in the testicular tubules.

sertraline (Zoloft) (Psych)—an antidepressant (a 5HT blocker) which inhibits the uptake of serotonin in the brain.

serumcidal—see *cidal.*

serum p24 antigen concentration—a marker used to monitor HIV serum levels.

Servo pump (Neuro)—used in cases of hydrocephalus to control intracranial pressure at desired levels.

sestamibi stress test (Radiol). The radioactive imaging agent ^{99m}TC sestamibi (Cardiolite) shows areas of myocardial infarction during a stress test.

Seton hip brace (Ortho).

setting sun sign. With increased intracranial pressure or irritation of the brain stem, the eyes can deviate downwards so that white sclera is seen above the iris.

Sever-L'Episcopo repair of shoulder.

Severin intraocular lens.

Sewell-Boyden flap (ENT).

Sewell retractor (ENT).

sexually transmitted disease (STD).

Sézary cell.

Sézary syndrome—exfoliative erythroderma, manifested by hyperkeratosis, edema, alopecia, and pigment and nail changes.

SF_6 (sulfur hexafluoride)—a gas used in pneumatic retinopexy (Oph).

SFA (subclavian flap aortoplasty).

SGA (small for gestational age) (Ob).

Sgambati's reaction; test ("zgahm-bah-tee"). This is a test for peritonitis. When the patient's urine is combined with nitric acid and chloroform, a resulting red tint is a positive sign of peritonitis.

SGIA stapling device; staples.

shagreen lesions of the lens (Oph).

shake test—tests the maturity of fetal lungs. See *foam stability test.*

Shapshay/Healy 20 cm phonatory and operating laryngoscope (ENT).

sharp and blunt dissection (Surg)—separating or cutting apart tissues with sharp instruments (scalpel, scissors) where necessary and with blunt instruments or fingers where possible. Separation of structures and development of tissue planes by blunt dissection is less traumatic and causes less bleeding.

Sharpey's fibers—collagenous fibers of a tendon, ligament, or periosteum buried in the subperiosteal bone.

Sharplan 733 CO_2 laser.

Sharpoint microsurgical knife.

sharps—operating room slang for suture needles, scalpel blades, hypodermic needles, cautery blades, and safety pins—all of which require special handling to avoid injury to healthcare personnel and to reduce their risk of acquiring bloodborne infections.

Sharrard-type kyphectomy (Ortho).

Shaw scalpel—an electrical scalpel. A dictator mentioning this instrument will usually give settings in degrees of temperature.

Shea drill (Oto).

Shearing intraocular implant lens.

Sheehy incus replacement prosthesis (ENT).

Sheehy syndrome—rapidly advancing sensorineural hearing loss in younger age groups.

sheet sign—psychological despair in AIDS patients shown by hiding under bedcovers and refusing human contact.

Sheets (Implens) **intraocular lens.**

Shepard intraocular lens implant.

Shepard-Reinstein intraocular lens forceps (Oph).

Shepherd technique (Oph)—a technique for intraocular lens insertion using a 3-4 mm incision and closure with suture knots covered with conjunctiva.

Shiatsu therapeutic massage.

Shier total knee prosthesis.

shift to the left (white blood cells)—means there are increased numbers of immature neutrophils which may indicate presence of infection. The term refers to a white blood cell differential counted manually; the technician uses a diagram which places the younger, developing cells on the left side of the page. A rise in the number of these cells, a shift to the

shift to the left *(cont.)* left, is a sign of the body's reaction to an infection, or of leukemia.

shift to the right—means that there are increased numbers of older neutrophils present in the blood. Cf. *shift to the left.*

shifting dullness on percussion—an indication of the presence of ascites. The abdomen is percussed with the patient lying in the supine position, then with the patient lying on each side. If the area of dullness shifts, this is an indication of the presence of ascitic fluid, rather than edema or cyst.

shill, protrusio (Ortho).

shim coil; shimming—MRI terms.

shin splints—painful spasm of shin muscles due to strain, usually as a result of running.

Shirodkar procedure (cervical cerclage) (Ob-Gyn).

shock blocks—blocks placed under the foot of a bed to elevate it manually for a patient in shock.

shocky—in shock, or showing signs (tachycardia, pallor, diaphoresis, restlessness) suggestive of shock.

shoe, WACH—a cast shoe used in orthopedics. (WACH, **w**edge **a**djustable **c**ushioned **h**eel.

Shohl's solution—used in treatment of renal tubular acidosis.

ShortCut knife (Oph)—an ophthalmic knife with a unique rounded tip and short length for intraocular incisions. Also, A-OK ShortCut knife.

shorthand vertical mattress stitch—rapid skin everting suture technique (Surg).

short-limb dwarfism—a form of dwarfism in which the extremities are abnormally short, as differentiated from the true, or normal, dwarf, in which the only abnormality is the small size.

short TR/TE (or "T1-weighted")—MRI terms. TR (repetition time); TE (echo time).

shotty nodes, as in B-B shot. *Not* to be confused with "shoddy," as in "shoddy merchandise."

Shouldice hernia repair (Surg)—used for either direct or indirect hernias; a variation of the Halsted-Bassini repair.

shunt
- Cordis-Hakim
- Denver hydrocephalus
- Denver pleuroperitoneal
- Denver peritoneal venous
- Gibson inner ear
- Gott
- Holter
- House and Pulec otic-perotic
- Javid
- LeVeen peritoneal
- PFTE (polyfluorotetraethylene)
- Pruitt-Inahara carotid
- Quinton-Scribner
- Spetzler lumboperitoneal
- Torkildsen
- Vitagraft arteriovenous
- Warren
- Winters

Shur-Strip (Deknatel)—a sterile wound closure tape.

SI—see *International System.*

SIADH (syndrome of inappropriate antidiuretic hormone secretion).

Sibley-Lehninger—test for serum aldolase.

sick building syndrome—nausea, headache, and some other symptoms experienced by people who work in some new buildings in which windows cannot be opened. Apparently

sick building syndrome *(cont.)*
caused by many of the chemicals found in carpeting, furniture, etc.

Sickledex—a screening test for sickle cell disease.

sick sinus syndrome—*sinus* refers to the sinoatrial node (Cardio).

SICOR—a computer-assisted cardiac catheterization recording system that automatically calculates, displays, and reports all hemodynamic parameters, valve areas and shunts, and then prints a report immediately after catheterization.

side-biting clamp (Surg).

side-cutting spatulated needle that comes in one-fifth circle and one-third circle and is threaded with 4-0 cable-type Supramid Extra suture material.

side entry access port (SEA)

siderotic nodules in the spleen—also called Gamna-Gandy nodules or bodies (Radiol). See *Gamna-Gandy bodies.*

sievert (Sv) (''sé-vert'') (Radiol)—the SI unit of radiation absorbed dose equal to 1 gray (Gy) or 1 joule (J) per kilogram, or 100 rem.

"sigh"—see *p.s.i.*

Sigma—method used in testing serum CPK. See also *Oliver-Rosalki.*

sigmaS (Oncol)—a serum tumor marker used to distinguish between early and advanced stages of breast cancer.

sigmoidoscope
Pentax flexible
Reichert

sign
Aaron's
alien hand
Apley
Allis's
Aufrecht's
Babinski

sign *(cont.)*
bagpipe
Bard's
Battle's
blue dot
Blumberg's
bow-tie
Branham's
brim
Brudzinski's
Chadwick's
chandelier
Collier's
Courvoisier's
Cullen's
Dalrymple's
Dance's
de Musset's
doll's eye
Dorendorf's
double bubble
drawer
Duroziez'
Ewart's
fabere
fadir
Fajersztajn's crossed sciatic
fat pad
Federici's
Finkelstein's
Froment's
frontal release
Galeazzi
Gauss'
Goodell's
Gowers
green tongue
Griesinger's
Hamman's
Hoehne's
Homans'
Jacquemier's
Jackson's
Joffroy's
Kernig

sign *(cont.)*
Lasègue's
long tract
Macewen's
main d'accoucher
McCort's
McMurray
Moebius'
Mulder
mute toe
obturator
oil drop change
Ortolani's
parrot's
Phalen's
Pinard's
Pins'
pivot-shift
puddle
pyloric string
Queckenstedt's
root
Rovsing's
sail
seat belt
Seguin's
setting sun
sheet
soft neurologic
Spurling's
steeple
Stellwag's
string
target
tenting
Terry fingernail
Tinel's
Trousseau's
Unschuld's
vital
von Graefe's
Warthin's
Weill's

signal intensity (Radiol)—in magnetic resonance imaging, the strength of the signal or stream of radiofrequency energy emitted by tissue after an excitation pulse.

signal-to-noise ratio (S/N)—MRI term.

signet-ring pattern—a cellular change wherein the cell has a ring-like configuration; seen in gastric carcinoma.

Sigvaris compression stockings (Vasc Surg)—for treatment of venous disease in ambulatory patients.

Silastic bead embolization (Cardio)—used as therapy for some types of arteriovenous fistulae fed by several small arteries in areas not amenable to surgical repair, or if the vessel is not a critical artery which may be obliterated without fear of causing distal ischemia. (See *Gianturco coil,* used for the same purpose.)

Silastic H.P. tissue expander.

Silastic silo reduction of gastroschisis. See *Silon tent.*

silent—without symptoms or signs, as in silent gallstones, silent myocardial infarction.

silicon—a chemical element present in sand and various types of rock. Cf. *silicone.*

silicone—an organic compound used in the manufacture of various medical devices such as breast implants, catheters, drains, etc. Cf. *silicon.*

silicone flexor rod—placed in the sheath of the flexor tendon for reconstruction of a finger (Ortho, Hand Surg).

silicone ring.

Silon tent—used in an operative procedure for gastroschisis. The tent is placed over the abdominal opening and the intestines are gradually reduced back into the abdomen by ligating the top of the tent progressively. See also *Silastic silo.*

silver wire effect (Oph)—effect created by narrowing of arterioles in the retina.

Simcoe (Oph)
aspirating needle
intraocular implant lens
II posterior chamber lens

simkin analysis *(not* named for a person). It is **sim**ulation **kin**etics analysis to determine serum acetaminophen levels.

Simplex cement; adhesive (Ortho).

Simpson atherectomy catheter—used for atherectomy in atherosclerotic peripheral vascular disease (removal and retrieval of atheroma) (Cardio).

Simpson peripheral AtheroCath. See *Simpson atherectomy catheter.*

Simpulse system (Ortho)—high-pressure, high-volume pulsed lavage used in joint replacement procedures.

simultaneous volume imaging—MRI term.

simvastatin (Zocor) (Cardio)—used to lower levels of LDL in patients with hypercholesterolemia which has not responded to dietary measures. Other therapeutic actions include raising levels of HDL and lowering triglyceride levels. This drug belongs to the class known as HMG-CoA reductase inhibitors.

Sinding-Larsen-Johannson disease—of the patella (Ortho).

sine-wave pattern—in electrocardiogram, in patients with hyperkalemia. *(Not* sign-wave, but pronounced that way.)

Singer-Blom valve (Surg, ENT)—used for esophageal speech in patients who have had laryngectomies.

singer's node (ENT)—not an eponym, but a small white nodule which is often seen on the vocal cords of singers, or others who use their voices excessively.

Singh-Vaughn-Williams classification of arrhythmias (Cardio).

single photon emission computed tomography (SPECT).

SingleStitch PhacoFlex lens (Oph)—a silicone intraocular lens which folds for easy insertion through the small incision used for cataract surgery. The tiny opening can then be closed with one stitch (hence, SingleStitch).

single-stripe colitis (SSC) (GI)—a single stripe of ulcerated mucosa seen on colonoscopy is diagnostic of colitis.

singultus—hiccups. "The patient was observed to have multiple episodes of singultus during his emergency room stay."

sinoatrial node (SA or S-A node)—the pacemaker of the heart and what is referred to in "sinus rhythm." See *Flack's node* and *Koch's node* (which are synonymous).

Sinskey (Oph)
hook
intraocular lens forceps
posterior chamber lens

Sinskey/Sinskey modified blue loop intraocular lenses (Oph).

Sippy diet—named for Dr. Bertram Welton Sippy, who wrote on gastric and duodenal ulcers.

SISI (short increment sensitivity index) —used in hearing test (Audiol).

Sister Mary Joseph node—lymph node near the umbilicus. Named for the nurse who first observed that when she found such a node, the patient always had pancreatic carcinoma.

site—place or position, as "The site of the abscess was located quickly." Cf. *cite.*

situ—see *in situ.*

Sivash prosthesis (Ortho)—a total hip prosthesis that does not require use of cement.

6-AN protocol—topical cream (Derm).

6-mercaptopurine riboside (mercaptopurine).

6-MP (mercaptopurine).

6-MPR (mercaptopurine).

Sjögren's syndrome ("sho-grenz")—a symptom complex marked by keratoconjunctivitis sicca.

Skeele chalazion curet (curette) (Oph).

skeletonize—in *Webster's,* meaning "to produce in or reduce to skeleton form." Rarely found in medical dictionaries, although doctors use the word in dictation.

SKF (skilled nursing facility).

skilled nursing facility (SKF).

skills, sensorimotor *(not* sensory motor).

Skil Saw—an electric saw you will run into (figuratively speaking) in orthopedic surgery transcription in reference to the etiology of an injury.

skin depth—MRI term.

skin graft. See *graft, skin.*

Skin Skribe—trade name for a surgical marking pen used in Plastic Surgery.

Skinny dilatation catheter (Cardio)—used during cardiac catheterization. Skinny is a trade name.

skinny needle. See *Chiba needle* and *fine-needle biopsy.*

SkinStat pre-formed skin staple.

Skiodan (methiodal sodium)—a myelographic contrast medium (Radiol). May also be used in other areas, including the urinary tract.

"skir-us"—phonetic rendering of *scirrhous.*

Skoog release of Dupuytren's contracture (Ortho).

SK-SD, SKSD (streptokinase-streptodornase)—skin test for immune function.

Skribe, in *Skin Skribe*—a surgical marking pen used in plastic surgery.

skull plate, tantalum.

skull tongs, Gardner-Wells.

SKY epidural pain control system.

skyline view of patella (Radiol)—radiographic study of the knee region in which the patella is visualized above the distal femur and appears like a rising (or setting) sun.

SLAC wrist (scapholunate arthritic collapse) (Ortho)—in which a fracture deformity has healed in a rotated position and eroded the radioscaphoid joint.

Slant lens (Oph)—a single-piece intraocular lens with a new design which incorporates slanted haptics and a low profile for easy insertion through the longer scleral tunnel and more acute angle of entry now used in intraocular lens surgery. Slant is a trademark. Also, Cilco Slant haptics lens.

SLAP lesion (superior labrum [or labral] anterior posterior) (Ortho). "He has a SLAP lesion where the labrum is detached superiorly. We used a bur in order to get down to good bloody bone in that area, in an attempt to get the SLAP lesion to heal down to bloody bone."

sleep apnea—a disorder associated with snoring, irregular heartbeat, and wakefulness in which soft tissues in the throat can obstruct breathing. In severe cases, this can cause death.

sleep deprivation. On the average, adults require from 6 to 9 hours of sleep per night, with older people

sleep deprivation *(cont.)* thought to require less than younger ones. Sleep deprivation may be categorized as lack of total sleep, rapid eye movement (REM) sleep, or nonrapid eye movement (NREM) sleep. Fatigue, irritability, difficulty remembering, difficulty in concentrating, and problems with muscle coordination may be manifestations of sleep deprivation.

slim disease—This is the term used for AIDS in some countries in Africa; so-called because of the great loss of weight seen in this disease.

sling and swathe (Ortho)—used for immobilization of fractured humerus if comminution is not extensive.

sling, cardiac—see *cardiac sling.*

Slinky catheter (Cardio)—PTCA (percutaneous transluminal coronary angioplasty) catheter for use in invasive catheterization procedures.

slit-lamp biomicroscopy (Oph)—allows well-illuminated microscopic examination of eyelids and anterior segment of the eyeball in a three-dimensional cross-section view. See *Haag-Streit slit lamp.*

Sloan abdominal incision.

Slo-Phyllin Gyrocaps (Pulm)—used to treat bronchial asthma.

slow-channel blocking drugs (Cardio) —another name for calcium channel blockers.

SLRT ("slert") (straight leg raising test) (or tenderness).

Sluder-Jansen mouth gag (ENT).

Sluyter-Mehta thermocouple electrode (Neuro).

Sly disease—a form of mucopolysaccharidosis, with onset at the age of one to two years, manifested by cardiac anomalies, mental retardation, short stature, pectus carinatum, and facies seen in Hurler's syndrome.

SMA (superior mesenteric artery).

SMAC (Sequential Multiple Analyzer plus Computer) ("smack")—automated serum chemistry panels (profiles) comprising multiple tests.

SMA-6 (sequential multiple analyzer) test for sodium, potassium, chloride, bicarbonate (CO_2), blood urea nitrogen (BUN), and creatinine.

SMA-12 (sequential multiple analyzer) test for calcium, phosphorus, glucose, BUN, uric acid, cholesterol, total protein, albumin, total bilirubin, alkaline phosphatase, LDH, and SGOT.

SMA-20—automated serum chemistry panels (profiles) comprising 20 tests: glucose, BUN, creatinine, sodium, potassium, chloride, calcium, phosphorus, uric acid, cholesterol, total protein, biirubin, alkaline phosphatase, LDH, SGOT, SGGT, direct bilirubin, triglycerides, albumin, iron.

small-bowel enteroscopy (SBE) (GI)—a technique used to visualize the small bowel in patients with idiopathic gastrointestinal bleeding.

small-bowel transit time (Radiol)—on upper GI series, the time required for swallowed contrast medium to pass through the small bowel and appear in the colon.

Small-Carrion penile prosthesis. Small is a proper name, not a size.

small for gestational age (SGA).

SmallPort needle (Oph)—a phacoemulsification needle used in cataract extraction to remove the nucleus and polish the capsule. It has a smaller opening at the tip than other phacoemulsification needles.

Sm antigen—Smith antigen, in systemic lupus erythematous (SLE).

SmartNeedle (Cardio)—needle hooked to a Doppler which emits an audio signal that helps locate femoral, subclavian, or internal jugular vessels for catheterization.

SMAS ("smass") (superficial musculoaponeurotic system)—a term referring to a layer of the face, used in plastic surgery in rhytidectomies.

Smead-Jones type closure.

SMF (streptozocin, mitomycin, fluorouracil)—chemotherapy protocol.

smile, or smiling, incision. If you're going to have an incision at all, I suppose it's better to have a smiling one.

Smith intraocular implant lens (Oph).

Smith-Petersen gouge (Ortho).

Smith-Petersen osteotome (Ortho).

SMo—stainless steel with molybdenum; used in orthopedic appliances; causes minimal tissue reaction.

SMO (supramalleolar orthosis) (Ortho, Pod)—allows for plantar flexion and dorsiflexion. Orthosis for ambulation in children with cerebral palsy and myelomeningocele.

SMV (superior mesenteric vein).

SMZ/TMP (sulfamethoxazole and trimethoprim). These two agents are combined in Bactrim and Septra, familiar trade name drugs for use against urinary tract infections, now also used against *Pneumocystis carinii* pneumonia.

SNA, SNB—measurements in orthodontics. S stands for sella, N for nasion (nasal point), A and B are reference points.

SNAP (sensory nerve action potential) (Neuro).

snap gauge band (Urol)—a band made of elastic fabric and Velcro. It has three snaps, designed to open at progressively higher degrees of penile rigidity. Used to test for organic vs. psychogenic impotence. See *Dacomed snap gauge.*

Snellen chart—a test for visual acuity, using progressively smaller letters or symbols.

SNHL (sensorineural hearing loss) (ENT). Note: *Not* sensory neural.

snowball opacities (Oph).

snowbanks (Oph)—aggregation of inflammatory cells seen on the anterior inferior retina; characteristic of pars planitis.

snowstorm shadow, on chest x-ray—one of the indications for diagnosis of neurogenic pulmonary edema.

Sn-protoporphyrin (Neonat)—a drug for neonates that decreases elevated bilirubin levels faster than phototherapy. It acts by inhibiting an enzyme necessary for the production of bilirubin.

S/N ratio (signal-to-noise) (Radiol)—used in magnetic resonance imaging.

snuffbox, anatomical—see *anatomical snuffbox.*

SOAP note—refers to a format setup of clinic, hospital, and physician chart notes or progress notes. Acronym for Subjective, Objective, Assessment, Plan, which are paragraph subheads of the report.

Soave abdominal pull-through procedure—surgical treatment for Hirschsprung's disease. This procedure does not require pelvic dissection. Instead, the aganglionic rectal musculature is not removed, but the rectal mucosa *is* removed, and the normal ganglionic segment is then brought down through the rectal muscular cuff.

SOB (short of breath).
sodium tetradecyl sulfate (Sotradecol) (GI)—used to treat bleeding esophageal ulcers.
Soehendra dilator (GI)—used to dilate the cystic duct.
Soemmering's area or ring—an oval, yellowish spot located exactly in the center of the posterior part of the retina.
Softgut—a surgical chromic suture.
soft neurologic signs—nonlocalizable signs.
Sof-Wick dressings; drain sponges.
solar keratosis—horny skin growth in some individuals, caused by overexposure to sunlight.
Solcotrans drainage/reinfusion system (Ortho)—used as a blood-saving system, especially in spinal fusion procedures.
Solitaire needle (Oph)—slightly curved needle used for closure following small-incision cataract surgery.
soluble CD4—a drug used to treat AIDS.
Soluset—a volume control device for administering intravenous solutions.
solution—see *medication.*
Solvang graft (Plas Surg)—a tip graft to the nose.
somatomedin levels for growth hormone testing.
somatosensory evoked potential (SEP). See *SEP.*
somatosensory evoked response (SER).
somatuline (Oncol)—a drug given to patients with metastatic prostatic cancer that has not responded to castration or reduction of naturally occurring levels of male hormones, a condition termed androgen-resistant.
Somer uterine elevator (Ob-Gyn).
Somogyi effect (''so-mo'-jee'').
Somogyi units—results of serum amylase testing are expressed in Somogyi units.
"somophagia"—see *psomophagia.*
"sonameter"—see *centimeter.*
Sondergaard's cleft—the interatrial groove (Cardio).
Sondermann's canal.
S 10036 (fotemustin)—a chemotherapy drug to treat advanced gastric carcinoma.
Sones selective coronary arteriography.
Sonksen-Silver acuity cards (Oph)—to test visual acuity in children age 3 and up or those with communication problems.
sonography, Acuson computed.
sonolucent (Radiol)—offering relatively little resistance to ultrasound waves (as air or fluid) and hence generating few or no echoes. Cf. *radiolucent; translucent.*
SONOP—an ultrasonic aspiration system (Neuro).
Soonawalla uterine elevator.
Sophy programmable pressure valve—used in neurosurgery in the management of hydrocephalus.
Sorbothane heel cushions (Ortho).
Sorbsan topical wound dressing (Surg)—used to treat decubitus ulcers.
"sore-a-len"—see *psoralen.*
sotalol (Betapace) (Cardio)—a structurally unique antiarrhythmic drug that combines the qualities of a beta blocker with prolongation of the repolarization phase of the myocardium. Used to prevent or treat life-threatening arrhythmias.
Sotradecol (sodium tetradecyl sulfate).
souffle (''soo'-f'l'')—not the cheese or chocolate kind; this is a soft blowing sound heard on auscultation.

Southwick osteotomy (Ortho).

sparfloxacin—used to treat MAC infection in AIDS patients.

spatula, Castroviejo cyclodialysis.

Speare dural hook (Neuro).

speckle, laser. See *laser speckle.*

SPECT (single photon emission computed tomography)—a cardiac imaging technique using a single gamma camera which moves in a series of positions around the chest of the patient, receiving radionuclide signals from many angles. This provides a three-dimensional image and helps to localize regions of poorly perfused myocardium by eliminating image overlap. This is a thallium study.

Spectrax programmable Medtronic pacemaker (Cardio).

speculum
- Amko vaginal
- Fanta eye
- Guyton-Park eye
- Hardy-Duddy weighted vaginal
- Landoldt pituitary
- Park-Maumenee lid
- Yankauer pharyngeal

speech mapping (of the brain).

speech reception threshold (SRT).

Speedy balloon catheter (Cardio)—used during percutaneous transluminal coronary angioplasty.

Spence, tail of; also called *tail of the breast.* It is the tail-like segment of mammary gland tissue that extends to the axillary region.

SPEP ("S-PEP")—serum protein electrophoresis.

Spetzler lumboperitoneal shunt (Neurosurg).

SpF Spinal Fusion Stimulator (Ortho, Neuro)—a fully implantable stimulator. Used to increase the rate of healing after spinal fusion.

sphincterotome, Wilson-Cook (modified) **wire-guided.**

spica bandage (Ortho).

spica cast (Ortho).

spiking fever—a fever characterized by recurrent sudden brief elevations, which look like a row of spikes on a temperature graph.

spin density; echo—MRI terms.

spin-echo image (SE) (Radiol)—a magnetic resonance image obtained by the spin-echo technique. With this technique, T2 is determined indirectly, as a function of TE (echo time).

spin-lattice relaxation time—MRI term.

spin-warp imaging—MRI term.

spiral band of Gosset—the second palmar layer in the hand (Ortho, Hand Surg). Sometimes referred to in dictation of operative procedures for Dupuytren's contracture.

spirals, Curschmann's.

spirometry, incentive.

spiramycin (Rovamycin)—a drug used to treat cryptosporidal diarrhea in AIDS patients.

Spitz-Holter valve—old type of valve (used in the late 1950s) for ventriculoatrial shunting in hydrocephalus.

Spivack valve—a technique used in performing a Depage-Janeway gastrostomy (Surg).

splint
- air
- Aquaplast
- birdcage
- buddy
- Budin toe
- Bunnell
- Bunnell active hand and finger
- Bunnell knuckle-bender with outrigger
- Bunnell modified safety-pin

splint *(cont.)*
Darco medical-surgical shoe and toe alignment
Delbet
Denis Browne clubfoot
Denver nasal
Donjoy (or DonJoy) knee
Futura wrist
Hydro-Splint II
inflatable
Link Stack Split
plaster slab
polyvinylalcohol
Rolyan foot drop
Sam
shin
Stader's
sugar-tong plaster
talipes hobble
Thomas

splinter hemorrhage—a short linear hemorrhage under a fingernail or toenail, longitudinally oriented and looking somewhat like a splinter; often due to trauma but sometimes a sign of infective endocarditis.

splinting—stiffening of muscles to avoid pain in a part or extremity (Pulm, Ortho). Examples: "She is splinting rather markedly, and on this basis appears to be short of breath." "This may be associated with a certain amount of splinting and a reluctance to take deep inspirations."

splinting material—polyvinylalcohol.

Splintrex—an instrument used for rapid removal of wood or metal splinters; consists of forceps and a loupe.

split sheath catheter.

spondylophyte impaction set—used for correction of bony impingements of neural structures (Neuro).

sponge
Custodis
Helistat absorbable collagen hemostatic
Lapwall laparotomy
Lincoff
Merocel
peanut
pledgets
Ray-Tec x-ray detectable surgical
Sof-Wick
Vistec x-ray detectable
Weck-cel

sponge dissector (dissecting sponge)—used in surgery. Also called *peanut* or *cherry*. Cf. *spud dissector*.

spontaneous bacterial peritonitis (SBP)

Sporanox (itraconazole)—an antifungal drug used to treat histoplasmosis, blastomycosis, aspergillosis, and cryptococcal meningitis in AIDS patients.

Sporicidin—a glutaraldehyde-phenate cold sterilizing solution for disinfecting surgical instruments, endoscopes, respiratory therapy equipment, etc.

spot
ash leaf
café au lait
Campbell de Morgan
De Morgan's
Koplik's
Roth's

spotting—scanty vaginal bleeding, menstrual or otherwise.

Sprague-Dawley rats—a strain of rats used in laboratories.

spud dissector—used in surgery.

spun urine sediment—urine specimen centrifuged to concentrate sediment (cells, casts, crystals, and other formed elements) before microscopic

spun urine sediment *(cont.)* examination. "Spun urine sediment demonstrated 15-20 white cells."

Spurling's sign (Neuro).

Spurling-Kerrison up-biting and down-biting laminectomy rongeurs (Neuro).

spurring (Radiol)—formation of one or more jagged osteophytes, as in osteoarthritis.

squamous cell carcinoma (SCC).

square knot—an easy and reliable knot used for tying most suture materials, including surgical gut, collagen, silk, cotton, and stainless steel sutures. May also be indicated in Ethilon (nylon), Ethibond (polyester), and Prolene (polypropylene) sutures.

S-ROM total hip modular system with Poly-Dial Insert System (Ortho).

SRT (speech reception threshold) (ENT).

SSC (single-stripe colitis).

SSEP (somatosensory evoked potential) (Neuro). See also *SEP,* which is synonymous.

SSFP (steady state free precession)—MRI term.

SSKI (saturated solution of potassium iodide).

S-sleep (synchronized sleep).

Staar lens (Oph)—a foldable intraocular lens.

stacked scans (Radiol)—in computed tomography, a series of scans without intervals of unexamined tissue between them. Same as *contiguous images.*

Stader's splint (Ortho)—a metal bar with pins at right angles to the bar; the pins are driven into the fragments of the fractured bone, and the bar holds the pieces in alignment.

Stadie-Riggs microtome (Surg).

Stadol NS (butorphanol tartrate)—synthetic analgesic used to treat migraines. Previously available only by injection for moderate to severe pain as a preoperative and postoperative medication. Now available as a nasal spray, hence the "NS" in the trade name. One metered spray is the equivalent of a 1 mg dose.

stages, breast fibrocystic disease. See *breast fibrocystic disease.*

stages of labor (Obs)
- first stage—dilatation of the cervix until it is fully dilated and flush with the vagina
- second stage—expulsion of infant
- third stage—expulsion of placenta and membranes, and contraction of the uterus

staging—see *classification.*

Stahl calipers ("stall") (Oph)—used in measuring orbital implants.

stain
- Alcian blue
- auramine-rhodamine
- Congo red
- elastic fibers
- elastica-van Gieson's
- Giemsa-Wright
- Gram's
- Hansel's
- H&E (hematoxylin & eosin)
- HPS (hematoxylin, phloxine, safranin)
- immunoperoxidase
- Kinyoun
- Kleihauer-Betke
- Leder
- Mallory-Azan
- Mallory's
- meconium
- Nissl's
- oil red O
- PAS (periodic acid-Schiff)
- PTAH (phosphotungstic acid-hematoxylin)

stain *(cont.)*
Sudan
toluidine blue
von Kossa
Weigert
Wright's
Ziehl-Neelsen

STA-MCA bypass procedure (superficial temporal artery-middle cerebral artery).

Stamey needle (Urol)—a single-prong ligature carrier used in the Stamey bladder suspension procedure.

Stamey test—a test used in evaluating patients thought to have renovascular hypertension. The prognosis after corrective surgery is better in patients with a positive Stamey test. The test: a differential ureteral catheterization in which urinary flow rate and creatinine or PAH (paraaminohippuric acid) concentrations are measured from each kidney on diuresis. Patients with renal hypertension caused by obstruction of the renal artery will have a significantly decreased flow rate and a significantly increased creatinine or PAH concentration on the same side, as compared with the normal kidney on the other side.

Stamm gastrostomy.

Stammberger antrum punch (ENT).

Stanmore shoulder arthroplasty.

***Staphylococcus aureus* septicemia**—seen in AIDS patients.

Staphylococcus epidermidis—skin flora (formerly *Staph. albus).*

stapler
Appose disposable skin
Auto Suture Multifire Endo GIA 30
Auto Suture Premium CEEA
Auto Suture surgical
CEEA circular (curved EEA)
EEA (end-to-end anastomosis)

stapler *(cont.)*
Endopath ES reusable endoscopic
GIA (GI anastomosis)
ILA surgical
PI surgical
Precise disposable skin
Premium CEEA circular
Proximate flexible linear
SGIA
TA-55
TA-90
Watt's skin closure

star figure (Oph)—a star-shaped folding or pleating of the retina due to edema.

star, macular.

stare, thyroid—see *Collier's sign.*

Starr-Edwards aortic valve prosthesis.

starry-sky pattern (Path), as "There was a starry-sky pattern with phagocytosis of tumor cells."

stat, STAT (L. *statim*)—immediately. Often used in a request for an emergency lab report or x-ray, or a rush report from Transcription, in which case it means "I need it yesterday." Dictionaries show a period after *stat* because it is an abbreviation, but most medical personnel do not treat *stat* like an abbreviation and do not place a period after it. Often it appears in all caps.

Statak—soft tissue attachment device by Zimmer for use as alternative to conventional transosseous techniques.

Statham electromagnetic flow meter—flow measurements in blood vessels.

Stat 2 Pumpette—disposable I.V. pump that maintains flow rate under changing conditions.

status post—the condition or fact of having sustained an injury or illness or having undergone a surgical procedure, as in status post appendectomy.

stavudine (d4T, didehydrodideoxythymidine)—used to treat patients with AIDS and ARC and HIV-positive patients.

Stayoden 9000F TENS—see *TENS.*

stay sutures—see *retention sutures.*

STD (sexually transmitted disease).

steady state free precession (SSFP)—MRI term.

Stecher arachnoid knife (Neuro).

Steell, in *Graham Steell murmur.*

steel-winged butterfly needle.

steeple sign—on chest x-ray.

Steffee plates and screws (Ortho, Neuro)—used in lumbar fusion.

Stein intraocular implant lens.

Steinmann pin (Ortho). These pins come in both threaded and non-threaded configurations.

steinstrasse (Ger., stone street)—urinary sand and stone fragments which result from extracorporeal shock-wave lithotripsy (ESWL) of kidney stone.

Stellwag's sign—in exophthalmos, the upper lid is retracted and there are spasms of the lid as the patient looks upward, and the patient winks less than normally.

stem-cell marrow harvesting—for autologous frozen stem-cell marrow storage. This is done in patients with acute lymphoblastic leukemia while in relative remission, for use in relapse when an HLA-matched compatible donor is not available.

Stensen's duct.

stent
  Double-J indwelling catheter
  Gianturco expandable biliary
  Hood stoma
  Palmaz
  Palmaz-Schatz
  Palmaz vascular

stent *(cont.)*
  Percuflex
  Strecker
  T-Y
  Wall
  Wiktor cardiac
  Wiktor coronary
  Z

Stenver's views (Radiol).

stepping of vessels—abrupt change in the direction of retinal vessels passing over the brim of an abnormally deep optic cup (Oph).

stereognosis (Neurol)—relates to the ability to perceive, recognize, and understand the form of objects only by touching and manipulating them; a test of the function of the parietal lobes of the cerebral cortex.

stereotactic needle biopsy (Radiol)—a nonsurgical breast biopsy.

stereotaxy—the use of the Leksell stereotaxic device, modified for use with the CT scanner, for localizing areas of the brain for implanting radioactive sources, or implanting brain electrodes (Neuro).

Steri-Drape—trade name of a plastic incise drape.

sterilely (*not* sterilly or sterily).

steroid—adrenocortical steroid.

stethodynia—chest pain.

Stevens tenotomy scissors (Oph).

Stewart-Treves syndrome—lymphangiosarcoma.

stick tie—in some operating rooms, this is a suture ligature (or transfixion suture); in others it is a long strand of suture clamped on a hemostat.

Stifcore aspiration needle (GI, Pulm)—used to obtain gastric or bronchial biopsies.

Stille cranial drill (Neuro).

Stille-Mayo scissors (Thor Surg).

Stilling-Türk-Duane syndrome—see *Duane's syndrome.*

Still's disease—juvenile rheumatoid arthritis.

stimulation, stimulator
AME bone growth
Axostim nerve
dorsal column
EBI SPF-2 implantable bone
electrogalvanic
faradic (electrical)
Hilger facial nerve
magnetic
OrthoPak II
Osteo-Stim implantable bone growth
photic
Pisces spinal cord system
Reese
SpF Spinal Fusion
TENS (transcutaneous electrical nerve)

STIR—acronym for short-tau (pronounced "taw") inversion recovery, a term used in magnetic resonance imaging (Radiol).

St. Jude Medical
aortic valve prosthesis
bi-leaflet tilting aortic disk valve prosthesis

stockinette (stockinet) (Ortho, Surg)—a knitted, elastic material, used for wrapping over dressings.

stockings
Jobst
Sigvaris compression
TED
thigh-high antiembolic
Vairox high compression vascular

stone basket (Urol)
Dormia
Ellik
Pfister

stone extractor, Glassman (Urol).

STOO—Series Ten Thousand Ocutome probe and vitreous cutter (Oph).

stooling (Peds)—defecation; used generally of infants not yet toilet-trained.

Storz Calcutript—see *Karl Storz Calcutript.*

Storz flexible ureteropyeloscope—see *Karl Storz flexible ureteropyeloscope.*

Storz infant bronchoscope.

Storz radial incision marker (Oph)—used during cataract surgery.

Stoxil (idoxuridine).

Straatsma intraocular implant lens.

strabismus—the deviation of one eye from parallelism with the other. Types: A-pattern, concomitant, incomitant, nonconcomitant.

straddling embolus—same as *saddle embolus.*

Strampelli implant cataract lens.

strandy infiltrate (Radiol)—on chest x-ray, a pulmonic infiltrate that appears as strands or streaks of increased density.

strangury—slow, painful urination, caused by spasm of the urinary bladder and urethra (Urol). "He has no dysuria, but does have some chronic urinary urgency and frequency. There is no strangury."

Strecker stent (GI)—a tantalum-metal mesh, self-expanding stent which is placed on a balloon catheter and inserted and positioned endoscopically. Covered with a gelatinous layer which dissolves in one to two minutes, the stent then expands and remains expanded due to special memory metal fibers in the stent.

strep throat—streptococcal infection of throat. *(Not* strept throat.)

Streptococcus milleri—a recently identified microaerophilic gram-positive organism; thought to be a significant pathogen in childhood appendicitis.

streptokinase-streptodornase (SK-SD) skin test for immune function.

streptozotocin—antineoplastic agent.

stress cystogram—a radiographic study of the bladder intended to demonstrate stress incontinence. Contrast medium is instilled into the bladder and films are taken while the patient coughs and bears down.

stress test, sestamibi.

striatal nigral degeneration (Neuro)—a form of atypical parkinsonism; the name comes from the corpus striatum which is adjacent to the foramen of Monro.

string sign—long, severe stenosis of the distal segment of the internal carotid artery.

stripper, Dunlop thrombus.

stroma-free hemoglobin solution—may be used in the future for transfusions.

Strong-Campbell Vocational Interest Inventory (SCVII) (Psych).

Struempel-Voss ethmoid sinus forceps.

struma—see *Riedel's struma.*

Struycken nasal cutting forceps.

Stryker leg exerciser—device that provides continuing passive motion to the leg to help restore a patient's range of motion postoperatively (Ortho, Phys Ther).

Stryker Surgilav machine (Ortho). See *Surgilav.*

Stuart factor. See *blood coagulation factors.*

stump pressure (Vasc Surg); pressures measuring retrograde flow.

sty, stye—see *hordeolum* (Oph). I had always thought that there was a differentiation—that *stye* was a hordeolum and that *sty* was an enclosure for pigs, but dictionaries list both spellings for *hordeolum.*

subarachnoid hemorrhage (SAH).

subclavian flap aortoplasty (SFA) (Cardio)—a technique used to correct aortic coarctation in children.

subclavian peel-away sheath. See *Littleford/Spector introducer.*

subclavian steal syndrome—cerebrovascular insufficiency caused by obstruction of the subclavian artery proximal to the vertebral artery, reversing the blood flow through the vertebral artery. The subclavian artery thus, in effect, "steals" cerebral blood, causing cerebral or brain stem ischemia (Neuro, Vasc Surg).

subcortical atherosclerotic encephalopathy (SAE).

subcu or subQ—could mean either*subcutaneous* or *subcuticular.* Subcutaneous is the deeper layer, and subcuticular the more superficial layer. This may help in determining which is meant.

subcutaneous emphysema (Radiol)—air or gas in subcutaneous tissues.

subcutaneous fat lines (Radiol)—the edges or borders of the subcutaneous fat layer as seen on an x-ray film.

suberosis—extrinsic allergic alveolitis caused by exposure to oak bark or cork dust.

Subjective, Objective, Assessment, and Plan (SOAP). See *SOAP.*

suboptimal (Radiol)—not as good as might have been expected; usually referring to technical factors in an x-ray study, such as positioning, film quality, and patient cooperation.

Sub-Q-Set—see *CSQI.*

subset, as in "T-cell subset studies," a group within a group (T-4 cells, T-8 cells).

subtraction films (Radiol). A scout film is taken first, before the dye is in-

subtraction films *(cont.)* jected. The scout negative is made into a positive (darkens it). Then the angiogram is taken (this is a negative). Then a scout positive is taken and put under the dye-injected negative (the patient, not the film has had the dye injection), which screens out the bone, so that all that is then visible are the arteries and veins.

Suby's solution G—used as an irrigant to dissolve some types of kidney stones. Also referred to as "Suby G."

succimer (Chemet)—a drug to treat lead poisoning in children. A chelating agent which forms a water-soluble complex when it encounters lead in the blood stream. This complex is then excreted by the kidneys. Can be given orally, an advantage over the standard treatment with calcium disodium edetate which had to be given intramuscularly because it was poorly absorbed from the stomach. Treatment lasts 19 days and is monitored by serum lead levels.

succussion splash.

sucralfate (Carafate)—a medication used for coating duodenal ulcers.

suction-assisted lipectomy (SAL) (Plas Surg). Fat is removed by a suction device, rather than by sharp dissection.

Suction Buster catheter (GI)—a combination duodenal decompression tube and feeding tube with multiple holes down the side of the tube. Also called Moss Suction Buster tube.

suction punch, DyoVac.

suction, Seroma-Cath.

Sudan stain—an iodine compound used as a test for stool fat. It colors the droplets of fat, thus making them visible under the microscope. If there is excessive fat in the stool (steatorrhea), it may indicate liver disease, small bowel malabsorption problems, or pancreatic problems. If, on the other hand, the stool fat is extremely low, that may mean a vitamin D deficiency (since vitamin D is fat soluble).

Sudeck's atrophy—acute osteoporosis.

sugar-tong plaster splint (Ortho); used for immobilization in Colles' fracture.

Sugita aneurysm clip (Neuro).

Sugiura procedure for esophageal varices (Vasc Surg); esophageal transection with paraesophagogastric devascularization.

SUI (stress urinary incontinence).

Suit, in *Fletcher-Suit applicator.*

Sulamyd (sulfacetamide sodium) (Oph) —a sulfonamide used for treatment of conjunctivitis, etc.

sulfate, dextran.

sulfur hexafluoride (SF_6)—a gas used in pneumatic retinopexy (Oph).

sulindac (Clinoril) (Oncol)—a nonsteroidal anti-inflammatory drug used to treat osteoarthritis, rheumatoid arthritis, bursitis, and gout, as well as to prevent colorectal adenocarcinoma in patients with multiple polyposis.

summation gallop (S_3 and S_4)—in cardiac examination.

sumatriptan (Imitrex) (Neuro)—a drug for migraine headaches. It is chemically related to the neurotransmitter, serotonin, whose levels have been found to be decreased during migraines. Sumatriptan stimulates serotonin receptors in the brain to constrict blood vessels and relieve the migraine pain.

sundown syndrome (Psych)—a complex of symptoms such as disorientation, agitation, and emotional stress

sundown syndrome *(cont.)* which appear in elderly patients about the time of sunset. The hypothesized causes include decreasing light levels which increase disorientation in patients whose sight is already impaired, dehydration, or progressive fatigue. The patient afflicted with this syndrome is termed a sundowner, a pejorative term.

Sundt-Kees clip—for clipping aneurysms (Neuro).

sunrise view of the patella (Ortho, Rad).

sunset eyes (Neuro)—an abnormal appearance of the eyes in which the pupils lie at or below the level of the lower lids; seen in infantile hydrocephalus and due to retraction of the upper lids.

Superblade—a small blade used in ophthalmology; made by Medical Workshop in Holland.

superconducting magnet—MRI term.

superficial musculoaponeurotic system (SMAS).

Superglue (cyanoacrylate)—a tissue adhesive.

superior mesenteric vein (SMV).

supernate—the liquid material that rises to the top, after the solid material, or sediment, has settled to the bottom. Also *supernatant.* Cf. *infranate.*

supernumerary—more than the usual number, as of digits, or parathyroid glands.

Super PEG tube (GI)—a percutaneous endoscopic gastrostomy tube. Super is a trade name.

Super Pinky—a pink rubber ball with attached elastic headband. The ball is applied over the closed eyelids to lower intraocular pressure prior to surgery on the eye.

Supprelin (histrelin acetate)—used to treat children with precocious puberty.

suppressor cell, or T-8 suppressor cell, lymphocytes, part of the immune system. These are different from the T-4 lymphocytes attacked by the virus, but they need to interact with T-4 cells for the immune system to function correctly. Also called *cytotoxic cells.*

Supramid ptosis sling.

Supramid suture—a multiple monofilament nylon stranded suture in a nylon sheath; used for intestinal anastomoses.

suprasellar—above the sella turcica.

supratentorial symptoms—a way for physicians to indicate confidentially that there might be a functional overlay to an illness. The tentorium lies at the base of the cerebrum in the brain; hence, by definition, activity the patient can control is above this point. It can also be used in a somewhat pejorative sense or whenever physicians want to indicate among themselves, without being understood by laymen reading the record or overhearing, that the patient might have an element of hypochondriasis to his complaints. Using *lues* for syphilis is another example.

supraventricular tachycardia (SVT), or tachyarrhythmia.

suramin—an anti-infective agent used to treat infections in immunocompromised patients. Marketed under various trade names, including Fourneau 309, Germanin, Moranyl, Naganol, and Naphuride.

surcingle (''sur-single'')—a girdle; also a band, belt, or girth passing over a

surcingle *(cont.)* horse's back or saddle. See *Von Lackum surcingle.*

SureBite biopsy forceps (GI)—a flexible tube with a cup biopsy tip for gastrointestinal biopsies.

surface coil (Radiol)—in magnetic resonance imaging, a simple flat coil placed on the surface of the body and used as a receiver.

surf test—medical slang for surfactant test of amniotic fluid.

surfactant (Neonat)—a combination of the phospholipids lecithin and sphingomyelin which coats the alveoli. In premature infants, surfactant levels are so low and the resulting surface tension of the alveoli so high that the lungs collapse with each breath. Surfactant derived from amniotic fluid (Human Surf) or from cows' lungs (Infasurf) can be used to correct the deficit.

Surfit adhesive ("sure-fit").

Surgairtome (Ortho)—by Zimmer.

surgeon's knot (also friction knot)—suggested use in tying Vicryl and Mersilene sutures.

surgical gut—catgut; may be made from the serosal layer of beef intestine or the submucosal layer of sheep intestine; this is an absorbable suture.

Surgical Nu-Knit—an absorbable hemostatic material (like a loosely-knitted fabric, but thicker and more closely woven than Surgicel)—oxidized regenerated cellulose.

Surgical Simplex P radiopaque bone cement (Ortho).

Surgicel—an oxidized regenerated cellulose product that will be absorbed by body tissues; used for hemostasis.

Surgidev intraocular lens.

Surgidine—a germicidal solution. "The left leg was prepared with Surgidine and draped."

Surgilav machine (Stryker) used in washing the acetabulum or other operative area in orthopedic surgery.

Surgilene—a monofilament polypropylene suture material.

Surgilon—braided nylon suture material. Cf. *Surgilone.*

Surgilone—a monofilament polypropylene suture material. Cf. *Surgilon.*

Surgiport—disposable surgical trocar and sleeve to be used during endoscopic procedures.

Surgi-Prep (Surg)—Betadine (povidone-iodine) surgical preparation solution.

Surgitek mammary prosthesis.

Surgitek penile prosthesis.

Surgitron—portable radiosurgical unit; it has four therapeutic currents, as well as bipolar capabilities for microsurgical procedures.

sursumduction—upward movement of only one eye in testing for vertical divergence (Oph). Also, supraduction, superduction, supravergence, sursumvergence. Cf. *circumduction.*

Survanta (beractant; modified bovine surfactant extract) (Neonat)—used to treat RDS (respiratory distress syndrome) in premature infants. See also *Exosurf, RDS, surfactant.*

Susadrin—a nitroglycerin preparation.

Sussman four-mirror hand-held gonioscope (Oph).

Sutherland or Sutherland-Grieshaber scissors—manufactured by Grieshaber & Co.

Sutter-Smeloff prosthetic heart valve (ball valve type). If this sounds familiar, it is because we have had the Cutter-Smeloff heart valve for years.

Sutter-Smeloff valve *(cont.)*
What you will hear now is Sutter-Smeloff, named for Sutter Memorial Hospital in Sacramento where it was developed. You may still hear the old name in histories of patients who had that valve inserted years ago.

suture (material, technique, type)
absorbable
atraumatic
blanket
braided Ethibond
braided Mersilene
braided Nurolon
braided silk
bridle
bunching
catgut
chromic catgut
coated Vicryl
collagen
Connell
Connell inverting
continuous
continuous blanket
continuous Lembert
continuous locked
continuous mattress
cotton
coupled
Cushing
Deklene
dermal
Dermalene
Dermalon
Dexon
DG Softgut
double-armed
Endoloop
Ethibond
Ethiflex
Ethilon
Ethilon monofilament nylon
Exon II
figure-of-8

suture *(cont.)*
fixation
Flexon
funicular
Gambee
Gillies horizontal dermal
guy
Halsted
Halsted interrupted mattress
Herculon
interrupted
interrupted Lembert
interrupted mattress
interrupted near-far, far-near
Kessler
Lembert
mattress
Maxon
Mersilene
monofilament
multifilament
nonabsorbable (or unabsorbable)
Novafil
Nurolon
nylon
over-and-over
PDS (polydioxanone)
Perlon
Perma-Hand braided silk
Perma-Hand silk
Polydek
polydioxanone (PDS)
polypropylene
Prolene
pursestring, purse-string
retention
running lock
Sabreloc (spatula needle)
shorthand vertical mattress
silk
Softgut
stainless steel
stay
stick tie (suture ligature or transfixion suture)

suture *(cont.)*
Supramid
Supramid Extra
surgical gut
Surgilene
Surgilon
Surgilone
suture ligature (stick tie or transfixion suture)
swaged-on
tension
Thirsch
Ti-Cron
transfixion (stick tie or suture ligature)
twisted cotton, dermal, linen
Tycron
unabsorbable (or nonabsorbable)
undyed braided polyglycolic acid
U-shaped continuous
Vicryl
wing
wire

suture ligature—see *stick tie* and *transfixion suture.*

Suture Strip Plus—a stretch wound closure strip (Surg).

Suture/VesiBand organizer (Surg)—attaches to drape or skin within the sterile field to eliminate entanglement of multiple sutures and silicone bands.

suturing, coupled.

SVT (supraventricular tachycardia, or supraventricular tachyarrhythmia).

swaged-on (rhymes with "wedged") **suture.** The suture and needle are fused together. Also called *atraumatic suture.*

Swan-Ganz catheter—used to monitor pulmonary capillary wedge pressure.

Swann-Morton surgical blade.

Swanson PIP joint arthroplasty (Hand Surg). "A Swanson PIP joint arthroplasty of the right ring finger and extensor pulley reconstruction, for boutonnière deformity, was performed, using a Swanson prosthesis."

swathe. See *sling and swathe.*

sweat chloride levels. An elevated level of chloride in perspiration is a sign of cystic fibrosis. One method of measurement is the pilocarpine iontophoresis method.

Swede-O braces (Ortho).

"sweetheart"—operating room slang for Harrington retractor. See *Harrington retractor.*

Swenson papillotome (GI)—used to perform a papillotomy during an endoscopic transpapillary catheterization of the gallbladder in patients with symptomatic gallstones.

Swenson pull-through procedure—for Hirschsprung's disease.

swimmer's view (Radiol)—an oblique view of the thoracic spine in which the arm nearer to the x-ray source hangs at the patient's side and the opposite arm is upraised.

switch, duodenal.

Symbion J-7-70-mL-ventricle—total artificial heart (Cardio).

Syme amputation (Ortho)—ankle disarticulation. "The patient should consider talking with other amputees about the likelihood of a below-knee amputation prosthesis, as I don't feel that a Syme amputation would be indicated in this patient."

symmetrical phased array—term used in B-scan, Doppler, and color Doppler imaging. See *B-scan.*

Synarel (nafarelin).

SynchroMed infusion system—an implanted programmable pump and catheter used to deliver morphine into the epidural space. It is used to treat cancer patients with unrelieved pain. This pump has also been ap-

SynchroMed infusion system *(cont.)* proved to deliver certain chemotherapy drugs, clindamycin (to treat osteomyelitis), and baclofen (to treat chronic muscle spasticity).

synchronized sleep (S-sleep, or non-REM [NREM] sleep). S-sleep precedes desynchronized sleep and is the time when the muscles begin to relax, and is the time when fatigue is relieved. There are also changes in electrical activity on EEG. Cf. *REM* and *desynchronized sleep.* See *polysomnogram.*

syncytial knot formation (''sin-sish-al'')—a placental layer which proliferates and folds on itself, producing tangles of tissue.

syndactyly—a congenital anomaly in which the webbing between two (or more) digits extends to fusing the fingers to each other.

syndrome (See also *disease; sign.*)
- Aarskog
- acute tumor lysis (ATL)
- alien hand
- apallic
- Bartter's
- Bazex
- Beckwith-Wiedemann
- Behçet's
- Blackfan-Diamond
- Bloom
- blue diaper
- blue rubber-bleb nevus (BRBNS)
- blue toe
- Boerhaave's
- brain death
- Brown's
- Brown's tendon sheath
- Budd-Chiari
- buried bumper
- capillary leak
- carpal tunnel (CTS)
- cat's cry

syndrome *(cont.)*
- cauda equina
- Chilaiditi
- chronic fatigue
- Cobb's
- CPD (chorioretinopathy and pituitary dysfunction)
- CREST
- cri du chat
- CRST
- CTS (carpal tunnel)
- cubital tunnel
- Cushing's
- Dandy-Walker
- de Morsier's
- de Morsier-Gauthier
- DiGeorge
- DIMOAD
- Duane's
- Duane's retraction
- dumping
- dysplastic nevus
- Eagle-Barrett
- EEC
- Ehlers-Danlos
- empty nest
- empty sella
- eosinophilia-myalgia
- failed back surgery (FBSS)
- fat embolism (FES)
- Fitz-Hugh and Curtis
- fragile X
- Gastaut's
- Gerstmann's
- Gianotti-Crosti's
- Gilles de la Tourette's
- Goldenhar's
- Guillain-Barré
- Halbrecht's
- Hamman-Rich
- Harada's
- HEE (hemiconvulsion, hemiplegia, epilepsy)
- HELLP
- Henoch-Schönlein

syndrome *(cont.)*
HVS (hyperventilation)
ICE (irido-corneal-endothelial)
impaired regeneration (IRS)
Ivemark's
Josephs-Blackfan-Diamond
Kasabach-Merritt
Kaznelson's
Kearns-Sayre-Shy
Klinefelter's (XXY)
Koerber-Salus-Elschnig
Landry-Guillain-Barré-Strohl
large vestibular aqueduct
LAS (lymphadenopathy)
Laurence-Moon-Biedl
lazy leukocyte (LLS)
Lejeune's
Lennox-Gastaut
Leriche
Lesch-Nyhan
LLS (lazy leukocyte)
locked-in
locker-room
Löffler's (Loeffler's)
Louis-Bar's
Lowe's
Lown-Ganong-Levine
Marcus Gunn's jaw-winking
MEN (multiple endocrine neoplasia)
MEN I (type I)
MEWD (multiple evanescent white dot)
micrognathia-glossoptosis
Miege's
monosomy 7
mucocutaneous lymph node (MLNS)
multiple endocrine neoplasia type 2b
Munchausen
myalgic encephalomyelitis (ME)
nephrotic
Nezelof
organic brain
otospongiosis/otosclerosis

syndrome *(cont.)*
painter's encephalopathy
Parinaud's
Penderluft
Peutz-Jeghers
Pierre Robin
Plummer-Vinson
POEMS
Poland's
postviral fatigue
P pulmonale
prune-belly
13q-deletion
respiratory distress (RDS)
Reye's
Robin
Rothmund-Thomson
Saethre-Chotzen
Sandifer
Sanger-Brown
SAS (sleep apnea)
Schwachman's
Sertoli-cell-only
Sézary
Sheehy
SIADH
sick building
sick sinus
Sjögren's
Stewart-Treves
Stilling-Türk-Duane
subclavian steal
sundown
sundowner
tarsal tunnel
tethered cord
13-q-deletion
Tolosa-Hunt
Tourette's
translocation Down's
trisomy-D
Turner's
UGH+
VACTERL
VATER

syndrome *(cont.)*
Vogt-Koyanagi-Harada
wasting
white clot
Wiskott-Aldrich
Wolff-Parkinson-White (WPW)
XXY (Klinefelter's)
Zollinger-Ellison (ZES)

synechialysis (Oph).

synovial frost (Ortho).

Synthaderm—synthetic (polyurethane) occlusive wound dressing used on ulcerations, usually on the lower extremities.

Synthes compression hip screw (Ortho)—American version of the German A-O hip compression screw.

syntonic (Psych)—characterized by normal emotional response. "His affect was generally appropriate, and mood syntonic."

syringe, Raulerson.

system—see *device.*

systemic and topical hypothermia.

systemic lupus erythematosus—an inflammatory disorder of the connective tissues, characterized by a "butterfly" erythema over the malar area and the bridge of the nose, arthralgias, and it may include renal involvement, recurrent pleurisy, splenomegaly, as well as involvement of other body systems. It is thought to be an autoimmune disorder, and is seen predominantly in young women, but is also seen in children. Also called *disseminated lupus erythematosus* and *SLE.* See also *Farr test.*

systemic vascular resistance (SVR).

systolic anterior motion (SAM) on 2-D echocardiogram.

T, t

T (tesla)—SI unit of magnetic strength (used in MRI). The term *gauss* was formerly used.

TAC ("tack") (triamcinolone cream)—used in the treatment of psoriasis and other dermatological conditions.

TACE (chlorotrianisene).

tacrine (Cognex) (Psych, Neuro)—a drug used to treat Alzheimer's disease.

Tactilaze angioplasty laser catheter (Cardio)—a laser used to vaporize atherosclerotic plaque by means of an angioplasty catheter threaded through the artery.

TA-55 stapler (Neuro).

tag (Radiol)—in nuclear medicine to tag (or label) is to render a substance radioactive by incorporating a radionuclide in it; also, to cause a tissue or organ to take up radioactive material. Cf. *label; sensitize.*

Tagamet (cimetidine).

TAG system (tissue anchor guide).

tail—slender appendage, as in *tail of Spence, tail of the breast.* Cf. *cauda.*

tail of the breast (Radiol)—in mammography, a wedge-shaped zone of breast tissue extending toward the axilla. Also known as the axillary tail of Spence.

tail of Spence—also called tail of the breast. It is the tail-like segment of mammary gland tissue that extends to the axillary region.

tailor's bunion (Ortho)—This gets its name from the days in the distant past when tailors sat cross-legged on the floor to do their sewing, and thus developed bunions on the fifth metatarsal (rather than the first metatarsal where they usually occur).

Takahashi forceps (ENT, Neuro).

Takata laser interferometer (from Eye Center of Louisiana State University).

Takayasu's arteritis—arteritis involving the aortic arch and its branches.

takeoff of a vessel (Radiol)—in angiography, the commencement (or origin) of a vessel as it branches off from a larger vessel.

talipes hobble splint. See *Denis Browne clubfoot splint.*

tamoxifen citrate (Nolvadex)—chemotherapy drug.

"T and C"—slang for Tylenol and codeine. When a physician dictates, "The patient was given T and C for pain," we should transcribe, "The patient was given Tylenol and codeine for pain."

tangential cut—a cut which is slightly off center, or glancing.

tangential speech—rambling, tending to go off on tangents.

TA–90 surgical stapler (Surg).

tanned red cells test (TRC).

Tanner Developmental Scale (Peds)—to stage secondary sexual characteristics on a scale of I to V, I indicating no development, V indicating full development; "breasts Tanner stage II," for example. Also, *Marshall and Tanner pubertal staging.*

Tanner mesher—a device used to mesh skin in preparation for grafting; permits the skin to stretch, thus covering a greater area (Plas Surg). See also *Tanner-Vandeput mesh dermatome.*

Tanner-Vandeput mesh dermatome (Plas Surg). This instrument cuts small parallel slits in split thickness skin grafts, permitting the graft to expand two to three times its original size. When the graft is applied, the slits expand and become diamond-shaped areas which then epithelialize from the surrounding skin edges.

tantalum bronchogram (using powdered tantalum).

tantalum mesh; plate; ring; wire. Tantalum is not an alloy; it is biologically inert, having great tissue acceptability and high tensile strength. In plate form it is used for skull plates.

Tao (troleandomycin).

tap—see *glabellar tap.*

tape

Elastikon elastic
Hy-Tape

tape *(cont.)*

lap
MaxCast
Microfoam surgical
Scotchcast 2 casting
Shur-Strip
Transpore surgical

taper—to reduce the dose of a medicine gradually; to change size gradually.

Tapercut needle.

TARA prosthesis (total articular replacement arthroplasty) (Ortho). See *Townley TARA prosthesis.*

tardy palsy—referred to in electromyograph reports and nerve conduction velocities, with reference to carpal tunnel syndrome. Example: "Impression: Slowing of ulnar nerve, slowing across the elbow, consistent with a tardy palsy."

target lesion—a skin lesion consisting of concentric rings of erythema. For example, target lesion (of Lyme disease). See *erythema migrans.*

target sign. If a cerebrospinal fluid leak is suspected, examination of the bloody fluid placed on porous paper will show a clear halo around the inner bloody residue if positive.

Targocid (teicoplanin).

Tarlov cyst ("tar-loff")—perineurial cyst.

tarsal cyst—see *chalazion.*

tarsal tunnel syndrome—a group of symptoms caused by compression of the posterior tibial nerve, or the plantar nerves, in the tarsal tunnel, resulting in pain, numbness and paresthesias of the plantar aspect of the foot (Ortho). "The left medial great toe pain was suggestive of tarsal tunnel syndrome." Cf. *carpal tunnel syndrome.*

Tart cells—named for the patient in whom the cells were discovered.

Tart cells *(cont.)*
They can be seen in some cases of rheumatoid arthritis or serum sickness.

TAT inhibitor—a drug used to treat HIV-positive patients.

Taussig-Bing anomaly—a congenital defect of the heart, characterized by complete transposition of the pulmonary artery in association with a ventricular septal defect. Symptoms may include cyanosis, dyspnea on exertion, severe pulmonary hypertension, systolic murmur, loud pulmonic second sound, and polycythemia. Right ventricular hypertrophy or incomplete bundle branch block may also be present.

Taylor pinwheel—used in sensory examination in neurologic testing.

Tazidime (ceftazidime).

TBSA (total body surface area).

TBT (transcervical balloon tuboplasty).

TCA (tricyclic antidepressant).

T-cell—thymus-derived lymphocyte, part of the immune system. See *B-cell, T-4, T-8.*

TcHIDA ("tek-high-dah")—see *HIDA; PIPIDA.*

TCN-P (triciribine phosphate)—chemotherapy drug.

TCPM pneumatic tourniquet system—for orthopedic procedures.

T-cuts—for corneal astigmatism (Oph).

TDD (thoracic duct drainage)—being evaluated as an adjunct to classical immunosuppression (preoperatively) in the prevention of early rejection of organ transplants.

TDR (thymidine deoxyriboside).

TDS (treadmill duration score).

TE (echo time) (Radiol)—in magnetic resonance imaging, the interval between the first pulse in a spin-echo examination and the appearance of the resulting echo.

tear—see *Mallory-Weiss tear; retinal tear.*

tear strips—see *Schirmer's tear strips.*

teboroxime scan (Radiol). The radioactive imaging agent ^{99m}TC teboroxime (known as CardioTek) shows areas of myocardial infarction on a cardiac scan. Used for emergency scans, it clears rapidly from the blood to allow subsequent scans, if necessary.

TEC (thiotepa, etoposide, carboplatin) —chemotherapy drug used to treat malignant glioma.

TECA study (technetium albumin).

teceleukin (recombinant interleukin-2) (Oncol)—a chemotherapy drug used to treat metastatic renal cell carcinoma.

TechneScan MAG3—renal diagnostic imaging agent that uses technetium-99m mertiatide to determine kidney function.

technetium—an element, an isotope of which Tc-99m (^{99m}Tc) is used as a diagnostic aid in liver, brain, lung, and kidney scans. See also *radioisotope.* Examples of technetium:
Cardiolite (^{99m}Tc sestamibi)
CardioTek (^{99m}Tc teboroxime)
Tc-99m albumin
Tc-99m albumin aggregated
Tc-99m albumin colloid
Tc-99m bicisate
Tc-99m colloid
Tc-99m disofenin
Tc-99m etidronate
Tc-99m ferpentetate
Tc-99m glucepate
TcHIDA
Tc-99m iron-ascorbate-DTPA (Renotec)

technetium *(cont.)*
Tc-99m lidofenin
Tc-99m macroaggregated albumin (^{99m}Tc-MAA)
Tc-99m medronate (Macrotec)
Tc-99m mertiatide (TechneScan MAG3)
Tc-99m oxidronate
Tc-99m penetate (Techneplex)
Tc-99m pertechnetate sodium
Tc-99m PIPIDA
Tc-99m pyrophosphate
Tc-99m sestamibi (Cardiolite)
Tc-99m siboroxime
Tc-99m sodium
Tc-99m succimer
Tc-99m sulfur colloid (^{99m}Tc-SC) (Tesuloid)
Tc-99m teboroxime (CardioTek)
Macrotec (^{99m}Tc medronate)
Renotec (^{99m}Tc iron-ascorbate-DTPA)
Techneplex (^{99m}Tc penetate)
technetium stannous pyrophosphate (TSPP)
Technescan MAG3 (^{99m}Tc mertiatide)
Tesuloid (^{99m}Tc-SC, sulfur colloid)

technetium macroaggregated albumin (Tc-99m MAA (or ^{99m}Tc-MAA)—a predictor of gastrointestinal toxicity during hepatic artery infusion.

technetium pertechnetate (Tc-99m)—a tracer used in radionuclide studies for active gastrointestinal bleeding; this material labels red blood cells. If bleeding occurs in a period of up to 24 hours that the labeled red blood cells remain in the circulating blood, the tracer will extravasate and accumulate at or near the site. It is also used to demonstrate the presence of a Meckel's diverticululm. See also *technetium sulfur colloid.*

technetium sulfur colloid (^{99m}Tc-SC) (Tesuloid)—a tracer used in radionuclide scans for active gastrointestinal bleeding. This material is cleared from the blood and concentrated in the reticuloendothelial system with a half-life of less than 2½ minutes. If GI bleeding occurs during this time, the tracer will accumulate at the bleeding site. See also *technetium pertechnetate.*

TEE (transesophageal echocardiography).

T-8 cell—also called suppressor/cytotoxic cell. See *suppressor cell.*

Teflon paste injection for incontinence (Urol)—a procedure in which injection of a Teflon paste (Polytef, Ethicon) into the periurethral tissues at the bladder neck is done on an outpatient basis to restore urinary control in incontinent women, particularly the elderly. The injection works by adding bulk to these tissues, compressing the urethral lumen and increasing the resistance to the outflow of urine.

Tegaderm transparent dressing—a waterproof dressing for wound and I.V. site coverage. Made by 3M.

Teicholz ejection fraction—used in echocardiogram.

teicoplanin (Targocid)—an antibiotic, effective against gram-positive bacteria.

telangiectasia, ataxia.

telecurietherapy—radiotherapy.

Tele-Sensor, Cosman ICP.

Teletrast (Neuro)—an absorbable surgical gauze which contains a plastic thread that has been impregnated with barium sulfide, thus making it radiopaque. Among other applications, it is used in microvascular decompression to displace a vessel that is compressing the trigeminal nerve.

Teller acuity cards (TAC)—used in eye testing (Oph).

telogen—the resting phase of hair growth. See *anagen.*

TEM (transanal endoscopic microsurgery).

temafloxacin (Omniflox)—a broad-spectrum oral antibiotic used to treat respiratory, genitourinary, and skin infections.

TEMP (tamoxifen, etoposide, mitoxantrone, Platinol)—chemotherapy protocol used to treat breast carcinoma.

temporal arcade.

temporomandibular joint (TMJ).

T.E.N.—see *Vivonex T.E.N.*

10-EDAM—see *EDAM.*

Tenckhoff peritoneal catheter.

tendinitis, *not* tendonitis.

tendo Achillis (or Achilles tendon).

tendon—the fibrous cord by which a muscle is attached. Cf. *tenon.*

teniposide (VM-26)—chemotherapy drug for childhood acute lymphocytic leukemia.

Tennant intraocular implant lens.

Tennison-Randall repair, for cleft lip.

Tennis Racquet catheter used in angiography (Rad). This is a trade name, and the catheter does look like a tennis racquet.

tenon (*not* tendon)—a projecting member in a piece of wood or other material for insertion into a mortise to make a joint. See *mortise.* Cf. *tendon.*

TENS (transcutaneous electrical nerve stimulation)—a nondrug, noninvasive, nonaddictive alternative for control of pain. It appears to enhance the concentration of beta-endorphins significantly. The TENS system consists of a small battery-powered stimulator with lead wires that attach to two or more surface electrodes. See *Eclipse TENS, Maxima II TENS, Stayoden 9000F TENS.*

Tensilon test—for myasthenia gravis.

tenting of hemidiaphragm (Radiol)—on chest x-ray, a distortion of the diaphragm by scarring, in which an upward-pointing angular configuration (like a tent) replaces all or part of the normal curved contour of a hemidiaphragm.

tenting sign—a simple test for severe dehydration; a pinched fold of skin will stay tented up.

Tenzel calipers (Plas Surg)—used to measure the lid crease. A modification of Jameson calipers.

terazosin (Hytrin) (Urol)—an $alpha_1$ antihypertensive also used to treat symptoms of benign prostatic hyperplasia (BPH).

terlipressin (Glypressin) (GI)—used to treat bleeding esophageal ulcers.

terodiline (Micturin) (Urol)—used to treat urinary incontinence.

teroxirone (alpha-TGI) (Oncol)—chemotherapy drug given intraperitoneally for advanced malignancies of the abdominal cavity.

Terrien's degeneration (Oph)—marginal thinning and degeneration of the upper nasal quadrants of the cornea.

Terry fingernail sign—see *Terry nails.*

Terry keratometer (Oph)—enables surgeons to measure astigmatism while the patient is still on the operating table after surgery, and while the final wound closure is being accomplished.

Terry-Mayo needle (Urol)—heavy, small Mayo needle.

Terry nails—white opaque ground-glass appearance of the nails proximally, with a normal pink area distally. Seen in cirrhosis of the liver, and certain other liver diseases. "Terry nails are present, and he has some clubbing."

tertiary contractions (Radiol)—on upper GI series, aberrant contractions of the esophagus, occurring after the primary and secondary waves of normal swallowing.

tertipara—a woman who has given birth three times (para III or para 3).

Terumo dialyzer—for hemodialysis.

Terumo guide wire (GI)—used to pass strictures encountered during ERCP.

tesla (T)—SI unit of magnetic strength (used in MRI). The term *gauss* was formerly used.

Tessier elevator (Plas Surg).

test; scale; score
- Abbreviated Injury Scale (AIS)
- AccuPoint hCG Pregnancy Test Disc
- affinity chromatography
- AFP (alpha-fetoprotein test)
- agarose gel electrophoresis (AGE)
- AGE (agarose gel electrophoresis)
- agglutination test
- AGI (apnea-hypopnea index)
- air conduction test
- AIS (Abbreviated Injury Scale)
- Alberts' Famous Faces Test
- Allen's circulatory test
- alpha-fetoprotein test (AFP)
- Amsler grid
- anti-RHO-D titer
- antistreptolysin titer (AST)
- APACHE II score
- APGAR questionnaire
- Apgar score
- apnea-hypopnea index (AGI)
- applanation tonometry
- apprehension test
- arginine tolerance (ATT)
- AST (antistreptolysin titer)
- ATT (arginine tolerance)
- Autoclix blood glucose test
- Autolet blood glucose test
- BAEP test (brain stem auditory evoked potential)

test *(cont.)*
- BAER test (brain stem auditory evoked response)
- Bang's horseshoe-crab blood test
- Barlow hip dysplasia
- Bayley Scales of Infant Development
- Bender Gestalt Test
- bentonite flocculation test
- benzalkonium chloride patch test
- Berens 3-character (eye) test
- Berkson-Gage breast cancer survival rates
- Bielschowsky's head tilt test
- Bing auditory acuity test
- Biocept-5 pregnancy test
- Biocept-G pregnancy test
- bone conduction test
- brain tests, noninvasive
- Brazelton Neonatal Assessment Scale
- breath hydrogen excretion test
- Brief Neuropsychological Mental Status Examination (BNMSE)
- caloric test
- caloric test of vestibular function
- capillary blood sugar test
- capillary electrophoresis test
- Cattell Infant Intelligence Scale
- cell assay
- Champion Trauma Score
- Chemstrip bG
- Cherry-Crandall serum lipase test
- chromohydrotubation
- CIE (countercurrent immunoelectrophoresis)
- CIWA-A (Clinical Institute Withdrawal Assessment–Alcohol)
- coin test
- cold water calorics test
- Colorgene DNA Hybridization
- concealed straight leg raising test
- complement fixation test
- copper-binding protein test (CBP)

test *(cont.)*
cover-uncover test
cracker test
cribogram
cross-cover test
cryocrit test
Cybex
dark-field microscopy
Denver Developmental Screening
DFA (direct fluorescent antibody)
Diagnex Blue
direct fluorescent antibody (DFA)
Dix-Hallpike test
Doppler test
Draw-a-Bicycle test (DAB)
Draw-a-Flower test (DAF)
Draw-a-House test (DAH)
Draw-a-Person test (DAP)
Dubowitz scale for infant maturity
duck waddle
duction
Dunlop synoptophore
EAST
EIA (enzyme-linked immunoassay)
electrotransfer test
ELISA (enzyme-linked immuno-sorbent assay)
Ellestad treadmill stress test
Entero-Test
Envacor
EP test (evoked potential)
ergonovine maleate
ER test (evoked response)
Esterman visual function score
$EtCO_2$
estrogen receptor
ExacTech blood glucose meter
exercise tolerance test
fabere test
fadir test
Fagan test
Farr test
F_ECO_2
FEF_{25-75}

test *(cont.)*
fern test
fetal-pelvic index
Fick cardiac output
finger-to-nose (F to N) test
Finkelstein's test
5'nucleotidase test
flocculation flow cytometry
Flu-Glow
fluorescein uptake test
Fluor-i-Strip
foam stability test
Folstein's Mini-Mental Status Test
free beta test
free thyroxine index (FTI)
French scale
FTA-ABS test (fluorescent treponemal antibody absorption test for syphilis)
gait and station
Galveston Orientation and Amnesia Test (GOAT)
gas chromotography
Gastroccult
GeneAmp PCR
GGTP liver function test
glabellar tap
Glasgow Coma Scale
Glasgow Outcome Scale
glial fibrillary acidic protein (GFAP)
GOAT (Galveston Orientation and Amnesia Test)
Gomori (or Grocott) methenamine silver (GMS) test
gonioscopy
Goodenough test
GRASS
Gravindex pregnancy
guaiac test
Hallpike caloric stimulation
Halstead-Wepman Aphasia Screening Test
heavy metal screening
heelstick hematocrit

test *(cont.)*
heel-to-shin test
Heinz body test
Hemoccult II
HemoCue
Heprofile ELISA
Herp-Check
H reflex electrodiagnostic test
Histoplasma capsulatum polysaccharide antigen
HI titer
HIVAGEN
HRL color vision test
ice water calorics
iliopsoas test
Incomplete Sentence Blank Test (ISB)
indirect fluorescent antibody test (IFA)
Injury Severity Score
ink potassium hydroxide test
INVOS 2100 breast cancer test
Ishihara color vision test
islet cell antibodies screening (ICA)
Jaeger's test
Jamar grip test
Karnofsky rating scale
Kleihauer-Betke test
Kleihauer test
Krimsky's test
Kruskal-Wallis test
Kveim test
Lachman test
LAL (Limulus amoebocyte lysate)
Landolt's ring test
LAP (leucine aminopeptidase) test
LAP (leukocyte alkaline phosphatase) test
latex agglutination test
Lezak's Malingering Test
LFT (liver function) test
Limulus amoebocyte lysate (LAL)
litmus test
L/S ratio

test *(cont.)*
Lysholm knee score
Maddox rod test
Mancini plates test
Mantoux tuberculosis test
Master's two-step test
maternal serum alpha-fetoprotein test (MSAFP)
McNemar's test
mental status test
Mentor BVAT test
MEP test (multimodality evoked potential)
MHA-TP (microhemagglutination test for *Treponema pallidum*)
Micral chemstrip
microsomal TRC (tanned red cells)
Minnesota Multiphasic Personality Inventory (MMPI)
MOBS (Montefiore Organic Brain Scale)
modified rapid urease (RUT) test
Monojector blood glucose test
multiple sleep latency (MSLT) test
Myers-Briggs Personality Inventory
Nardi (morphine-prostigmine) test
Naughton cardiac exercise treadmill test
Neurobehavioral Cognitive Status
O&P (ova and parasites)
OCT (oxytocin challenge test)
octopus peripheral vision test
octopus visual field test
Oliver-Rosalki serum CPK test
ophthalmoscopy
ophthalmodynamometry
osmolality
Ouchterlony double diffuse test
Outerbridge scale
ox cell hemolysin test
oxytocin challenge test (OCT)
Paragon immunofixation electrophoresis
past-pointing test

test *(cont.)*
patellar apprehension test
Pathfinder DFA test
Patrick's (fabere) test
PBPI (penile brachial pressure index)
PCR (polymerase chain reaction)
peak expiratory flow rate (PEFR)
P_ECO_2
PEFR (peak expiratory flow rate)
penile brachial pressure index (PBPI)
pentagastrin stimulated analysis
periodic acid-Schiff (PAS) test
PHA skin test
Phalen's test
pilocarpine iontophoresis
pivot-shift
Polatest vision test
PPD skin test
PPL skin test
PRA test (plasma renin activity)
Protocult
P300 dementia
Pylori Fiax assay
Pylori Stat assay
Queckenstedt test
quellung reaction
radioallergosorbent (RAST) test
Raji cell assay
Randot test
rapid plasma reagin (RPR)
RAST (radioallergosorbent test)
refraction test
Reitman-Frankel SGOT and SGPT test
renin test
Rey and Taylor Complex Figure Test
Rey Auditory Verbal Learning Test
Rinne test
RISA (radioactive iodinated serum albumin) test
Romberg test
Roos test
Rorschach test

test *(cont.)*
Rotazyme diagnostic test
RPR (rapid plasma reagin) test
RPR-CT (rapid plasma reagin—circle card test)
RUT (rapid urease test)
Schiller test
Schiötz tonometry
Schirmer's test
Schwartz test
SCVII
sed rate
sedimentation rate
Seidel test
SEP test (somatosensory evoked potential)
SER test (somatosensory evoked response)
serum protein electrophoresis
Sgambati's test for peritonitis
shake test
Sibley-Lehninger serum aldolase test
Sickledex
Sigma CPK test
simkin analysis
SK-SD (streptokinase-streptodornase) skin test
slit-lamp test
SLRT (straight leg raising test)
SMAC test
SMA-6 test
SMA-12 test
SMA-20 test
Snellen chart
Sonksen-Silver acuity cards
Stamey test
straight leg raising test (SLRT)
streptokinase-streptodornase (SK-SD) test
Strong-Campbell Vocational Interest Inventory (SCVII)
surf (surfactant) test
sweat chloride test
tanned red cells (TRC) test

test *(cont.)*
Tanner Development Scale
TAT (Thematic Apperception Test)
Teller acuity cards test
Tensilon test
Tes-Tape urine glucose
TestPackChlamydia (no spaces)
thallium stress test
Thayer-Martin gonorrhea test
Thematic Apperception Test (TAT)
thin-layer chromatography screen
Thompson test
Thorn test
thyrocalcitonin for pheochromocytoma test
thyroxine radioisotope assay (T_4 RIA)
tine test
Titmus test
T-lymphocyte subset ratio
Toxocara ELISA
Tracer Blood Glucose Micro-monitor
Trail Making Test
TRC (tanned red cells) antibody titer
treadmill test
T water fructose intolerance test
tyramine test for pheochromocytoma
tyrosine tolerance test
Tzanck test
Uricult dipslide
Urocyte diagnostic cytometry
van den Bergh's test
VDRL test
VEP test (visual evoked potential)
VER test (visual evoked response)
Vineland Social Maturity Scale
ViraPap
Visidex, Visidex II
visual analogue scale
visual field test
V/Q (ventilation/perfusion)
von Kossa calcium test
Wada test

test *(cont.)*
Weber test
Wechsler Adult Intelligence Scale—Revised (WAIS-R)
Wechsler Memory Scale; Test
Well-Cogen latex agglutination test
Westergren sedimentation rate
Western blot electrotransfer test
Wilcoxon rank sum test
Wirt stereo test
Wood's light test
Worth four-dot test (W4D)
Wroblewski serum LDH test
Yergason test
zona hamster egg test
Zung Depression Scale

Tes-Tape—trade name of a reagent strip used in testing urine for glucose.

TestPackChlamydia (no spaces)—a doctor's office quick test for *Chlamydia* based on enzyme-linked immunosorbent assay.

"tet spell"—medical slang for a ''spell typical of tetralogy of Fallot.''

tethered cord syndrome (Neuro)—seen when an area of the spinal cord is firmly caught up in scar tissue or between vertebrae.

tetracycline (Pulm). This common oral antibiotic can also be given by intrapleural injection to sclerose lung tissues and reduce the chance of repeat pneumothorax.

tetrahydrocannabinol—see *THC.*

tetralogy of Fallot (''fal-lo')—complex of four congenital cardiac anomalies: pulmonary stenosis, ventricular septal defect, dextroposition of the aorta, and right ventricular hypertrophy. Cf. *Fallot's pentalogy, Fallot's trilogy.* See also *pink tetralogy of Fallot.*

Texas Scottish Rite Hospital (TSRH).

TFL (tensor fasciae latae).

T-4 cell—the cell specifically attacked by the HIV virus. Called helper/inducer T-cell.

T_4 RIA—thyroxine radioisotope assay.

T4, soluble recombinant human—a drug used to treat HIV-positive patients.

TFT (tight fingertip dilated), as in "The cervical os was TFT."

TGA (transposition of the great arteries) (Cardio).

THA (total hip arthroplasty) (Ortho).

thalidomide (Oncol)—used to prevent graft-versus-host disease in patients undergoing bone marrow transplant. Well known in the past as the drug which caused seal limb deformities in babies whose mothers took it for morning sickness.

thallium stress test (Radiol)—used to reveal the presence and extent of coronary artery disease by comparing blood flow in the heart during treadmill exercise with the blood flow at rest. Thallium is taken up by the heart in direct proportion to the blood flow, and images of areas of the heart showing thallium retention delineate the areas of arterial blockage. The radioisotope used is thallium-201 (Tl-201).

thalamotomy, parafascicular.

Thal repair of esophageal stricture.

Thayer-Martin culture medium—used in testing for *Neisseria gonorrhoeae.*

THC (tetrahydrocannabinol)—the active ingredient in marijuana; used for treatment of nausea and vomiting secondary to chemotherapy, and for reducing pressures in glaucoma.

THC:YAG laser (thulium-holmium-chromium:YAG laser).

THE (transhepatic embolization).

theca cell—a cell found in the ovary after ovulation; it is derived from nurse cells surrounding the developing egg.

thelarche—the beginning of breast development.

Thematic Apperception Test (TAT)—mental status examination.

Theocon (Pulm)—trade name for extended release theophylline.

TheraCys (Urol)—injected directly into the bladder to treat patients with recurrent bladder tumors. Contains an attenuated strain of *Mycobacterium* known as bacille Calmette-Guérin (BCG), after the two French bacteriologists, Albert Calmette and Camille Guérin, who first weakened the bacillus through many series of cultures.

TheraSeed (Rad Oncol)—an alternative permanent implant with a 17-day half-life. Used in the treatment of rapidly growing tumors. A palladium-103 (Pd-103) active isotope in a titanium capsule.

thermistor—a type of thermometer that registers very small changes in temperature. "Respiratory parameters were monitored by nasal and oral thermistor and abdominal and chest wall strain gauges."

thermistor-plethysmography (Cardio).

thermodilution catheter (Cardio)—a specially designed, triple-lumen Swan-Ganz catheter. One lumen is used to inject a cold solution to measure cardiac output. See *thermodilution technique.*

thermodilution technique (Cardio). Following injection of a cold solution (saline, 5% dextrose in water, or autologous blood) into the right atrium,

thermodilution technique *(cont.)* a change in temperature of the circulating blood can be detected by a temperature-sensitive catheter in the pulmonary artery. The numerical values obtained are then used to calculate cardiac output.

Thermophore—moist heat pads used for external application of heat, to relieve pain (Phys Ther).

Thermoscan Pro-1-Instant thermometer. Using infrared technology, this new thermometer is able to obtain a reading in just two seconds. Using a special speculum which fits into the ear canal, the thermometer accurately reflects the body core temperature because of its closeness to the tympanic membrane. An aural temperature reading is unlike oral readings which can be affected by eating, drinking, or smoking.

THI needle—used in cardiac surgery to express air from the ventricle.

thianamycin—an antibiotic.

Thiersch-Duplay urethroplasty (Urol).

Thiersch suture.

thigh-high antiembolic stockings (Ortho).

thin-layer chromatography screen—an analytic technique used to screen serum or urine samples for poisons or drugs of abuse.

ThinPrep processor and system (Lab)—for Pap smears and other cytologic samples. Assures uniformity of slide samples.

third spacing—movement of fluids in the body into the third space (not the vascular space, in the blood vessels, and not inside cells, in the intracellular space). This interstitial fluid can be in one organ or systemic, and can be caused by lymphatic blockage, increased capillary permeability, or lowered plasma proteins.

13-cis-retinoic acid, 13-CRA — see *isotretinoin.*

13q-deletion syndrome (46 Dr or 46 Dq)—due to a deletion of the long arms of chromosome 13 (one of the group D chromosomes). The syndrome may include mental retardation and physical retardation, broad nasal bridge, large and prominent low-set ears, facial asymmetry, hypertelorism, ptosis, epicanthus, microcephaly, microphthalmia, imperforate anus, and a number of other anomalies.

Thomas splint (Ortho).

Thom flap (ENT)—laryngeal reconstruction.

Thompson test (Ortho)—"The Achilles tendon is intact by Thompson test." With the foot at rest, compression of the calf (gastrocnemius) muscle causes ankle flexion if the Achilles tendon is intact.

thoracic duct drainage (TDD).

Thoracoseal drainage (Pulm).

Thora-Drain III three-bottle chest drainage unit—an underwater seal drainage system.

Thora-Klex chest drainage system.

Thorel's bundle—a bundle of muscle fibers in the heart that connects the sinoatrial and atrioventricular nodes (Cardio).

Thorn test—(1) a test of uric acid excretion, (2) a test to help in the diagnosis of Addison's disease.

Thornton 360° arcuate marker (Oph)—used during corneal surgery and during keratotomy for astigmatism.

THR (total hip replacement) (Ortho).

3DFT magnetic resonance angiography (three-dimensional Fourier transform) (Radiol)—a noninvasive vascular imaging technique.

three-pillow or two-pillow orthopnea—refers to the number of pillows a patient must use to prop himself up in bed to sleep comfortably without difficulty breathing.

throat, strep (streptococcal). *(Not* strept.)

thrombocytopenia, HIV-associated.

thromboembolic disease (TED).

ThromboScan MRU (Radiol)—an imaging agent combined with molecular recognition units (MRUs) to produce better scans.

thrombosis, but *thrombus.*

thrombosis, deep venous (DVT).

thrombotic thrombocytopenic purpura (TTP)—complication in AIDS patients.

thrombus, but *thrombosis.*

thrombus stripper, Dunlop.

thulium-holmium-chromium:YAG laser—see *THC:YAG laser.*

thumb, gamekeeper's.

thumbprinting (Radiol)—indentations that look like thumbprints, seen radiographically on the surface of the colon in a barium enema. They are indicative of ischemic colitis or of hematoma formation on the bowel wall.

thunderclap headache (Neuro)—a sudden, extremely painful, high-intensity headache (not migraine, tension, or cluster headache). The name is very descriptive. May indicate a brain aneurysm and impending rupture.

thymic humoral factor—a drug used to treat HIV-positive patients.

thymidine deoxyriboside (TDR) (Oncol)—chemotherapy drug.

thymopentin (Timunox)—a drug used to treat HIV-positive patients.

thymostimuline (TP-1)—drug used to treat patients with AIDS.

thyrocalcitonin—test for pheochromocytoma.

thyroid stare—see *Collier's sign.*

thyroid storm—episode of heightened thyroid hormone activity due to sudden release of an abnormal amount of hormone into the circulation. A thyroid storm may be induced by stress or infection, or it may occur spontaneously. Symptoms are anxiety, rapid pulse, fear, high fever, restlessness, breathing problems, exhaustion. In severe cases, which may prove fatal, the patient may be delirious and then become comatose. Also, thyroid crisis.

thyroxine radioisotope assay (T_4RIA).

TI (inversion time)—MRI term.

TIA (transient ischemic attack)—cerebrovascular occlusion, in which the symptoms resolve within 24 hours (Neuro). Cf. *CVA.*

tiagabine—an anticonvulsant drug for epilepsy.

tibial plateau (Radiol)—a flattened surface at the upper end of the anterior aspect of the tibia.

tic—involuntary repetitive muscle movement. See *Tourette's syndrome* and *Gilles de la Tourette's syndrome.* Cf. *tick.*

ticarcillin–clavulanate potassium (Timentin)—an antibiotic administered parenterally and said to be more active than ticarcillin alone against bacterial species such as penicillinase-producing *Staphylococcus aureus, Klebsiella, Haemophilus influenzae, Escherichia coli,* and *Bacteroides fragilis.*

Tice (intravesical BCG).

tick—a small bloodsucking arthropod; the lesion produced by its bite may cause anything from a small papule to a large ulcerating wound, with acute pain and swelling. See *Lyme disease,* which is transmitted by the deer tick. Cf. *tic.*

Ticlid (ticlopidine).

ticlopidine (Ticlid)—a drug used to prevent initial and recurrent strokes in patients with transient ischemic attacks. Because it causes neutropenia and agranulocytosis, it is used only in patients who cannot tolerate aspirin therapy.

Ti-Cron—see *Tycron.*

tidal volume (Pulm)—the amount of air exchanged with each breath.

Tiemann Meals tenolysis knife (Plas and Hand Surg).

"tie-sis"—see *phthisis.*

tie, stick (suture ligature).

Tiersch graft—a delayed pedicle skin graft.

Ti-Fit modular hip system by Richards (Ortho).

tight asthmatic—an asthmatic with extreme difficulty breathing, that is, with extreme bronchospasm. "Examination revealed a very tight asthmatic, using accessory muscles, and breathing at 28. He had tight inspiratory and expiratory wheezing."

tight fingertip dilated (TFT). See *TFT.*

TIL (tumor-infiltrating lymphocytes).

Tilade (nedocromil)—inhaled drug used to treat reversible obstructive airway disease.

Tilderquist needle holder (Oph).

time
- acquisition
- activated coagulation time (ACT)
- Duke bleeding
- echo (TE)

time *(cont.)*
- interpulse
- inversion time (TI)
- Ivy bleeding
- relaxation
- repetition time (TR)
- tincture of time (TOT)

Timentin (ticarcillin-clavulanate potassium).

TiMesh (ENT)—a titanium mesh used for rigid fixation of bone fractures.

Timunox (thymopentin)—a drug used to treat HIV-positive patients.

tine test—a tuberculin skin test in which a multiple-puncture device is used. The blades resemble the tines of a fork, hence the name. Not as reliable as the Mantoux test but a good mass screening test.

Tinel's sign (Neuro)—positive if there is tingling and numbness at the distal end of a limb when percussion is performed over the site of a divided nerve. The fact that there is some sensation indicates that the nerve has not been completely divided, or that there is some regeneration of the nerve.

Tischler cervical biopsy punch forceps (Ob-Gyn).

tissue expander—see *expander.*

tissue plasminogen activator (t-PA).

Tis-U-Sol (Oph)—a balanced saline solution, used in eye surgery to keep the eye tissues moist.

Tis-u-trap—endometrial suction catheter.

titer
- anti-RHO-D
- anti-teichoic acid
- HI (hemagglutination inhibition)
- microsomal TRC antibody

Titmus test (Oph)—for stereo acuity. The test pattern can be seen in three

Titmus test *(cont.)* dimensions only when both eyes are working together. Cf. *litmus test.*

TI-23—a cytomegalovirus monoclonal antibody used to treat CMV retinitis.

t.i.w.—three times a week.

TKO-type I.V. (to keep open, the vein) —an intravenous infusion given as slowly as possible to keep the blood from clotting in the needle, but not to give the patient any fluid volume. Also, *KVO-type I.V.* (keep vein open).

TLC G-65 (gentamicin liposome)—a drug used to treat MAI infections in AIDS patients.

T-lens—therapeutic contact lens.

TLI (total lymphoid irradiation)—used previously for cancer, now used with organ transplant patients to suppress T cells and decrease organ rejection. It may even allow transplant patients to avoid taking immunosuppressive drugs.

TLSO (thoracolumbosacral orthosis) (Ortho)—a semirigid plastic jacket (brace) used to treat scoliosis in children. The jacket is worn during the years of growth to prevent or slow further progression of the curve beyond 30°.

T-lymphocyte subset ratio—used to measure an AIDS drug's ability to improve immune function.

TMA (transmetatarsal amputation).

"T-max"—slang for temperature maximum, the highest recorded temperature.

TMJ (temporomandibular joint) (Oral Surg).

TMP-SMZ (trimethoprim-sulfamethoxazole) (Bactrim, Septra)—antibiotic often used in treating the first episode of *Pneumocystis carinii* pneumonia.

TMST (treadmill stress test).

TNB (Tru-Cut needle biopsy).

TNF (tumor necrosis factor) (Oncol)—a chemical toxin released from a gene (introduced by genetic engineering into human white blood cells) and toxic to malignant tumors. Therapy currently used to treat patients with malignant melanoma and ARC. Certain white blood cells known as tumor-infiltrating lymphocytes (TIL), which the body naturally produces to fight malignancies, are removed from the patient's body and genetically altered to include the gene that produces tumor necrosis factor. These cells are then given back to the patient. They migrate to the tumor site and begin manufacturing TNF.

TNM classification of malignant tumors: *T* represents the size of the tumor, *N* the clinical status of the nodes, and *M* metastasis.

- T1 Direct extension of primary tumor.
- T2 Direct extension of primary tumor to specific organs.
- T3 Direct advanced extension of tumor, unresectable.
- TX Direct extension of tumor, not assessed.
- N0 Regional lymph nodes not involved.
- N1 Regional lymph nodes involved.
- NX Regional lymph nodes not assessed.
- M0 No distant metastases.
- M1 Distant metastases present.
- MX Distant metastases not assessed.
- Stage I, T1-2, N0, M0, No extension or node involvement.
- Stage II, T3, N0, M0, Advanced extension, unresectable.
- Stage III, T1-3, N1, M0, Node involvement.
- Stage IV, T1-3, N0-1, M1, Distant metastases present.

tobramycin sulfate (Nebcin).

tocainide (Tonocard) (Cardio)—an oral antiarrhythmic.

Todd-Wells guide—used in stereotaxic procedures (Neuro). Cf. *BRW CT stereotaxic guide.*

toeing in, toeing out—turning the forefoot in or out in walking.

Toennis anastomosis scissors.

togavirus—a subgroup of arboviruses (**ar**thropod-**bo**rne viruses) that includes viruses carried by mosquitoes and ticks. The togavirus is the cause of hemorrhagic fever, and is so-called because it wears a covering (or toga).

Toldt ligament; line.

Tolentino ring (Oph). Also, Klein-Tolentino ring.

tolerogen—a substance that the immune system recognizes as "self," and not a foreign substance. Tolerogens are made by chemically linking fragments of DNA with specific protein molecules which the body already recognizes as "self." Tolerogens have potential in the control of autoimmune diseases such as systemic lupus erythematosus, rheumatoid arthritis, myasthenia gravis, etc.

tolmetin—a nonsteroidal anti-inflammatory drug (NSAID).

Tolosa-Hunt syndrome—painful ophthalmoplegia.

tolrestat (Alredase) (Oph)—a drug used in treating diabetic retinopathy.

toluidine blue stain.

Tom Jones closure—heavy retention suture closing all layers together (instead of in separate layers) except for the skin.

tomography
computed (CT)
computerized axial (CAT)

tomography *(cont.)*
dynamic computerized
positron emission (PET)
single photon emission computed (SPECT).
ultrasonic

T1 (Radiol)—in magnetic resonance imaging, the time it takes for protons to return to their orientation to a static magnetic field after an excitation pulse.

T1 weighted image (Radiol)—in magnetic resonance imaging, a spin-echo image generated by a pulse sequence using a short repetition time (0.6 seconds or less). Also called short TR/TE.

tongs
Crutchfield
Gardner-Wells skull
sugar-tong plaster splint
Trippi-Wells traction
Vinke

tonic-clonic seizure—the newer name for grand mal seizure.

tonometer
Draeger
Goldmann applanation
Mackay-Marg
Perkins
Schiötz
Tono-Pen

tonometry *(not* tenometry) (Oph)—measurement of intraocular pressure in the diagnosis of glaucoma. See *applanation tonometry; Schiötz tonometry.*

Tono-Pen tonometer (Oph)—used in measuring intraocular pressure.

tonsil snare, Neivert.

topotecan (Oncol)—used to treat advanced carcinoma of the pancreas, prostate, stomach, or head and neck, and also small-cell lung carcinoma,

topotecan *(cont.)* but not leukemia. Previously known as hycamptamine.

Toprol XL (metoprolol succinate).

Toradol (ketorolac tromethamine).

TORCH screening (titer)—an acronym:

T toxoplasmosis
O other
R rubella
C cytomegalic inclusion disease
H herpes
Also:
TO **to**xoplasmosis
R **r**ubella
C **c**ytomegalovirus infections
H congenital **h**erpes

Torcon NB selective angiographic catheter (Rad).

Torkildsen shunt procedure—ventriculocisternostomy (Neuro).

Tornalate (bitolterol).

Tornwaldt's bursitis.

Toronto parapodium (Ortho)—has one lock for both hip and knee joints. Orthosis for ambulation in children with cerebral palsy and myelomeningocele.

TORP (total ossicular replacement prosthesis)—used in otological surgery.

torque guide, Lunderquist-Ring.

torr—a unit of measurement that relates to pressure in the patient in neurosurgery, when hypothermia and hypotension are used: "The pressure was kept at 70 torr and then dropped to 60 torr."

torsade de pointes (Cardio)—a very rapid ventricular tachycardia in which there is waxing and waning of amplitudes in the QRS complexes as seen on the electrocardiogram. It could be self-limiting or could go on to ventricular fibrillation. It is said to have been named by a cardiologist who thought the EKG tracing looked like a ballet step (dancing on point, on toes).

Torula histolytica—the cause of torulosis, the old name for cryptococcosis.

TOT (tincture of time), as in "Given tincture of time, we may soon see a resolution of his symptoms." Physicians say that aggressive treatment may cure only a small number of illnesses, and that tincture of time (watchful waiting) cures a large proportion of curable illnesses.

total lymphoid irradiation—see *TLI.*

Tourette's syndrome (*maladie des tics*)—a disorder of tics, throat sounds, generalized jerking movements, and the uncontrollable use of obscene language. Also, Gilles de la Tourette's syndrome.

tourniquet
Digikit finger
Medi-quet surgical
Rumel
TCPM pneumatic

Towne projection in x-rays—occipital view of the skull.

Townley TARA prosthesis (Ortho). See *TARA prosthesis.*

Townsend knee brace (Ortho)—made of lightweight titanium and graphite.

toxic—showing signs of toxemia or septicemia, such as fever, tachycardia, flushing, and mental confusion.

***Toxocara* ELISA**—test for endophthalmitis (Oph).

Toxoplasma gondii—can cause central nervous system toxoplasmosis in patients with AIDS.

t-PA (tissue plasminogen activator) (Activase, alteplase)—given intravenously to dissolve a thrombus.

TPDCV (thioguanine, procarbazine, DBC [mitolactol], CCNU, vincristine)—chemotherapy protocol used to treat brain tumors.

TP-5 (thymopentin).

TP-40 (Oncol)—a chemotherapy drug given intravesically to patients with unresectable superficial bladder carcinoma.

T-piece oxygen—administration of humidified oxygen through a tube connected to a T-shaped connector attached to an endotracheal tube.

TPN line (total parenteral nutrition).

TP-1 (thymostimuline)—used to treat AIDS.

TPPN (total peripheral parenteral nutrition).

TR (repetition time) (Radiol)—in magnetic resonance imaging, the interval between one spin echo pulse sequence and the next.

TRA (all-trans-retinoic acid) (Oncol)—a form of vitamin A given orally to patients with malignant solid tumors unresponsive to other chemotherapy.

trabecula (pl., trabeculae)—thin fibrous band of tissue.

trabeculectomy, Pearce.

trabeculoplasty (Oph)—brief laser treatment which produces tightening of the outflow mechanism in glaucoma patients by placing a number of pinpoint lesions directly over the drain. Usually performed on an outpatient basis under topical anesthesia. Also, argon laser trabeculoplasty (ALT).

Tracer Blood Glucose Micro-monitor for self-testing by diabetics.

tracheal tug—a downward impulse imparted to the trachea by an aortic aneurysm, synchronous with heartbeat.

tracheal tube, Dumon-Harrell.

trachelotomy (Ob-Gyn)—incision into, or excision of, the neck of the uterus (cervix uteri); also called cervicectomy. Cf. *tracheotomy.*

tracheostomy tube, Kistner.

tracheotomy—incision of the trachea. Cf. *trachelotomy.*

track—the path along which something has moved and left a mark, e.g., needle track. This word is not often used in medical dictation. Cf. *tract.*

Tracker-18 Soft Stream catheter (Cardio)—a microcatheter used to deliver drugs to lyse intracoronary thrombi. The holes in the sides of the catheter deliver a soft stream which does not injure the blood vessel.

tract—a collection of nerve fibers that have a common origin, function, and termination—as in spinal tract; or a group of organs that are arranged serially and together perform a common function—as in gastrointestinal tract; or an abnormal passage through tissue—as sinus tract, fistulous tract. Cf. *track.* See *Bachman tract.*

traction
Bryant's
Buck's
Cotrel
Crutchfield skeletal
halo
halter
Russell's
skeletal

TRAIDS (transfusion related AIDS, acquired immunodeficiency syndrome).

Trail Making Test—neurological test.

TRAM flap (transverse rectus abdominis myocutaneous)—used in breast reconstruction (Plas Surg). In this technique to reconstruct the breast, tissue is transferred from the central portion of the abdomen onto the chest wall, or tunneled beneath the

TRAM flap *(cont.)* skin to the breast. See *tummy tuck flap.*

transanal endoscopic microsurgery (TEM) (GI)—a minimally invasive technique for resection of sessile adenomas and some rectal carcinomas.

transcervical balloon tuboplasty (TBT) (Ob-Gyn)—a procedure used to open blocked fallopian tubes which have been the cause of infertility. Anesthesia is obtained with a paracervical block and a catheter is inserted into the blocked fallopian tube under fluoroscopic guidance. The procedure is less expensive than standard surgery for blocked tubes or in vitro fertilization. Also called recanalization.

transcutaneous electrical nerve stimulation (TENS).

transcutaneous oxygen level ($TcPO_2$).

transferrin (as in *ferr*ous)—a glycoprotein. Also called iron binding protein.

transfixion suture—suture ligature; used to suture a large blood vessel closed; secures against slippage of the knot; sometimes called *stick tie.*

transform, fast-Fourier—MRI term.

transfusion, autologous.

transhepatic embolization (THE).

transient ischemic attack (TIA).

translocation Down's syndrome—caused by an extra 21st chromosome that moves from the 21st chromosome pair to either the 13th or 15th pair, resulting in 13/21 or 15/21 translocation Down's syndrome.

transnasal endoluminal ultrasonography—a method used to study the anatomy of the GI tract.

transplantation—see *orthotopic transplantation.*

Transpore surgical tape.

transposition of the great arteries (TGA).

transtracheal oxygen catheter—can replace a nasal cannula for better patient comfort and aesthetics. Inserted at the base of the neck through a small, permanent, surgically created tract into the trachea. The catheter is connected to tubing to a portable oxygen tank.

transverse magnetization; orientation—MRI term.

trap bottle—used for suction in surgery.

Traube's space—the gastric bubble, which causes a different tympanitic note from percussion over the lungs.

Travasorb MCT—a medium chain triglyceride food supplement.

Travenol infuser—a disposable device for the delivery of continuous parenteral drug therapy to patients who can be ambulatory.

TRC (tanned red cells) (microsomal TRC antibody titer)—a test used in the study of thyroid antibodies.

treadmill testing—stress testing of cardiac response, in which the patient progressively increases walking speed, and the incline of the treadmill is also increased. The test is continued until signs of ischemia are noted, or when the target heart rate is reached. The test is discontinued when the patient becomes fatigued, short of breath, or notes claudication, vertigo, etc.

tremor, pill-rolling.

Trendelenburg position.

trephine
- Arruga lacrimal
- Cardona corneal prosthesis
- Castroviejo
- D'Errico skull

trephine *(cont.)*
Hessburg-Barron vacuum
Katena

trepopnea—a preference for the recumbent position, because breathing is easier in that position.

Triad, O'Donohue's Unhappy (OUT).

triamcinolone cream. See *TAC.*

triatriatum, cor.

triazolam (Halcion).

trichiasis—inversion of the eyelashes so that they rub against the cornea, causing continual irritation of the eyeball.

trichinosis—infection with trichinae; caused by eating undercooked pork and some other meats containing *Trichinella spiralis.* Cf. *trichocyst, trichosis.*

trichocyst—a cell structure which is derived from the cytoplasm. Cf. *trichinosis, trichosis.*

trichosanthin (compound Q)—a drug used to treat patients with AIDS and ARC. See *GLQ223.*

trichosis—a disease of, or abnormal growth of, the hair. Cf. *trichinosis, trichocyst.*

Trichosporon beigelii—seen in postsurgical soft tissue infections (Lab).

trichotillomania—compulsive tugging at one's hair (Psych). "Her symptoms included rather depressive features, and trichotillomania."

triciribine phosphate (TCN-P) (Oncol) —a drug used to treat non-small-cell lung carcinoma.

tricorrectional bunionectomy—see *bunionectomy, tricorrectional.*

tricyclic antidepressant (TCA).

trigger point—a localized zone of tenderness, especially in a muscle.

trilogy, Fallot's. See *Fallot's trilogy, Fallot's pentalogy, tetralogy of Fallot.*

trimethoprim-sulfamethoxazole—see *TMP-SMZ.*

trimetrexate gluconate—used to treat various carcinomas and also *Pneumocystis carinii* infection in AIDS patients.

tripe palm (Oncol)—a cutaneous marker for internal malignancy which produces a rugose or corrugated thickening of the skin of the palm.

Triphasil—triphasic contraceptive (levonorgestrel and ethinyl estradiol).

"triple A" (AAA) (medical slang for abdominal aortic aneurysm).

triple antibiotics.

Trippi-Wells tongs—used for traction (Neuro, Ortho).

tripoding (Neuro)—Gowers' sign, classical sign of Duchenne muscular dystrophy.

triquetrum (Ortho)—the triquetral bone in the wrist; between the pisiform and lunate bones; os triquetrum, also called the triangular bone.

trisodium phosphonoformate—see *phosphonoformate trisodium; foscarnet.*

trisomy-D syndrome—manifested by the following clinical features: apneic spells, apparent deafness, capillary hemangioma, cardiac defects, characteristic dermal pattern, cleft lip and palate, death in early infancy, ear malformation, polydactyly, scalp defects, and severe central nervous system defects.

trisomy-G—a genetically determined disorder; one of a group of such disorders associated with increased risk of leukemia.

Triumph VR pacemaker (Cardio)—a single chamber adaptive rate pacemaker by CPI.

Trocan disposable CO_2 trocar and cannula.

Troisier's node—see *sentinel node.*

troleandomycin (Tao)—an antibiotic in the macrolide class of drugs, similar in effectiveness to penicillin and erythromycin but with fewer side effects.

Trousseau's sign—the occurrence of carpal spasm, in latent tetany, when the upper arm is compressed (as with the use of a tourniquet).

TR/TE, long—see *T2 weighted image.*

TR/TE, short—see *T1 weighted image.*

Tru-Cut needle—used for liver biopsy.

true vertigo (Neuro)—as differentiated from dizziness; a feeling that everything is revolving around the patient, or that he himself is revolving.

trumpet, Iowa (Surg).

Trumpet Valve hydrodissector—see *Nezhat-Dorsey Trumpet Valve hydrodissector.*

TRUS (transrectal ultrasonography)—to evaluate prostate carcinoma.

T-Span tissue expander.

TSPP rectilinear bone scan (technetium stannous pyrophosphate).

TSRH Crosslink (Texas Scottish Rite Hospital) (Ortho)—a spinal instrumentation system used to stabilize the rods used in correction of scoliosis. Also, *Cotrel-Dubousset.*

TTP (thrombotic thrombocytopenic purpura).

T2 (Radiol)—in magnetic resonance imaging, the time it takes for protons to go out of phase after having been shifted in their orientation by an excitation pulse.

T-2 protocol (Oncol)—for treatment of Ewing's sarcoma.

T2 weighted image (Radiol)—in magnetic resonance imaging, a spin-echo image generated by a pulse sequence using a long repetition time (2.0 seconds or more). Also called long TR/TE.

tube
- Abbott-Rawson
- Adson suction
- Amsterdam
- Argyle-Salem sump
- Atkinson endoprosthesis
- Axiom double sump
- Baron suction
- Blakemore-Sengstaken
- Cantor
- Castelli
- Celestin latex rubber
- Christopher-Williams
- Cilastin
- Cope nephrostomy
- Corpak feeding
- Dennis
- Dobbhoff feeding
- Dumon-Harrell tracheal
- fenestrated tracheostomy
- Feuerstein myringotomy drain
- fil d'Arion silicone
- Flexiflo Stomate low-profile gastrostomy
- germ
- germination
- glutaraldehyde-tanned bovine collagen
- Guibor Silastic
- Hodge intestinal decompression
- Holter tubing
- Jergesen
- Keofeed
- Kistner tracheostomy
- K-Tube
- Lanz low-pressure cuff endotracheal
- Lepley-Ernst
- Levin
- Linton
- Mallinckrodt feeding
- Mallinckrodt Laser-Flex
- MIC gastroenteric
- Micron
- Miller-Abbott
- Minnesota
- Molteno seton

tube *(cont.)*
Moss Suction Buster
nasogastric (NG)
nasojejunal (NJ)
Newvicon vacuum chamber pickup
Nuport PEG
Nyhus/Nelson feeding
O'Dwyer's
Olympus One-Step Button
Osmolite feeding
Pedi PEG
PEG (percutaneous endoscopic gastrostomy)
Pitt talking tracheostomy
Portex tracheostomy
Quickert-Dryden
Quinton
RAE endotracheal
Replogle
Reuter bobbin
Ring-McLean sump
Rubin Brandborg biopsy
Sacks-Vine PEG
Sandoz suction/feeding
Saticon vacuum chamber pickup
Sengstaken-Blakemore
Super PEG
Tygon
Vidicon vacuum chamber pickup
Vivonex Moss

Tube-Lok tracheotomy dressing.

tuber cinereum (Neuro)—part of the hypothalamus.

tubercle—see *Gerdy's tubercle.*

Tubex injector—a closed injection system to protect doctors and nurses against needle-stick injuries.

tuboplasty, transcervical balloon.

Tuffier rib retractor (Thor Surg).

tularemia (also Valley fever)—first described in Tulare, California. The vector (carrier) is thought to be *Ixodes pacificus* (a common deer and cattle tick).

Tulevech lacrimal cannula (Oph).

tulip probe (Neuro).

Tum-E-Vac—gastric lavage kit for use in emergency situations.

tummy tuck flap (Plas Surg)—a method of breast reconstruction in which the transverse rectus abdominis muscle (TRAM) is used to create a myocutaneous flap which is tunneled beneath the skin to the breast. Similar in procedure to an abdominoplasty, hence the name tummy tuck flap. Also called TRAM flap.

tumor
cerebellopontile angle
Krukenberg
nonseminomatous germ cell (NSGCT)
Pott's puffy
Warthin's
Wharton's

tumor blush—vascularization seen on angiography. Increased vascularization is a clue to the presence of a tumor and may represent a malignancy rather than hypertrophy.

tumor-infiltrating lymphocytes (TIL).

tumor marker—a biochemical indicator that, when found in the blood, urine, or serum, indicates the presence of a tumor. Examples of these markers are carcinoembryonic antigen (CEA) as a marker for carcinomas of the colon, breast; prostate-specific antigen (PSA) for cancer of the prostate; alpha-fetoprotein (AFP) for hepatomas and teratomas, Paget's disease of the bone and Hodgkin's disease, etc. Examples: CA 15-3, CA 19-9, CA 72-4.

tumor necrosis factor—see *TNF.*

tumor plop—the sound made by a pedunculated myxoma in a cardiac chamber when the patient is rolled over.

tunnel views (Radiol).

Tuohy needle (Neuro)—used to insert a lumbar subarachnoid catheter.

Tuohy-Bost introducer—used to introduce balloon, electrode, and closed-end catheters.

Turner's mosaicism (syndrome).

Turner-Warwick method (GI)—uses the right gastroepiploic artery as the vascular supply for a pedicle graft in a bowel reconstruction procedure.

Turner-Warwick urethroplasty.

T water test—for fructose intolerance.

twenty-nail involvement (or 20-nail) in patient with psoriasis; all the fingernails and toenails are involved in the disease process.

21-channel EEG (electroencephalogram).

twig—smaller than a branch, e.g., in vessel or nerve. "There is a possibility that a neural branch or twig was injured, and should the sensory symptoms persist, she was advised to return."

Twisk needle holder/forceps/scissors—a combination instrument used in microsurgery.

twist drill catheter.

2-CdA (2-chlorodeoxyadenosine) (Oncol)—a chemotherapy drug used to treat acute myeloid leukemia. Cf. *CDA*.

2-chlorodeoxyadenosine (2-CdA).

two-dimensional echocardiography (sector scan)—a technique which has become, as one physician puts it, "the noninvasive 'gold standard' for diagnosis, [and] catheterization has been deemed unnecessary for some cardiac lesions."

two-flight dyspnea—difficulty breathing that occurs on climbing two flights of stairs. (But what is a flight? Ten steps? Twenty steps?)

T-Y stent—a tracheobronchial stent which has both T-shaped and Y-shaped sections. Used to maintain a patent airway after burns or trauma.

"Tyco #3"—medical slang for Tylenol and codeine.

Tycron suture—a nonabsorbable polyester fiber surgical suture. Note: Tycron and Ti-Cron are sold by different manufacturers but appear to be the same material.

Tygon tubing—used in venovenous bypass for transplantation of the liver. It probably has many other uses.

tylosis—callosities (Derm). See *hypertylosis*.

Tympan-O-Scope, Madsen.

Tyndall effect (Oph). See *aqueous flare*.

typhlitis—inflammation of the cecum; also, cecitis.

tyramine test—for pheochromocytoma.

tyrosine tolerance test.

Tzanck preparation ("zank").

U, u

UAC (umbilical artery catheter) (Neonat, Ped).

UBC brace—University of British Columbia brace.

"u-cerin"—see *Eucerin.*

UC strip—catheter tubing fastener.

U-87201E—used to treat HIV-positive patients. Manufactured by Upjohn.

Uendex (dextran sulfate).

UGH+ syndrome (Oph)—a syndrome with symptoms of uveitis, glaucoma, hyphema, plus vitreous hemorrhage.

UHMWPe ball liner (ultra-high molecular weight polyethylene) (Enduron acetabular liner).

Uhthoff's phenomenon; sign (Oph) (pronounced ''oot'-hoff'')—nystagmus seen in patients with multiple cerebrospinal sclerosis.

ulcer
  Curling's
  decubitus
  Hunner's
  Martorell hypertensive
  trophic

ulegyria—destruction of the cortex in a deep sulcus of a gyrus.

"U-lexin"—see *Eulexin.*

Ultec hydrocolloid dressing.

Ultradol (etodolac) (Ortho)—an analgesic and nonsteroidal anti-inflammatory drug.

Ultra-Drive bone cement removal system (Ortho)—used in total hip revision surgery to remove old cement without damage to the cortical wall. Uses ultrasonically tuned tool tips to provide audible and tactile feedback in order to differentiate between cement and bone.

ultrafast CT—see *cine CT.*

Ultramark 4 Ultrasound.

ultrasonography (Radiol)—a means of visualizing internal structures by observing the effects they have on a beam of sound waves. The sound used for this procedure is at a higher frequency (pitch) than the human ear can detect. Ultrasound waves pass through air, gas, and fluid without being reflected; however, they bounce back from rigid structures such as bone and gallstones, creating an ''echo'' that can be detected by a receiver. Solid organs such as the liver and kidney partially reflect ultrasound waves in predictable patterns. Waves are also reflected from

ultrasonography *(cont.)*
the interface between two structures. Ultrasonography might be compared to taking a flash photograph. Light from the flashbulb bounces off the patient and comes back to create an image on film of the surface contours of the patient; however, the echo must be converted electronically to a visible image before it can be interpreted. Sophisticated electronic equipment permits ultrasound scanning of a body region with generation of a two-dimensional picture of internal structures. In practice, the same device that generates the sound waves (called a transducer) also acts as the receiver. Although it emits signals at a rate of 1000 per second, the transducer is actually functioning as a receiver 99.9% of the time.

ultrasound (US)
ADR
Aloka
ATL real-time
BladderScan
duplex
endoscopic (EUS)
frequency domain imaging (FDI) in NeuroSectOR
real-time
transcervical tuboplasty
transnasal endoluminal
transrectal
TRUS (transrectal ultrasound)

ultrasound transcervical tuboplasty (Ob-Gyn)—unblocks obstructed fallopian tubes, without exposing the patient to abdominal surgery, x-rays, or x-ray dyes. A cervical cannula is positioned, and Doppler ultrasound is used (instead of fluoroscopy) to thread a catheter into the blocked tube, where normal saline is injected to check catheter position. Then a flexible wire is threaded through the catheter to break up the obstruction.

Ultratome (GI)—a small sphincterotome manufactured by Microvasive.

Ultravate (halobetasol propionate).

umbrella cell—found on the surface of the urothelium.

undyed braided polyglycolic acid suture (Thor Surg).

unenhanced scan (Radiol)—a scan made without the use of a contrast material.

ungual tuft—tip of the nail.

Unicard (dilevalol) (Cardio)—a beta blocker used to treat mild to moderate hypertension.

Uniflex—polyurethane adhesive surgical dressing.

Unilab Surgibone (Neuro, Ortho)—nonantigenic, sterile, specially processed mature bovine bone. Used instead of autologous or homologous bone for implantation into humans to fill cavities from which tumors or cysts have been removed. There are also specially prepared onlay grafts that have cancellous bone on one side and cortical bone on the other, and also load-bearing cancellous bone blocks and dowels.

UNILINK system (Hand Surg)—a mechanical anastomotic device, designed for work under the operating microscope, to anastomose small blood vessels. Introduced in Sweden.

unit (See also *measurement; radiation dosages; rem; unit of measurement.)*
Bessey-Lowry
BiLAP bipolar cautery
Bodansky
C-arm fluoroscopy
Eclipse TENS
Hounsfield
International
Keeler cryophake

unit *(cont.)*
King-Armstrong
Kreiselman
Maxima II TENS
Montevideo
mouse
pilosebaceous
postanesthesia care (PACU)
Respironics
rutherford (rd)
sievert (Sv)
Somogyi
Stayoden 9000F TENS

unit of measurement, prefixes

tera-	10^{12}	T
giga-	10^{9}	G
mega-	10^{6}	M
kilo-	10^{3}	k
hecto-	10^{2}	h
deca-	10^{1}	da
deci-	10^{-1}	d
centi-	10^{-2}	c
milli-	10^{-3}	m
micro-	10^{-6}	u
nano-	10^{-9}	n
pico-	10^{-12}	p
femto-	10^{-15}	f
atto-	10^{-18}	a

University of Akron artificial heart (Cardio)—fully implantable artificial heart that does not need to be connected to a machine outside the patient. Contains batteries to provide power and electromagnets to move the blood through its chambers.

Unna boot; paste; wrap (Ortho).

Unschuld's sign—a tendency to have cramps in the calves, an early indication of diabetes mellitus.

UPF prosthesis (universal proximal femur)—see *Bateman UPF prosthesis.*

upgoing toes—abnormal response to the Babinski test, in which the great toe curls upward when the sole of the foot is stroked. Diagnostic of disorders of the central nervous system.

Upper Hands—a self-retaining retractor used in liver transplantation.

UPPP (uvulopalatopharyngoplasty).

uptake (Radiol)—in radionuclide scans, the absorption or concentration of a radionuclide by an organ or tissue. Also, fluorescein uptake.

urachus, patent—in a neonate, incomplete closure of the umbilicus through which urine escapes; a urachal cyst may form and require surgical treatment.

uracil mustard—chemotherapy drug.

ureteroileal loop, Cordonnier.

ureteropelvic junction (UPJ).

ureteropyeloscope
Karl Storz Calcutript
Karl Storz flexible

ureterovesicoplasty, Leadbetter-Politano.

urethral sound, LeFort.

urethroplasty
Thiersch-Duplay
Turner-Warwick

Uricult dipslides (Urol)—used in testing urine for bacteria.

uridine rescue (Oncol)—a drug regimen which allows larger than usual doses of fluorouracil (5-FU) to be given to patients with metastatic colorectal carcinoma.

urinary reservoir, Mainz pouch.

urine, maple syrup.

Urocyte diagnostic cytometry system—noninvasive test for carcinoma of the urothelium.

urocytogram—study of estrogen effect on desquamated cells from the urogenital tract (used in investigation of precocious puberty).

urothelium—epithelium of the urinary bladder.

ursodeoxycholic acid (ursodiol)—used to dissolve stones. "To consider use of ursodeoxycholic acid in a person this young would not be appropriate, as he has a high possibility of recurrence, even after dissolution of the stones." See *Actigall.*

urushiol ("oo-roo-she-all") (Derm)—that component in poison oak, poison sumac, and poison ivy that causes the contact dermatitis in people who are sensitive to these plants.

USCI cannula (Surg).

Utah artificial arm—a myoelectric prosthesis for amputations above the elbow; it comes with either a hook or an artificial Myobock hand.

uterine prolapse repair, LeFort.

uterus didelphys—double uterus.

"u-thymic"—see *euthymic.*

"u-thyroid"—see *euthyroid.*

Utrata capsulorhexis forceps (Oph)—used in small-incision eye surgery. See also *Kraff-Utrata tear capsulotomy forceps.*

uveitides—plural form of *uveitis.*

V, v

V (ventricular).

VAC (vinblastine, actinomycin D, Cytoxan)—chemotherapy protocol.

Vabra aspirator—disposable system for endometrial screening (Gyn).

VAB-6 (Oncol)—a chemotherapy protocol used to treat testicular cancer.

VACA (vincristine, actinomycin D, Cytoxan, Adriamycin)—chemotherapy protocol.

VACAD (vincristine, Adriamycin, Cytoxan, actinomycin D, dacarbazine) —chemotherapy protocol.

vaccine
- AIDS
- gp120
- gp160
- HIB polysaccharide
- HIV
- influenza
- Melacine
- RG-83894
- r-gp160
- Rhesus diploid cell strain rabies v. (RDRV) (adsorbed)
- rp24
- vaccinia
- VaxSyn HIV-1
- zoster immune globulin (ZIG)

vaccinia vaccine (No, the physician who dictates this is not stammering.): "He received vaccinia vaccine last summer." This is a vaccine used infrequently, generally by those who have contact with smallpox virus in laboratories. It is no longer commercially produced.

VACP (VePesid, Adriamycin, Cytoxan, Platinol)—chemotherapy protocol.

Vac-Pak Pad (Ortho)—a pad used for immobilization during total hip surgery.

VACTERL syndrome
- V vertebral or vascular defects
- A anorectal malformation (imperforate anus)
- C cardiac anomaly
- TE tracheoesophageal fistula
- R renal anomaly
- L limb anomaly

Vacurette—suction curet (Ob-Gyn).

Vacutainer—rubber-stoppered vacuum tube used to draw blood.

VAD (ventricular assist device) (Cardiothoracic).

VAD (vincristine, Adriamycin, dexamethasone)—chemotherapy protocol.

VAD/V (vincristine, Adriamycin, dexamethasone, verapamil)—chemotherapy protocol.

vagal nerve implant (Neuro). A patient with epilepsy that cannot be controlled by drugs or surgery may be given a vagal nerve implant. The implant is placed subcutaneously under the collarbone, and two electrodes from it are placed on the vagal nerve. When patients sense the onset of a seizure, they activate the implant to stimulate the vagal nerve. This appears to interrupt epileptic activity in the brain.

vaginal birth after (previous) **cesarean section** (VBAC).

vaginal candle (Gyn, Oncol)—used in radium insertion.

vaginal interruption of pregnancy, with dilatation and curettage (VIP-DAC).

vaginalis
 Gardnerella
 Haemophilus

Vagistat (tioconazole).

VAI (vincristine, actinomycin D, ifosfamide)—chemotherapy protocol.

Vairox high compression vascular stocking (Vasc Surg).

Valergan (estradiol)—chemotherapy drug.

Valleylab (Surg)—laparoscopic and electrosurgical instruments.

Valtrac BAR (biofragmentable anastomotic ring) (GI).

valve
 Arenberg-Denver inner ear
 Beall Surgitool mitral
 Blom-Singer
 Carpentier-Edwards
 Cutter-Smeloff cardiac
 glutaraldehyde-tanned porcine heart

valve *(cont.)*
 Hall-Kaster mitral
 Hancock M.O. Bioprosthesis
 Heimlich
 Holter
 Ionescu-Shiley
 Kastec mitral
 Krupin-Denver eye
 LeVeen
 Medtronic Hall heart
 Passy-Muir tracheostomy speaking
 St. Jude Medical
 Singer-Blom
 Sophy programmable pressure
 Spitz-Holter
 Spivack
 Star-Edwards Silastic prosthetic heart
 Sutter-Smeloff prosthetic heart
 Veall Surgitool mitral
 Wada
 Xenotech prosthetic

valvotomy, percutaneous mitral balloon (PMBV).

valvulotome, Hall.

VAM (VP-16, Adriamycin, methotrexate)—chemotherapy protocol.

VAMP (vincristine, actinomycin-D, methotrexate, prednisone)—chemotherapy protocol used in treating acute leukemias in children.

Van Bogaert's disease—a rare familial disease, resulting in hepatomegaly secondary to very high concentrations of cholesterol esters.

van den Bergh's test—of the concentration of bilirubin in the blood. Normal range: direct bilirubin 0.0 to 0.1 mg per 100 ml of serum; total bilirubin 0.2 to 1.4 mg per 100 ml of serum.

Vandeput, in *Tanner-Vandeput mesh dermatome.*

Van Herick (Oph), as "Anterior chambers were deep by Van Herick."

van Heuven's anatomic classification—diabetic retinopathy (Oph).

van Loonen operating keratoscope (Oph).

Vannas capsulotomy scissors (Oph).

vanSonnenberg sump—used for percutaneous abscess and fluid drainage (PAFD). (No space in vanSonnenberg.)

vanSonnenberg-Wittich catheter—used for percutaneous abscess and fluid drainage (PAFD).

varicella zoster virus—see *VZV.*

Varidyne drain (ENT) (made by Surgidyne).

Vari/Moist wound dressing with nonadherent moisture vapor characteristics (Surg).

Varivas R (Vasc Surg)—denatured homologous vein harvested after saphenous vein stripping and used in various lengths for vascular access and bypass surgeries.

vasa deferentia—plural of vas deferens.

Vascor (bepridil).

vasoactive intestinal polypeptide. See *VIP.*

VAT (vinblastine, Adriamycin, thiotepa)—chemotherapy protocol.

VATER syndrome:

V vertebral and/or vascular defects
A anorectal malformation
TE tracheoesophageal fistula
R radial, ray, or renal anomaly

VaxSyn HIV-1—see *AIDS vaccine.*

VBAC (vaginal birth after [previous] cesarean section).

VBC (VePesid, BCNU, Cytoxan)—chemotherapy protocol.

VBG (vertical-banded gastroplasty).

VBMCP (vincristine, BCNU, melphalan, Cytoxan, prednisone)—chemotherapy protocol.

VBMF (vincristine, bleomycin, methotrexate, fluorouracil)—chemotherapy protocol.

VBP (vinblastine, bleomycin, cisplatin)—chemotherapy protocol.

VCUG (vesicoureterogram) (Urol).

VCUG (voiding cystourethrogram) (Urol).

VDRL (Venereal Disease Research Laboratory).

vectis (Obs)—a curved lever used for traction on the fetal head during delivery.

vectorcardiography—a noninvasive cardiac diagnostic procedure that presents the same diagnostic information as that given by electrocardiography, but in a different form. It gives a three-dimensional picture of the conduction of electrical impulses from the sino-atrial node, across the right atrium to the atrioventricular node, down the bundle of His, through the bundle branches to the apex, and upward into the Purkinje fibers, stimulating the myocardial muscle.

veil—see *Sattler veil.*

Veingard—a transparent dressing which is moisture-permeable, waterproof, and sterile. Used over an I.V. site, so the site can be monitored.

vein/graft holder, GraftAssist.

vein of Galen—vena cerebri magna, the great cerebral vein, formed by the two internal cerebral veins; named after the second century A.D. Greek physician.

vein of Labbé ("lab-bay").

vein stripping operation (Cardio).

VeIP (vinblastine, ifosfamide, Platinol)—chemotherapy protocol.

Veirs cannula; needle (Oph).

Velban (vinblastine).

Velcro rales.

Veley headrest (Neuro)—Light-Veley headrest used in neurosurgical procedures.

velolaryngeal endoscopy (ENT) (Surg) —endoscopy of the soft palate (velum palatinum) and laryngeal mechanisms.

Velpeau dressing or bandage—used for treatment of dislocation of the shoulder or other shoulder girdle injuries. It consists of bandaging the arm in such a manner that the injured arm is bent at the elbow over the patient's chest, with the palm of the hand at the uninjured shoulder, taking the weight off the injured shoulder.

Velsar (vinblastine).

Vena Tech LGM filter—an inferior vena cava filter used to prevent recurrent pulmonary embolism. Can be placed in the jugular or femoral artery. LGM is for Lehman, Gerofliea, and Metais—the French engineers who developed the filter.

venipuncture (*not* veno- or vena-).

Venocath (trade name).

venogram (*not* venagram).

venoscope, Landry Vein Light.

venous web disease (hepatic). See *hepatic venous web disease.*

Ventak AICD pacemaker (automatic implantable cardioverter-defibrillator).

venter (noun)—belly, or belly-shaped part. See *ventral.*

ventilate (verb)—(1) to express verbally, especially as a release for pent-up emotions; (2) to breathe for a patient either by means of a hand-held bag or mechanical respirator.

ventilation (Neonat)—high-frequency jet and high-frequency oscillation assisted respiration for premature infants.

ventilator; respirator
- BABYbird respirator
- Bennett PR-2 ventilator
- Bird respirator
- Bourns infant ventilator
- Bourns-Bear ventilator
- high-frequency jet ventilator
- high-frequency oscillation ventilator
- KinetiX ventilation monitor
- MVV (maximal voluntary ventilation)
- Monaghan 300 ventilator

ventral (adj.)—toward the belly, anterior. See *venter.*

ventricular assistance device—see *DMVA.*

ventricular ejection fraction (Radiol)—in multiple gated acquisition scan, or MUGA, that portion of the total volume of a ventricle that is ejected during ventricular contraction (systole); usually expressed as a percent rather than a fraction.

ventriculocisternostomy—Torkildsen shunt procedure.

ventroposterolateral thalamic electrode. See *VPL thalamic electrode.*

Venturi mask—used in the administration of oxygen.

VEP (visual evoked potential) (Neuro) —see *brain tests, noninvasive.*

VePesid (etoposide)—chemotherapeutic agent used in treatment of refractory testicular tumors.

VER (visual evoked response) (Neuro).

verapamil (Calan, Isoptin, Verelan) (Cardio, Psych)—a calcium channel blocker commonly used to treat angina, arrhythmias, and hypertension, and also used to treat manic-depressive disorder.

Verbatim balloon catheter (Cardio)—so named because the balloon expands precisely to preprogrammed sizes. Used in coronary angioplasty.

Verelan (verapamil).

Veress needle *(not* Verres)—used in laparoscopy for insufflation of carbon dioxide (Gyn).

vermian veins (Neuro)—veins of the cerebellar vermis.

Vernier calipers (Neuro)—used to measure the amount of intervertebral disk protrusion present, or for any other fine measurement.

VERP (ventricular effective refractory period).

Versadopp 10 probe (Ob-Gyn)—pen-size ultrasonic Doppler probe by Diagnostic Ultrasound.

Versa-Fx (Ortho)—femoral fixation system which requires removal of less bone.

VersaPulse holmium laser (Neuro)—for use in laser nucleotomy. See *laser nucleotomy.*

Versatrax cardiac pacemaker.

versions (Oph)—binocular voluntary movement of the eyes in conjugate gaze (in the same direction).

vertebrae, scalloping of.

vertebral body impactor (Neuro)—an instrument used in the management of thoracic and lumbar spine fractures, after first performing hemilaminectomy and resection of the pedicle on the side where there is most compression of the spinal canal. "With the impactor, the bone graft was securely seated."

vertex—top, generally used alone to refer to the top of the head, as in "vertex presentation," but also used in referring to the top or apex of other organs. Cf. *vortex.*

vertical-banded gastroplasty (VBG).

vesical (adj.)—pertaining to the bladder. Cf. *vesicle.*

vesicant—a drug or agent that causes blistering. "Serious tissue damage can result if vesicants leak from a previously punctured site."

vesicle (noun)—a small blister, a small bladder or sac containing liquid. Cf. *vesical.*

vesicoureterogram (VCUG).

vesicourethral suspension (Urol)—Marshall-Marchetti-Krantz procedure (MMK).

vessels, ghost (in cornea).

vestibular window—opening between the tympanic cavity and the scala vestibuli of the cochlea, into which the footplate of the stapes fits. Also called *oval window; fenestra ovalis; fenestra vestibuli.*

"V fib" (ventricular fibrillation).

Viasorb wound dressing (Surg).

Vibram—soled rockerbottom shoe used after foot surgery.

vibrissae ("vi-bris'-e")—the hairs that grow in the nostrils.

VIC (vinblastine, ifosfamide, CCNU)—chemotherapy protocol.

Vickers microsurgical instruments.

VID (vitello-intestinal duct) (Neonat)—a patent VID in neonates can produce a T-shaped prolapse of intestine through the umbilicus.

Vidal-Ardrey modified Hoffmann device (Ortho). See *Hoffmann external fixation device.*

vidarabine (adenine arabinoside, Ara-A, Vira-A)—an antiviral drug used to treat herpes simplex and herpes zoster infections.

video-laseroscopy—see *laparoscopic laser cholecystectomy.*

Videx (didanosine, dideoxyinosine, ddI)—approved by FDA to treat HIV-positive patients.

Vidicon vacuum chamber pickup tube for video camera used in arthroscopy.

VIE (vincristine, ifosfamide, etoposide)—chemotherapy protocol.

view
Arcelin's
Caldwell
Chausse's
dens
five-
Hughston
Law's
Low-Beer's
Mayer's
outlet
Owen's
Schuller's
Stenver's
sunrise
Towne
tunnel
Waters'

Vigilon—a synthetic (polyethylene) occlusive dressing, for use on ulcerations. These dressings relieve pain, cause debridement, and stimulate the formation of granulation tissue.

villose (adj.)—variant spelling of *villous.*

villous—shaggy with soft hairs; covered with villi; "villous adenoma." Also spelled *villose.* Cf. *villus.*

villus (pl., villi)—small vascular protrusion, particularly a protrusion from the surface of a membrane, commonly seen in small bowel. Cf. *villous.*

vilona (inosine pranobex)—a drug used to treat AIDS patients.

viloxazine (Vivalan).

VIMRxyn (hypericin).

Vincasar (vincristine)

Vincent's infection (Oral Surg)—necrotizing ulcerative gingivitis.

vincristine sulfate (Oncovin).

vindesine (Eldisine) (Oncol)—a drug used in treating acute lymphocytic and chronic myelocytic leukemia.

Vineberg cardiac revascularization procedure—mammary artery transplant to the heart for coronary insufficiency. (May no longer be performed.)

Vineland Social Maturity Scale—test used in psychiatry/psychology evaluation.

Vinke tongs—skull traction apparatus.

Vinson, in *Plummer-Vinson syndrome.*

violaceous ("vi-o-láy-shus) (Derm)—violet-colored. Usually refers to lesions on the skin.

VIP (vasoactive intestinal peptides). "Elevations of VIP are associated with bronchogenic carcinoma."

VIP (VePesid, ifosfamide, and Platinol)—a standard chemotherapy protocol used to treat recurrent testicular carcinoma.

VIP-B (VP-16, ifosfamide, Platinol, bleomycin)—chemotherapy protocol.

VIP-DAC—vaginal interruption of pregnancy, with dilatation and curettage (Ob-Gyn).

vipoma—an endocrine tumor that produces VIP. See *VIP* (vasoactive intestinal peptides).

Vira-A (vidarabine).

viral hepatitides—hepatitis A, B, C.

ViraPap—human papillomavirus detection test used along with the standard Pap smear (Lab).

Virazole (ribavirin).

Virchow's node—enlarged supraclavicular lymph node; often the first sign of a malignant abdominal tumor. Also called sentinel or signal node.

viroid—a virus-like unenveloped infective RNA particle.

virus—not a living organism, but a very small segment of genetic material (DNA or RNA) encased in a protective protein shell. Upon entering a living cell, the virus assumes control of that cell's function and reproduction. The normal operations of the cell are suspended and it becomes a factory for the synthesis of more virus. Finally the cell disintegrates, releasing hundreds of new virus particles, which can then invade other cells. Viral infection typically elicits an acute, self-limited inflammatory response, without suppuration or fibrotic reaction. Viruses show a predilection for skin and mucous membranes, and even those that cause systemic disease often produce eruptions of papules or vesicles (as in measles and chickenpox). Viruses cause the common cold, influenza, measles, mumps, chickenpox, warts, herpes simplex, hepatitis, poliomyelitis, AIDS, and rabies. Examples:
arbovirus
AIDS
Epstein-Barr (EBV)
hepatitis B (HBV)
herpesvirus
HIV
lentivirus
leukovirus
McKrae strain of herpesvirus
picornavirus
respiratory syncytial (RSV)
retrovirus
rotavirus
Rous sarcoma
togavirus
varicella zoster

virus-like infectious agent (VLIA)—a microbacterium.

virus-like particle—see *VLP.*

VISC (vitreous infusion suction cutter) (Oph).

viscera, plural form of *viscus.*

Viscoat (Oph)—a viscoelastic solution used to coat delicate tissues in eye surgery, to reduce risk of tears, to prevent further tearing of tissue, to prevent vitreous loss. It is indicated for use as a surgical aid in anterior segment procedures, including cataract extraction and intraocular lens implantation. It helps to maintain a deep chamber during anterior segment surgery, and protects the corneal endothelium and other ocular tissues. This solution also maintains the normal position of the vitreous face, thus preventing postoperative flattening of the chamber.

Viscoheel K (Pod)—orthosis used to reduce shock load to joints and spine, as well as to correct varus and valgus position of the heel and leg axis.

Viscoheel N (Pod)—orthosis used to reduce shock load to joints and spine.

Viscoheel SofSpot (Pod)—orthosis used to reduce heel spur pain and plantar fascial pain.

viscous—thick, not readily flowing. Cf. *viscus.*

viscus (pl., viscera)—an internal organ, particularly one in the abdominal or thoracic cavities. Cf. *viscous.*

Visi-Black surgical needle—a needle with a non-shiny finish and a slim, tapered point. The black finish is intended to provide greater visibility within the operative field. The manufacturer writes the name in all uppercase letters, but for ease in typing, I would suggest capitalizing only the two initial letters, as above.

Visidex, Visidex II (Lab)—blood glucose testing strips.

Visitec
cannula
cystitome
needle
nucleus hydrodissector

Vistec x-ray detectable sponge—a surgical sponge with radiopaque strands running through it for x-ray visualization (just in case the sponge count is incorrect!).

visual analogue scale—method often used in pain management to rate pain.

visual evoked potential (VEP).

visual field testing (Oph)—to test the function of retina, optic nerve, and optic pathways when both central and peripheral visual fields are examined.

Visulas Nd:YAG laser—Zeiss laser (Oph, Neuro).

visuscope (Oph)—an instrument used in testing the amblyopic eye.

VitaCuff (Cardio)—a subcutaneous attachable cuff containing silver, for use with central venous catheters, to decrease bacterial infections at the site of entry.

Vitagraft arteriovenous shunt.

Vital Cooley—microvascular needleholder.

Vitallium—trademark for an alloy used in prostheses and in skull plates. See *McKeever Vitallium cap prosthesis.*

Vital Ryder type microvascular needleholder.

vital signs—pulse, respiration, temperature. Sometimes a physician dictates, "Four vital signs are normal." In that case, blood pressure is the fourth sign.

Vital Vue—an illuminating suction and irrigation instrument.

Vitatron catheter electrode (Cardio).

vitelliform macular degeneration.

vitrectomy—surgical procedure used for bleeding inside the eye, usually caused by diabetic retinopathy. The blood-filled vitreous is removed and replaced with a clear solution. See *open-sky vitrectomy.*

vitrector probe (Oph)—used during cataract surgery to simultaneously aspirate, cut, and irrigate with balanced salt solution.

Vitreon (perfluorophenanthrene) (Oph)—a type of substitute solution for vitreous humor. Used to float and help facilitate removal of a dislocated intraocular lens.

vitreous
v. base—attachment to the ciliary epithelium (near the ora serrata).
v. body—a transparent jelly-like mass that fills the cavity of the eyeball.
v. face—anterior surface, that which is behind the lens.
v. space—vitreous body or the cavity it occupies.

vitreous cutter (Oph)—instrument used in eye surgery such as vitrectomy.

vitreous—see *persistent hyperplastic primary vitreous* (PHPV).

vitro—see *in vitro.*

Vitrophage Peyman System (Oph)—used with disposable handpieces.

Vivalan (viloxazine)—drug to treat sleep disorders such as narcolepsy.

vivo—see *in vivo.*

Vivonex HN (high nitrogen)—enteral feeding solution; administered via nasoenteric route, or via 16-gauge jejunostomy tube.

Vivonex Moss tube—a naso-esophagogastric decompression tube with duodenal feeding tube.

Vivonex T.E.N. (or TEN, total enteral nutrition)—used as a postsurgical liquid diet formula. In the Norwich

Vivonex *(cont.)* Eaton advertisement for the product, T.E.N. is written with periods.

VLCD (very-low-calorie diet)—a specific diet of nonfat milk with vitamins and mineral supplements.

Vleminckx's solution ("vlem-inks")—antiseptic used in patients with severe acne.

VLIA (virus-like infectious agent)—a microbacterium.

VLP—a virus-like particle believed to be the etiologic agent of enterically transmitted non-A, non-B hepatitis.

VMCP (vincristine, melphalan, Cytoxan, and prednisone)—chemotherapy protocol for treatment of multiple myeloma.

VMP (VePesid, mitoxantrone, prednimustine).

VM-26 (teniposide) (Oncol)—a drug used to treat leukemia.

vocal cord—*not* vocal chord.

Voerner's disease—rare form of hereditary epidermolytic palmoplantar keratoderma (PPK), which includes hyperkeratosis of the skin of the palms and soles, with fissuring and marked hyperhidrosis.

Vogt-Koyanagi-Harada disease.

Vogt, limbal girdle of (Oph).

Vogt lines (Oph)—seen on the cornea in keratoconus.

voice button, Panje.

voice, hot potato.

Volkmann's contracture—neurovascular contracture of an extremity due to arterial occlusion.

Volkmann's spoon—a small spoon used in removal of pancreatic calculi.

Volk Pan Retinal Lens for binocular indirect ophthalmoscopy (Oph).

Volk QuadrAspheric fundus lens—a diagnostic/therapeutic contact lens with four aspheric surfaces (Oph).

Voltaren (Oph)—an ophthalmic solution to prevent ocular inflammation following cataract surgery. It was previously known as a nonsteroidal anti-inflammatory drug to treat arthritis.

volume element (voxel)—MRI term.

Volutrol—control apparatus for intravenous infusion.

von Graefe muscle hook (Oph).

von Graefe's sign—in exophthalmos, the upper lid lags behind the lower, exposing the eyeball.

von Hippel-Lindau disease.

von Kossa staining—demonstrates the presence of calcium in tissues.

Von Lackum surcingle (Ortho)—a traction device using straps that apply contralateral pressure; for correction of scoliosis. See also *surcingle.*

von Recklinghausen's disease—neurofibromatosis.

von Rokitansky's disease—see *Budd-Chiari syndrome.*

von Willebrand's factor (vWF)—vWF antigen levels are most elevated in giant cell arteritis, but are also found in Sjögren's syndrome, choroiditis, and polymyalgia rheumatica. Elevation of the vWF antigen levels may help in the differential diagnosis of giant cell arteritis. Cf. *giant cell arteritis; von Willebrandt's knee.*

von Willebrandt's knee (Oph). Actually this has nothing to do with the knee; it is a group of optic nerve fibers, located in the anterior optic chiasm, that loop forward into the contralateral optic nerve and then back into the appropriate optic tract. Cf. *von Willebrand's factor.*

Voorhees needle. Cf. *Veress needle.*

vortex—a whorled pattern or arrangement, such as is found in fingerprints or the pattern of hair growth at the crown of the head. Cf. *vertex.*

Vozzle Vacu-Irrigator (Surg)—used for controlled irrigation and evacuation of body tissue and fluids during surgery.

VPCA (vincristine, prednisone, Cytoxan, Ara-C)—chemotherapy protocol.

VPL thalamic electrode (ventroposterolateral) (Neuro). This is used to alleviate intractable pain by deep brain stimulation, and is internalized in much the same way as a pacemaker. See also *electrode.*

VPP (Oncol)—a standard chemotherapy protocol used to treat small-cell lung cancer. Consists of the drugs VP-16 and Platinol.

VP-16 (etoposide).

V/Q scan (ventilation/perfusion). Also, VQ. (The *Q* stands for quotient.)

V tach (''vee-tack'')—medical slang for ventricular tachycardia, or ventricular tachyarrhythmia.

VTED (venous thromboembolic disease) (Ortho).

VT/VF (ventricular tachycardia/ventricular fibrillation) (Cardio).

vulvae—see *kraurosis vulvae.*

VZV (varicella zoster virus)—a virus often found in patients who have had bone marrow transplants.

W, w

WACH shoe (wedge adjustable cushioned heel) (pronounced "watch")—a cast shoe used in orthopedics.

Wada test—a test to determine hemispheric dominance.

Wada valve prosthesis (Cardiac Surg).

waddle, duck—see *duck waddle.*

wad, extensor—lateral humeral epicondyle.

WAIS (Wechsler Adult Intelligence Scale).

Waldenström's macroglobulinemia.

Waldhausen subclavian flap technique—in repair of coarctation of the aorta.

Wallach colposcope.

Wallach Colpostar-V6.

Wallach pencil (Oph)—a cryosurgery instrument, used for treatment of retinal tears and trichiasis.

Wallach Zoomscope.

wallerian degeneration—reaction resulting from a cut or injury to distal nerve fragments.

Wallidius knee prosthesis.

Wall stent (Cardio)—self-expanding arterial stents placed during percutaneous transluminal angioplasty to prevent mural thrombus formation.

Wall stent biliary endoprosthesis (GI)—a self-expanding metal stent used to treat bile duct strictures.

Walsham forceps—used in repair of facial fractures.

Wardill palatoplasty.

Warren splenorenal shunt.

Wartenberg pinwheel (Ortho, Neuro)—used in sensory examinations.

Warthin's cell; sign; tumor.

Warthin-Starry technique—a silver stain used to identify *Helicobacter pylori.*

Warthin's tumor—adenolymphoma. (Alfred S. Warthin, M.D., U.S. pathologist.) Cf. *Wharton's tumor.*

washerwoman's skin (Path)—the macerated appearance of the skin after long immersion in water. Used in autopsy dictation.

washout phase (Radiol)—in radionuclide scans, scintiscanning of the lungs at the conclusion of the inhalation phase of a lung scan, after an interval during which all inhaled radionuclide would be expected to have been exhaled.

wasting syndrome—a life-threatening weight loss, often seen in AIDS.

water brash—regurgitation of excessive saliva from the esophagus, often combined with some gastric juice; heartburn; pyrosis.

water hammer pulse (Cardio)—a very rapid upstroke and falloff, indicative of a number of cardiac problems, the common denominator being a low resistance of the runoff of blood.

Waters view (Radiol)—occipital film for view of the maxillary sinuses. For Charles Alexander Waters, M.D., U.S. radiologist.

Watson-Jones tenodesis (Ortho)—used to correct instability arising from injury of both the anterior talofibular ligament (ATFL) and calcaneofibular ligament (CFL).

Watt's skin closure staples.

Watzke Silicone sleeve (Oph)—used in scleral buckling procedures.

Waugh knee prosthesis (Ortho).

waves—see *Cannon waves.*

wean—to slowly decrease a person's dependence on something—a ventilator, for example; to discontinue a medicine by gradually reducing the dose.

weave—see *Pulver-Taft weave.*

Weber test (ENT). The Weber test uses bone conduction. The base of the activated (tapped or stroked) tuning fork is placed against the forehead, the vertex of the skull, or the front teeth, and the patient is asked in which ear he hears the sound best. In conductive hearing loss, the sound is referred to the deafer ear. In perceptive hearing loss, the sound is referred to the better ear. See *air conduction, bone conduction,* and *Rinne test.*

Webster needle holder (Plas Surg).

Wechsler Adult Intelligence Scale (WAIS)—mental status examination.

Wechsler Memory Scale or Test—mental status examination.

Weck-cel sponge.

Weck-Baggish Hystereroscopy System (Gyn).

Weck clip.

Weerda distending operating laryngoscope (ENT).

Wegener's granulomatosis.

Wehrs incus prosthesis (ENT)—used in ear reconstructive surgery.

Weigert stain—see *elastic fibers stain.*

Weill's sign (Ped)—indicative of pneumonia in an infant. During respiration, the subclavicular space on the affected side shows no expansion.

Weinberg retractor—also called Joe's hoe.

Weir excisions—alar excisions of the nose (Plas Surg).

Weir Mitchell's disease—erythermalgia or erythromelalgia; severe pains of the soles and palms. (Dr. Silas Weir Mitchell, Philadelphia neurologist.)

Welch Allyn AudioScope (Audioscope) —a new screening instrument for evaluating hearing loss in children; it is combined with the otoscope in a single device.

Well-Cogen ("well'-co-jen")—trade name of a number of latex agglutination tests by Burroughs Wellcome.

Wellcovorin (leucovorin calcium) tablets for prophylaxis and treatment of undesired effects of folic acid antagonists.

Wellferon (interferon alfa-nl)—a chemotherapy drug also used to treat Kaposi's sarcoma in AIDS patients.

wen—a sebaceous cyst or other bland swelling on, in, or under the skin.

Werdnig-Hoffmann disease—infantile motor neuron disease.

Wernicke's area of the brain (in the superior temporal gyrus) (Neuro)—im-

Wernicke's area of the brain *(cont.)* portant as the area involved in spoken language.

Wernicke's disease—a vitamin B_1 deficiency disease that causes memory loss.

Wertheim clamp.

Westcott tenotomy scissors (Oph).

Western blot (blotting) **electrotransfer test**, a second line AIDS test, more sensitive, given as a backup when the ELISA test is positive.

Westergren test—for sedimentation rate.

Westphal-Edinger nucleus. See *Edinger-Westphal nucleus* (Neurosurg).

wet field cautery *(not* Wetfield).

wet mount (Path)—a method of microscopic examination in which the specimen (a fluid or fluid suspension) is placed on a slide and then covered with a coverslip, rather than drying the specimen. "Wet mounts showed positive trichomoniasis."

wet prep (also wet mount) (Gyn). "Wet preps were taken, which were negative for yeast, but positive for *Trichomonas.*"

wet-to-dry dressings—sterile gauze is soaked in sterile normal saline, applied to a wound, and allowed to dry; when removed, it facilitates debridement.

Wharton's tumor (and duct)—a benign papillary cystadenoma of the submaxillary gland. Cf. *Warthin's tumor.*

wheal *(not* wheel). If you scratch the skin of your forearm with your fingernail, you may find, after a few minutes, a raised area appearing where you made the scratch. It may also become erythematous and may or may not itch. This is a *wheal.* A wheal may represent a positive reaction in skin tests (such as the tine test for PPD), and the diameter of the wheal is measured to determine whether the response is positive or negative. In tuberculin testing, a wheal of 8 to 10 mm in diameter 48 to 72 hours after injection is considered positive. Cf. *wheal and flare reaction.*

wheal and flare reaction—reaction to a test administered via injection. See *wheal.*

wheat weevil disease—extrinsic allergic alveolitis caused by exposure to wheat flour and weevils.

Wheeless method (GI)—for surgical construction of a J rectal pouch.

Whipple's disease—intestinal lipodystrophy. This is a rare chronic inflammatory disease, and intestinal disorder of malabsorption. It primarily affects the small intestine and the mesenteric lymph nodes, but it may affect other organs including the brain, spinal cord, and peripheral nerve plexuses. The onset is usually in middle age and occurs nine times more often in men than in women. Symptoms involve multisystems and may include ataxia, personality changes, seizures, memory deficits, ophthalmoplegia, and hearing loss.

Whipple procedure—pancreaticoduodenectomy—used for tumor of the distal common duct, or when severe pancreatitis is confined to the head of the pancreas.

white clot syndrome—spontaneous major arterial thrombosis in a patient receiving heparin therapy, usually preceded by thrombocytopenia (low platelet count).

whitlow, herpes—herpetic infection of the fingertips.

Whitnall's ligament (Oph).

whistletip ureteral catheter (Urol).

whole body hyperthermia—see *hyperthermia, whole body.*

Wiberg classification of patellar types (I, II, III) in relation to shapes of the inferior surface of the patella, and in association with chondromalacia patellae.

wick (usually gauze)—used for drainage of a wound. "A large amount of liquid pus was drained from the wound. The wound was packed with 1/2 inch plain gauze. He is to have the wick removed in two days."

Wies chalazion forceps (Oph).

Wiktor coronary stent (Cardio)—compressed stent made of tantalum wire which is inserted over the balloon of a coronary artery catheter and then expanded at the site of the angioplasty. Left in place, the stent remains expanded and prevents restenosis of the artery.

Wilcoxon rank sum test—used in legionnaires' disease.

Wild operating microscope.

Wilde incision (Oto).

Williams microsurgery saw.

Wills-Oglesby locking catheter.

Wilson-Cook (modified) **wire-guided sphincterotome**—used in endoscopic procedures.

Wiltse rods—used with bone graft in correcting and stabilizing vertebrae in spondylolisthesis (Ortho).

winged scapula (Ortho)—caused by a stretching injury to the long thoracic nerve. This results in weakness of the serratus anterior, with "winging" of the scapula.

wing sutures.

Winters arch bar (Oral Surg).

Winters shunt (Urol)—corpus spongiosum to corpus cavernosum (for priapism).

wire, wiring
- Compere fixation
- copper
- J-wire
- Killip
- ninety-ninety intraosseous
- olive
- Sadowsky
- tantalum

Wirt test (Oph)—for assessing stereoscopic acuity.

Wishard catheter—a catheter with one hole at the end; used for diagnostic purposes.

Wiskott-Aldrich syndrome—dysgammaglobulinemia.

Wissinger rod (Ortho)—used in correcting shoulder instability. "We inserted a Wissinger rod anteriorly, and we looked for the probe as it entered anteriorly."

Witzel duodenostomy.

Witzel enterostomy catheter.

Witzel tunnel (Surg)—for feeding jejunostomy.

Wolfe graft—used in hand surgery.

Wolfe mammographic parenchymal patterns (Rad).

Wolvek sternal approximation fixation instrument (Cardio)—used to close a sternotomy incision after cardiopulmonary bypass surgery.

Wood's light examination—of skin and hair for evidence of fungal infection.

wood pulp worker's lung disease—extrinsic allergic alveolitis caused by exposure to moldy logs.

word salad (Psych)—mixture of words and phrases that lack comprehensive meaning or logical coherence, commonly seen in schizophrenic states.

Woronoff's rings—in psoriasis (Derm).

Worst gonioprism contact lens (Oph)—a lens which allows the surgeon to

Worst gonioprism contact lens *(cont.)* directly examine synechiae (adhesions) which have formed around the haptics of an anterior chamber intraocular lens. The surgeon can then lyse these synechiae without having to cut the haptics of the intraocular lens. The intact intraocular lens can then be removed with less tissue trauma than if the haptics had been cut.

Worst intraocular lens (a name, not a criticism).

Worth four-dot test (W4D) (Oph)—for evaluating the ability of the two eyes to perceive images simultaneously.

Wound-Span Bridge II—trade name for a dressing that holds the ends of a wound together by spanning it rather than pressing on it.

WPW syndrome (Wolff–Parkinson–White).

Wright needle—used to fashion a fascia lata sling to repair ptosis (Oph).

Wright peak flow—a metered measurement used in testing pulmonary function. "The lungs are clear to percussion and auscultation. There is no wheezing. His Wright peak flow on three occasions was 525."

Wright's stain—used in the diagnosis of *Pneumocystis carinii* pneumonia. See *GMS, Gomori* or *Grocotti methenamine silver.*

Wrisberg, nerve of.

wrist drop—passive flexion of the wrist due to paralysis of extensor muscles.

Wroblewski method—of testing serum LDH.

WR-2721—see *ethiofos.*

Wurd catheter.

Wylie carotid artery clamp (Cardio).

Wyse pattern—for reduction mammoplasty (Plas Surg).

X, x

Xanar 20 Ambulase CO_2 laser—used in dermatologic and gynecologic surgery.

xanthelasma (Oph)—a flat or slightly raised yellowish tumor, found most frequently on the upper and lower lids, especially near the inner canthus.

X-body—see *Birbeck granule.*

xenograft (heterograft)—see *graft.*

Xenomedica prosthetic valve (Cardio).

xenon arc photocoagulator (made by Zeiss) (Oph).

xenon-133 scan (^{133}Xe)—a technique used in measuring cerebral blood flow by isolating the internal carotid artery and injecting the xenon-133. The cerebral blood flow is then calculated by automated cerebral blood flow analyzer.

Xenophor femoral prosthesis (Ortho).

Xenotech prosthetic valve (Cardio).

Xeroform gauze (''zero-form'').

xiphoid process (''zi'foid'') (Gr., sword-shaped)—the pointed cartilage and bone attached to the lower end of the sternum. Cf. *scyphoid.*

XMG (x-ray mammogram).

XMMEN-OE5 monoclonal antibody—used to treat patients in shock from a systemic gram-negative infection.

XomaZyme-H65 (Oncol)—a drug used to treat children and young adults with acute lymphoblastic leukemia.

x-ray (*not* X-ray)—roentgenogram or roentgen ray.

X-TEND-O knee flexer (Ortho)—provides patient-controlled flexion and extension exercises.

xylol pulse indicator.

Y, y

YAG (yttrium-aluminum-garnet).
YAG laser—neodymium:YAG (yttrium-aluminum-garnet).
Yankauer pharyngeal speculum.
Yasargil bayonet scissors.
years of potential life lost (YPLL).
Yeoman uterine biopsy forceps.
Yergason test—used in examining the shoulder to determine if subluxation of the long head of the biceps tendon is present.
Yersinia—genus of gram-negative rods. *Yersinia pestis* is the etiologic agent of plague.
Yorke-Mason incision.
YPLL (years of potential life lost)—used in mortality studies.
Y-shaped graft (Cardio).
yttrium-aluminum-garnet (YAG).
yuppie flu—see *chronic fatigue syndrome; myalgic encephalomyelitis.* Also, postviral fatigue syndrome.

Z, z

Zaditen (ketotifen) (Pulm)—an oral drug to prevent bronchial asthma attacks.

Zahn, line of. See *line of Zahn.*

Zancolli clawhand deformity repair.

ZDV (zidovudine).

ZEEP (zero end-expiratory pressure).

Zefazone (cefmetazole).

Zeiss—manufacturer of many ophthalmological instruments, cameras, and microscopes.

Zelsmyr Cytobrush—used to obtain material from endocervical canal for Pap smear, *Chlamydia* screen, and other lab tests.

Zenker's fixative—a mercury-containing solution used to harden and preserve tissue.

Zervas hypophysectomy kit (Neuro)—for stereotaxic procedures.

ZES (Zollinger-Ellison syndrome).

Zestoretic (Cardio)—a combination of the diuretic hydrochlorothiazide and the ACE inhibitor lisinopril. Used to treat hypertension.

zeugmatography—MRI term.

Zickel nail fixation (Ortho).

zidovudine (ZDV, Retrovir)—approved by the FDA for treating patients with AIDS and ARC. Previously known as azidothymidine (AZT).

Ziehl-Neelsen stain—for acid-fast bacilli.

ZIFT (zygote intrafallopian tube transfer) (Ob-Gyn)—used in cases of blocked fallopian tubes, to achieve pregnancy. This is a combination of techniques used in GIFT and IVF. In ZIFT, fertilization takes place in vitro (in a dish), and 18 hours later four of the zygotes that have formed are replaced in the fallopian tubes to work their way into the uterus. See *GIFT; IVF; zygote.*

ZIG vaccine (zoster immune globulin).

Zimmer low viscosity cement (Ortho).

Zimmer—manufacturer of various surgical instruments and products.

zipper scar (Surg).

Zirconia orthopedic prosthetic heads (Ortho)—made of zirconium oxide ceramic.

Zithromax (azithromycin)—an antibiotic drug for treating AIDS patients with MAC infection; also for strep pharyngitis, chlamydial infections, urethritis, toxoplasmosis, and cryptosporidiosis.

Zixoryn (flumecinol)—used to treat hyperbilirubinemia in newborns.
ZMC fracture (zygomatic-malar complex) (of the face) (Plas Surg).
ZMS intramedullary fixation system (Ortho)—a Zimmer fixation system that provides easy intramedullary passage over a guide wire through the fracture site without reaming.
Zocor (simvastatin) (Cardio)—used to lower levels of LDL in patients with hypercholesterolemia which has not responded to dietary measures. Other therapeutic actions include raising levels of HDL and lowering triglyceride levels. Belongs to the class of drugs known as HMG-CoA reductase inhibitors.
Zofran (ondansetron) (GI)—given to patients receiving certain types of chemotherapy drugs known to induce vomiting. The first drug which selectively blocks 5-HT_3 receptors in the central nervous system involved in the vomiting reflex. Given I.V. only.
Zoladex (goserelin).
Zollinger-Ellison syndrome (ZES)—gastric hypersecretion, peptic ulceration, pancreatic tumor syndrome, ulcerogenic tumor of pancreas syndrome.
Zoloft (sertraline).
Zomax (zomepirac sodium)—nonaddicting analgesic. Removed from market in 1984.
zona hamster egg test—used in male infertility to test the ability of spermatozoa to penetrate hamster ova, which approximate human ova.
zone—see *LLETZ* (large loop excision of the transformation).
zonula occludens—tight junction of endothelial cells.
zonulolysis (Oph)—dissolution of the ciliary zonule by use of enzymes, to permit surgical removal of the lens.
zoster immune globulin vaccine (ZIG).
Zovirax (acyclovir)—an antiviral drug which has been used to treat herpes simplex, herpes zoster infections, patients with AIDS and ARC, and is now approved for treating chickenpox in otherwise healthy children. It is found to cause faster healing of skin lesions with less scar formation.
Z stent (GI)—a self-expanding stent used to treat bile duct and esophageal stenosis, its wires are crisscrossed in a Z pattern. Also, Gianturco prosthesis; stent.
Zung Depression Scale (Psych).
Zweymuller prosthesis (Ortho)—cementless hip prosthesis.
Zyclast (Plas Surg)—collagen used for thinner wrinkles.
Zyderm I, Zyderm II (Plas Surg)—collagen injections.
zygote—a one-celled pre-embryo.
zymogen cell (peptic cell) of stomach.
zymogen granule—cellular granules consisting of inactive digestive enzymes awaiting secretion.
Z, Z′, Z″ (Ger., *Zuckung*)—chart notes for increasing degrees of contraction.

The Author

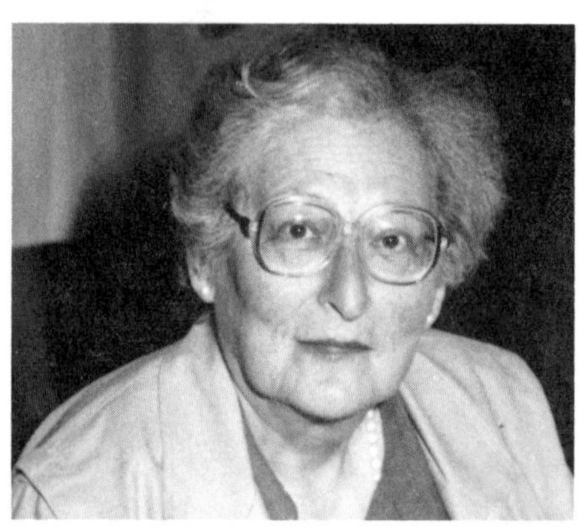

Vera Pyle is a certified medical transcriptionist (CMT) with over thirty years of medical transcription experience in private-practice medical offices and at the University of California Medical Center in San Francisco, where she was supervisor of medical transcription for many years. She also taught medical terminology and transcription at City College of San Francisco for eight years.

A founding member of the American Association for Medical Transcription (AAMT) in 1978, Vera Pyle served as a national director for six years, frequently speaking to audiences of medical transcriptionists and allied health professionals throughout the country, and writing articles and columns for AAMT publications, including a word list called "The AAMT Notebook" for ten years, now known as "Current Medical Terminology." She received the Distinguished Member Award in 1986 and has become known to medical transcriptionists and allied health professionals around the world through *Current Medical Terminology,* now in its fourth edition.

Semi-retired in recent years, she has been consulting editor to Health Professions Institute since 1985 on medical references and other publications and The SUM Program for Training Medical Transcriptionists.